G. Heusch · R. Schulz
Editors

New Paradigms of Coronary Artery Disease

Hibernation, Stunning, Ischemic Preconditioning

STEINKOPFF
DARMSTADT

Springer

Prof. Dr. Gerd Heusch
Dr. Rainer Schulz
Abt. für Pathophysiologie
Zentrum für Innere Medizin
Universitätsklinikum Essen

45122 Essen

ISBN 978-3-7985-1059-3 ISBN 978-3-642-53793-6 (eBook)
DOI 10.1007/978-3-642-53793-6

Die Deutsche Bibliothek –
CIP-Einheitsaufnahme

New paradigms of coronary artery disease :
hibernation, stunning, ischemic preconditioning /
G. Heusch ; R. Schulz, ed.
[Engl. ed.: James C. Willis]. –
Darmstadt : Steinkopff ; New York :
Springer, 1996
ISBN 978-3-7985-1059-3
NE: Heusch, Gerd [Hrsg.]

English editor: James C. Willis

Production: Holger Frey

Type-Setting: Typoservice, Griesheim

Printing: Vereinigte Buchdruckereien, Bad Buchau

FOREWORD

Detailed analyses of regional myocardial blood flow, function, metabolism and morphology in ischemic and reperfused myocardium have led to the identification of important phenomena, i.e., myocardial hibernation, myocardial stunning and ischemic preconditioning. Both the hibernating and the stunned myocardium characterize viable though dysfunctional as distinguished from necrotic tissue. With the advent of reperfusion procedures, the distinction between reversibly injured, hypofunctional myocardium from irreversibly injured, hypofunctional myocardium is of utmost clinical importance. The pathophysiological distinction of hibernating and stunned myocardium is controversial, but reperfusion is mandatory anyway. Ischemic preconditioning is the most powerful maneuver known so far to delay infarct development. Its clinical significance has been suggested from retrospective analyses of data from patients suffering a myocardial infarction as well as from controlled PTCA studies. Whether or not preconditioning can be achieved pharmacologically in the clinical setting remains to be established. The mechanisms and signal cascade underlying myocardial hibernation, myocardial stunning and ischemic preconditioning are not clear in detail.

Over the last year, focussed issues on myocardial hibernation, myocardial stunning and ischemic preconditioning were published in *Basic Research in Cardiology;* they have received great interest and a good response. Therefore, these focussed issues are now combined and published as a separate monograph.

We express our gratitude once more to all our colleagues who contributed to this monograph, to Ms. Ibkendanz of Steinkopff, and to Ms. Philipp and Mr. Heinrichs from Bayer AG Germany, who supported this additional publication.

Essen, March 1996 Gerd Heusch, Rainer Schulz

Foreword V

Myocardial Hibernation

I. Short-term hibernation: evidence for downregulation of contractile function and metabolic adaptation

C. S. Apstein, F. R. Eberli: Critical role of energy supply and glycolysis during short-term hibernation 3

J. M. Canty, Jr., J. A. Fallavollita: Hibernating myocardium represents a primary downregulation of regional myocardial oxygen consumption distal to a critical coronary stenosis . . 6

S. E. Downing: Myocardial hibernation: relationship to a model for segmental dyskinesis 10

K. P. Gallagher: Myocardial hibernation in terms of the flow- function relationship 13

A. Ilebekk, J. Offstad, K. Lande, K. A. Kirkebøen: Contractile pattern in acutely hibernating myocardium 17

E. Marban: Excitation-contraction coupling in hibernating myocardium 20

G. A. Pantely, J. D. Bristow: Hibernating myocardium: a hypometabolic state for energy conservation 24

J. D. Schipke: Myocardial hibernation 27

R. Schulz, G. Heusch: Acute adaptation to ischemia: Short-term hibernating myocardium . . . 30

II. Long-term hibernation

Hibernation vs. Stunning

H. Gewirtz: Myocardial hibernation: unresolved physiological and clinical issues . . 33

G. R. Heyndrickx: Hibernating myocardium 36

S. H. Rahimtoola: Hibernating myocardium: a brief article 39

J. Ross, Jr.: Myocardial hibernation, stunning, or both? 42

Morphology: Dedifferentiation vs. Degeneration

M. Borgers, J. Ausma: Structural aspects of the chronic hibernating myocardium in man 45

A. Elsässer, J. Schaper: Hibernating myocardium: adaptation or degeneration? 48

Clinical Identification

R. O. Bonow: The hibernating myocardium: identification of viable myocardium in patients with coronary artery disease and chronic left ventricular dysfunction 50

R. Ferrari: Commentary on hibernating myocardium and its clinical relevance . . . 53

W. Flameng, B. Shivalkar: Hibernating myocardium, a clinical entity 56

M. Schwaiger: Identification of "hibernating myocardium" by imaging approaches . . . 59

Myocardial Stunning

I. Definition and occurence

S. F. Vatner, G. R. Heyndrickx: Ubiquity of myocardial stunning 65

II. Methodological and conceptual problems

R. Bolli: Common methodological problems and artifacts associated with studies of myocardial stunning in vivo 69

D. J. Hearse: Stunning: Three questions and concerns 75

III. Excitation-contraction coupling

G. J. Gross: Do ATP-sensitive potassium channels play a role in myocardial stunning? 78

E. Marban, W. D. Gao: Stunned myocardium: a disease of the myofilaments? 81

W. Schaper: Stunned myocardium, an opinionated review 85

IV. Metabolism

R. Lerch: Myocardial stunning: the role of oxidative substrate metabolism 88

B. Renstrom, A. J. Liedtke: Adjustments in competitive substrate utilization in stunned myocardium during early reperfusion 91

V. Coronary blood flow alterations

L. C. Becker: Is stunned myocardium ischemic on a microvascular level? 94

P. G. Camici: Absolute myocardial blood flow in chronic left ventricular dysfunction . 97

L. Mandinov, P. Kaufmann, O. M. Hess: Coronary vasomotion of the stunned myocardium 100

VI. Pharmacotherapy

Y. Birnbaum, R. A. Kloner: Therapy for myocardial stunning 103

R. Schulz, T. Ehring, G. Heusch: Stunned myocardium: inotropic reserve and pharmacological attenuation 106

VII. Clinical relevance: hibernation vs. stunning

G. Ambrosio: The elusive difference between hibernation and stunning in patients . . 109

R. Ferrari: Commentary on myocardial stunning and its clinical relevance 112

L. H. Opie: Chronic stunning: The new switch in thought 115

Ischemic Preconditioning

I. Ischemic preconditioning: the concept

K. A. Reimer, R. B. Jennings: Ischemic preconditioning: a brief review . . . 119

L. M. King, L. H. Opie: Preconditioning – a reappraisal of protection . . . 123

W. Schaper: Ischemic preconditioning, remembrances of things past and future . . . 126

M. Connaughton, D. J. Hearse: Three questions about preconditioning . . . 130

II. Triggers and mediators of ischemic preconditioning: adenosine, bradykinin, nitric oxide and K_{ATP}-channels

A. C. Cave, C. S. Apstein: Preconditioning-induced protection against post-ischemic contractile dysfunction: Inhibitory effect of tissue washout . . . 134

T. Miura: Adenosine and bradykinin: Are they independent triggers of preconditioning? . . . 138

M. Kitakaze, T. Minamino, K. Node, K. Komamura, M. Hori: Activation of Ecto-5′-nucleotidase and cardioprotection by ischemic preconditioning . . . 141

J. R. Parratt, A. Vegh: Endothelial cells, nitric oxide and ischaemic preconditioning . . . 145

G. J. Gross, D. A. Mei, J. J. Schultz, T. Mizumura: Criteria for a mediator or effector of myocardial preconditioning: Do K_{ATP} channels meet the requirements? . . . 149

III. The controversial role of protein kinase C in ischemic preconditioning

J. M. Downey, M. V. Cohen: Preconditioning: Markers vs. epiphenomena . . . 153

D. M. Van Winkle: Limitation of infarct size by myocardial ischemic preconditioning . . . 156

K. Przyklenk, R. A. Kloner: Role of protein kinase C in ischemic preconditioning: in search of the "pure and simple truth" . . . 159

IV. Trigger mechanisms other than ischemia: stress and stretch

P. D. Verdouw, B. C. G. Gho, D. J. Duncker: Cardioprotection by organs in stress or distress . . . 162

P. Whittaker: An alternative perspective on ischemic preconditioning derived from mathematical modeling . . . 165

V. Ischemic preconditioning vs. myocardial hibernation

R. Schulz, G. Heusch: Ischemic preconditioning and myocardial hibernation: Is there a common mechanism? . . . 168

VI. Second window of protection

G. F. Baxter, D. M. Yellon: Delayed myocardial protection following ischaemic preconditioning . . . 171

R. Bolli: The early and late phases of preconditioning against myocardial stunning and the essential role of oxyradicals in the late phase: an overview . . . 175

Myocardial Hibernation

3–5
© Steinkopff Verlag 1996

C. S. Apstein
F. R. Eberli

Critical role of energy supply and glycolysis during short-term hibernation

Key words Glucose – insulin – ischemia – diastolic dysfunction – ATP – calcium

The terms "acute hibernation" and "short-term hibernation" may seem oxymoronic since "hibernation" implies a prolonged period of dormancy and subsequent reawakening. Nonetheless, the concept of acute hibernation has provided a useful framework for research studies involving relatively brief periods of low flow or moderate ischemia which depress myocardial function but do not cause homogeneous irreversible injury; therefore significant recovery or "reawakening" of the ischemically depressed myocardium can occur with reperfusion. The sequence of relatively brief ischemia followed by reperfusion has obvious relevance to clinical scenarios of unstable angina, acute coronary thrombosis and impending myocardial infarction which is treated with thrombolytic therapy, and the ischemia-reperfusion sequence which accompanies cardiac surgery. The mechanisms regulating acute hibernation during low-flow ischemia and recovery during reperfusion merit serious investigation because of their clinical relevance and potential for beneficial therapeutic manipulation.

Central to the concept of hibernation is the principle that myocardial function is depressed in parallel with the severity of the ischemic state to reduce energy utilization and conserve a limited energy supply. There is little experimental data to support or refute the concept of a long-term perfect balance between an ischemic reduction in oxygen supply and concomitant "downregulation" of contractile function which is maintained in a true steady-state of chronic hibernation over months or years; such a state of apparent chronic hibernation could also be the result of repetitive "stunning" (1). However in short-term or acute hibernation a matching between levels of myocardial perfusion and contraction over a wide range of flow reduction has been described (2). Such a "downregulation" of energy demand is critical for preserving cellular viability in the face of a decrease in energy availability.

However, even with a depressed level of contractile function, hibernating myocardium has significant energy requirements, and below a critical point of flow reduction energy supply is insufficient to maintain cell viability, despite contractile downregulation. For example, in isolated blood-perfused rabbit hearts subjected to a moderate degree of low-flow ischemia, Marshall and Zhang have shown that contractile function decreases to a proportionally greater extent than the decrease in oxygen availability such that relatively high levels of ATP are maintained during the low-flow ischemic state of acute hibernation. Nonetheless, at a critically low level of perfusion, myocardial high energy phosphate levels decreased markedly (3). Therefore, interventions which provide small but critical amounts of energy have the potential to create a successful hibernating state in ischemic myocardium which would otherwise undergo irreversible ischemic injury.

Supported in part by USPHS grant HL 48175

C. S. Apstein, M.D. (✉) · F. R. Eberli
Cardiac Muscle Research Laboratory
Whitaker Cardiovascular Institute
Boston University School of Medicine
Boston, Massachusetts 02118, USA

Importance of small amounts of oxygen

The importance of small increments in oxygen delivery in preserving the ability of ischemic myocardium to hibernate successfully is illustrated by a series of experiments in which groups of isolated buffer perfused normothermic rat hearts were subjected to 30 minutes of either zero flow ischemia or varying degrees of low-flow ischemia (4). Hearts which received no coronary flow or 3 % of baseline coronary flow had very poor post-ischemic recovery. However, increased coronary flows which provided only a very small amount of oxygen delivery during the ischemic period, e.g. 12 μlO_2/min/gm equivalent to 0.07 ml/min/gm of coronary blood flow, were associated with complete recovery of contractile function after 30 min of ischemia. In addition to providing additional oxygen delivery, the higher buffer coronary flow rates also provided significant lactate washout which may also have contributed to a successful hibernating state.

Importance of glycolytic metabolism

An active glycolytic pathway can also be critical in protecting against acute ischemic irreversible injury and facilitating successful short-term hibernation (5 – 7). Isolated rat hearts subjected to brief three-minute periods of total global zero flow ischemia recovered completely with reperfusion if the glycolytic pathway was active, but glycolytic blockade accelerated the fall in ischemic contractility, caused irreversible contracture after 30 seconds of ischemia, and recovery of contractile function was extremely poor. Thus during the first three minutes of severe ischemia glycolysis exerted a net beneficial effect on myocardial function, despite significant tissue lactate accumulation (5). The benefits of an active glycolytic pathway have also been demonstrated in protocols of sustained low-flow ischemia and short-term hibernation. Eberli et al. subjected isolated normothermic isovolumic blood-perfused rabbit hearts to 2 1/2 hours of severe low-flow ischemia with coronary flow reduced to a level of 11 – 13 % of baseline. The group which received high glucose and insulin during the period of low-flow ischemia had greater LV contractile function during ischemia and increased recovery during reperfusion, preserved diastolic function during both ischemia and reperfusion, and less loss of coronary vasomotor function. Oxygen consumption was similar in the two groups; thus the increased glycolytic flux that preserved glycogen stores and high-energy phosphate levels prevented cell contracture and cell death in otherwise fatally underperfused myocardium (7). The results of these experiments are summarized in figure 1. In a similar protocol in blood-perfused rat hearts, using 31P-NMR spectroscopy, Cave et al. have demonstrated that the high glucose and insulin substrate resulted directly in higher ATP levels during the acute hibernation (low-flow) ischemia state by a mechanism of enhanced glycolytic ATP synthesis rather than an increase in oxidative phosphorylation (8). Recently Vanoverschelde et al.

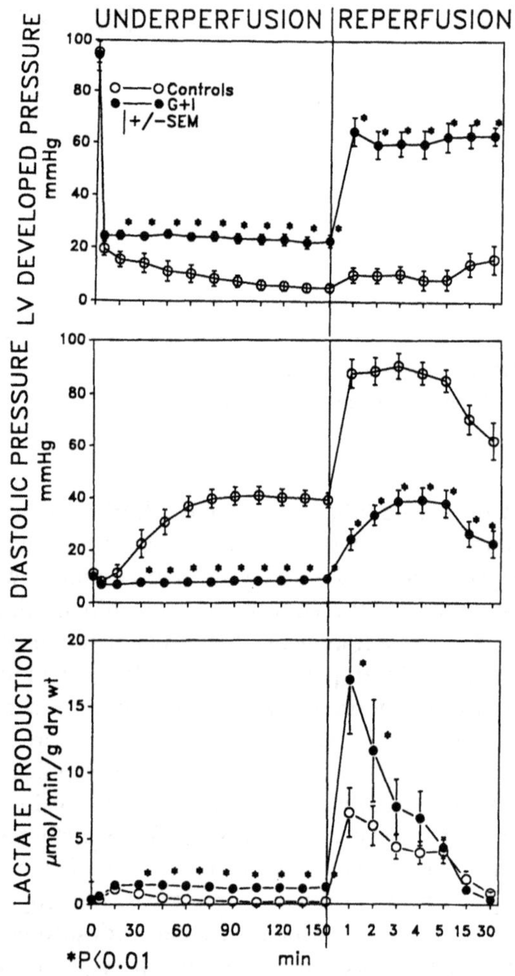

Fig. 1 Graphs showing left ventricular developed pressure, left ventricular diastolic pressure and lactate production of isolated red-cell perfused rabbit hearts exposed to 150 minutes of low-flow ischemia and 30 minutes of reperfusion, simulating an evolving myocardial infarction followed by reperfusion. After reduction of coronary perfusion pressure from 100 to 8 mmHg coronary blood flow decreased to 11 – 13 % of initial flow and a prompt decrease of developed pressure occurred. In the control group (Controls; n = 8; open circles) glycolytic flux, as assessed by lactate production started to decrease after 30 min of low-flow ischemia concomittant with the decrease in developed pressure and the development of contracture. In contrast, when glycolytic flux was enhanced by glucose and insulin infusion (G+I; n = 8; closed circles) hearts maintained an increased lactate production throughout the ischemic period and showed a greater lactate washout during reperfusion. No contracture developed in G+I hearts during underperfusion and hearts showed a better recovery of diastolic and systolic function during reperfusion. In addition, increased glycolytic flux decreased coronary resistance during underperfusion and increased coronary flow during reperfusion. Adapted from Eberli FR et al., Circ Res 1991; 68: 466–481.

have reported similar results demonstrating a protection of the myocardium during the low-flow ischemic "hibernating" state by several metabolic interventions which increased glycolytic flux (9).

Taken together these results suggest that significant clinical benefit might be gained by metabolic manipulations which increase glycolytic flux in patients with acutely ischemic myocardium. Interventions such as glucose and insulin have the potential to convert potentially fatal ischemic injury to a state of short-term hibernation and significantly increase recovery when such hibernating myocardium is "reawakened" with reperfusion.

References

1. Vanoverschelde J-LJ, Wijns W, Depré C, Essamri B, Heyndrickx GR, Borgers M, Bol A, Melin JA (1993) Mechanisms of chronic regional postischemic dysfunction in humans. Circulation 87: 1513–1523
2. Ross J Jr (1991) Myocardial perfusion-contraction matching. Implications for coronary heart disease and hibernation. Circulation 83: 1076–1083
3. Marshall RC, Zhang DY (1988) Correlation of contractile dysfunction with oxidative energy production and tissue high energy phosphate stores during partial coronary flow disruption in rabbit heart. J Clin Invest 82: 86–95
4. Apstein CS, Deckelbaum L, Mueller M, Hagopian L, Hood WB Jr (1977) Graded global ischemia and reperfusion. Cardiac function and lactate metabolism. Circulation 55: 864–872
5. Apstein CS, Deckelbaum L, Hagopian L, Hood WB Jr (1978) Acute cardiac ischemia and reperfusion: contractility, relaxation, and glycolysis. Am J Physiol 235: H637–H648
6. Apstein CS, Gravino FN, Haudenschild CC (1983) Determinants of a protective effect of glucose and insulin on the ischemic myocardium. Circulation Research 52: 515–526
7. Eberli FR, Weinberg EO, Grice WN, Horowitz GL, Apstein CS (1991) Protective effect of increased glycolytic substrate against systolic and diastolic dysfunction and increased coronary resistance from prolonged global underperfusion and reperfusion in isolated rabbit hearts perfused with erythrocyte suspensions. Circ Res 68: 466–480
8. Cave AC, Eberli FR, Ngoy S, Rose J, Ingwall JS, Apstein CS (1993) Increased glycolytic substrate protects against ischemic diastolic dysfunction: ^{31}P-NMR studies in the isolated blood perfused rat heart. Circulation 88 (Suppl I): I-43
9. Vanoverschelde J-LJ, Janier MF, Bakke JE, Marshall DR, Bergmann SR (1994) Rate of glycolysis during ischemia determines extent of ischemic injury and functional recovery after reperfusion. Am J Physiol 267: H1785–H1794

6–9
© Steinkopff Verlag 1996

J. M. Canty Jr.
J. A. Fallavollita

Hibernating myocardium represents a primary downregulation of regional myocardial oxygen consumption distal to a critical coronary stenosis

Key words Chronic hibernation – stunned myocardium – ischemia – flow reserve

This brief review will focus on the hypothesis that hibernating myocardium represents a primary downregulation of regional myocardial oxygen consumption in response to repetitive ischemia distal to a critical coronary stenosis. This not only maintains a balance between resting oxygen delivery and demand, but also permits relative increases in function to occur without producing metabolic evidence of a supply-demand imbalance. A key point is that the presence of both reductions in regional resting flow and oxygen consumption distinguish this adaptation from stunned myocardium (2, 9).

Criteria for hibernating myocardium

Hibernating myocardium is a clinically defined entity that, as of yet, does not have a suitable animal model. Thus, it is difficult to clearly distinguish this response from the effects of acute ischemia or post-ischemic stunning. Nevertheless, one could argue that such differences are somewhat semantic from a clinical standpoint since the major concern in managing patients is to identify dysfunctional myocardium associated with myocyte viability regardless of the cause.

J. M. Canty, Jr., M.D. (✉) · J. A. Fallavollita
State University of New York at Buffalo
Clinical Center Rm. CC-172
462 Grider Street
Buffalo, New York 14215, USA

At the present time, the gold standard for determining dysfunctional but viable myocardial tissue is to demonstrate that function improves following revascularization. Noninvasive predictors of improvement include preserved thallium uptake or a mismatch pattern between ^{18}F-2-deoxyglucose and perfusion using positron emission tomography (PET). Recently, functional improvement with inotropic stimulation has shown promise in identifying reversibly dysfunctional myocardium; however, the responses to inotropic stimulation may be difficult to interpret since superimposed acute ischemia could actually produce functional deterioration in otherwise viable tissue.

Despite the utility of these clinical criteria to define myocardial viability, they may not always adequately distinguish hibernation from stunning or nontransmural infarction. Because of this, we propose the following additional criteria to distinguish these three entities:

1.) Since hibernation represents a primary downregulation of function, both regional flow and oxygen consumption should be depressed in comparison to simultaneously measured values in a normally perfused region, in the absence of ongoing or recent (within 24 hours) symptomatic ischemia.
2.) To distinguish hibernation from stunning, the downregulation in function should be chronic and therefore not normalize unless there is a restoration of blood flow by revascularization.
3.) Myocardial fibrosis to an extent that could explain the reduction in function, flow and oxygen consumption on the basis of an admixture of normal and fibrotic tissue should be absent.
4.) Normalization of flow, function and metabolism after revascularization should occur over a longer time period than that usually associated with stunned myocardium produced by demand-induced ischemia.

5.) Finally, since regional function is downregulated as the primary adaptation, sustained submaximal increases in myocardial oxygen consumption above the depressed basal level should be maintainable without concomitant metabolic evidence of ischemia.

Potential importance of regional downregulation in relation to coronary flow reserve

The major advantage of an intrinsic myocardial adaptation that would result in chronic regional reductions in contractile function and oxygen consumption is illustrated in Figure 1. The graph on the left shows the relation between flow and distal coronary pressure in a region that is not hibernating distal to a chronic 90 % stenosis. The graph on the right depicts the circumstance when the stenotic region is hibernating. Oxygen extraction is assumed to be maximal at rest and thus, reductions in resting flow are directly proportional to reductions in regional myocardial oxygen consumption. At a normal level of resting flow and oxygen consumption the stenosis will reduce resting coronary pressure to a level approaching the lower limit of autoregulation (4). This, in effect, reflects a critical stenosis that causes subendocardial ischemia with any small increase in oxygen consumption. The graph on the right shows the same stenosis in a circumstance where there is heterogeneous left ventricular oxygen consumption due to regional hibernation. Because oxygen consumption is downregulated distal to the stenosis, there is a concomitant reduction in resting blood flow. Now, under resting conditions, the coronary pressure distal to the stenosis is actually higher than that in the panel on the left. In addition, modest relative increases in demand above the depressed baseline are possible since regional coronary flow reserve has been improved. Thus, hibernating regions can hypothetically increase their relative oxygen demand (from a depressed baseline) in response to global determinants that increase myocardial oxygen consumption during submaximal stress without actually producing metabolic evidence of a supply-demand imbalance. Obviously, with more severe stress, subendocardial ischemia will still occur. Teleologically, such an adaptation would act to preserve myocyte viability at the expense of a reduced level of contractile function. It would also reduce the frequency of superimposed acute ischemia and the associated reversible injury and resynthesis of myocardial proteins that occur with myocardial stunning (6).

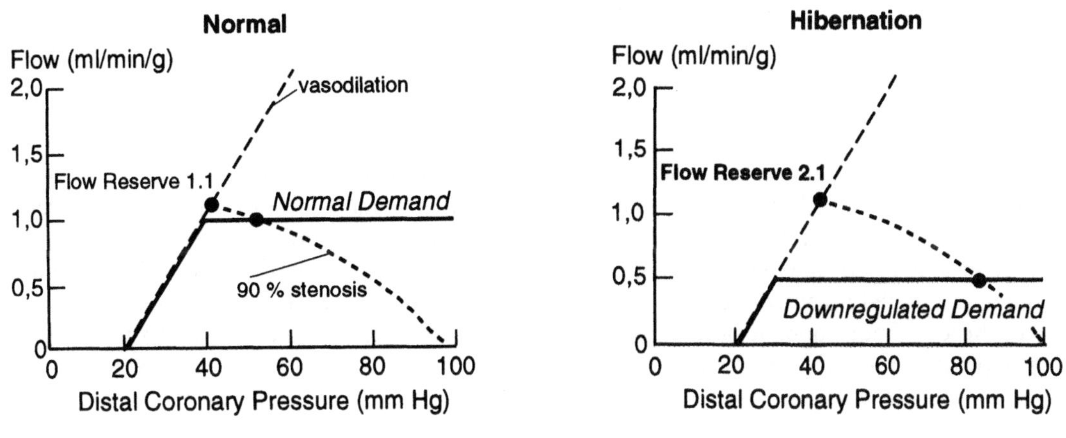

Fig. 1 Relation between resting oxygen demand and coronary flow reserve in normal and hibernating myocardium. The dashed line indicates the relationship between coronary pressure distal to the stenosis and coronary flow during maximum pharmacological vasodilation. The solid line shows the autoregulatory relation as distal coronary pressure is varied with coronary vasomotor tone intact. The dotted line shows the nonlinear relationship between flow across the coronary stenosis and distal coronary pressure. When demand is normal, the flow reserve (ratio of vasodilated to resting flow) distal to the stenosis is 1.1 and small changes in demand result in regional ischemia. When regional oxygen consumption is downregulated, resting coronary flow falls which results in a higher resting distal coronary pressure since there is less viscous pressure drop across the stenosis. Because of this, coronary flow reserve (i.e. the relationship between flow with vasodilation and resting flow) actually improves. Thus, moderate stress-induced increases in oxygen consumption can occur from the downregulated level in response to increases in external cardiac workload without immediately resulting in subendocardial ischemia. See text for further discussion.

Experimental evidence that hibernating myocardium is associated with reduced flow and oxygen consumption

The most clear cut evidence that hibernation is a distinct entity from other dysfunctional states comes from studies examining regional flow, function and metabolism in patients and animals with total coronary artery occlusions and collateral-dependent myocardium where coronary flow reserve is severely reduced. Several of these studies will be reviewed below.

In 1984, Arani et al. (1) described a group of patients with symptomatically stable angina, isolated left anterior descending coronary artery occlusion and angiographically visible collateral vessels. These patients also had mildly depressed anterior wall motion on ventriculography without symptoms of active ischemia and without electrocardiographic evidence or a history of myocardial infarction. Using inert gas washout techniques to quantify perfusion, they found that resting flow in the collateral dependent region was depressed to 0.38 ml/min/g versus 0.51 ml/min/g for the mixed normal and collateral dependent regions. Interestingly, selective measurements of great cardiac venous blood showed normal values for pO_2 (consistent with a depressed basal oxygen consumption) and normal lactate extraction.

More recently, Vanoverschelde and colleagues (10) used PET to study flow and metabolism in a similar patient population. They found that myocardial perfusion was depressed to 0.77 ml/min/g in collateral dependent regions versus 0.96 ml/min/g in normally perfused nonstenotic regions from the same patients. The magnitude of resting dysfunction was inversely related to collateral flow reserve. Metabolic imaging with positron emission tomography showed a mismatch between flow and ^{18}F-2-deoxyglucose uptake in collateral dependent regions along with resting reductions in regional oxygen consumption assessed by ^{11}C-acetate. Perhaps of most significance was the fact that biopsies obtained in selected patients undergoing revascularization showed only minor increases in replacement of myocytes with fibrosis. This provided the first direct evidence that physiological abnormalities consistent with a clinically defined hibernation could not be explained by an admixture of normal tissue and scar.

Existing animal models have had limited success in duplicating the physiology of hibernation on a chronic basis. This appears to largely relate to differences in collateral flow reserve following occlusion. Our laboratory attempted to circumvent this using an ameroid model where epicardial collaterals were ligated at the time of surgery in dogs (3). Prolonged relative reductions of regional function occurred in this model via two mechanisms. Prior to total ameroid occlusion, function was depressed without a change in subendocardial perfusion and consistent with findings in stunned myocardium (2, 9). Following ameroid occlusion, both subendocardial flow and function were depressed in relation to the corresponding control region. Although consistent with hibernation, these latter abnormalities were not sustained for more than a few weeks and returned to normal at the end of the study. Recently Mills and colleagues (8) have demonstrated chronic reductions in flow distal to a chronic anterior descending stenosis in pigs. Although function was not assessed, regional oxygen consumption was reduced in comparison to a historical control group suggesting that metabolic demand was downregulated. While each of these studies has limitations, they suggest that intrinsic myocardial adaptations consistent with chronic hibernation can be produced in some experimental circumstances. Based upon recent clinical studies (10), it appears that the level of flow during maximum pharmacological vasodilation is probably the most important determinant of whether the adaptation of hibernation is produced.

Clinical problems in identifying mechanisms for chronic regional dysfunction

One of the major problems in distinguishing specific mechanisms for chronic regional dysfunction is the fact that these areas all have severely reduced coronary flow reserve. It seems very unlikely that areas of pure hibernation actually exist since the limitation in flow reserve will predispose these regions to acute ischemia as well as to post-ischemic stunning. In fact, it seems quite plausible that the triggers for a primary adaptation at the myocyte level are related to the severity and frequency of ischemia and/or stunning. Although the hallmark of stunned myocardium is depressed regional function in the setting of normal perfusion (2, 9), stunned areas could have depressed flow and oxygen consumption if there was an admixture of normal and infarcted tissue. Thus, without direct biopsy quantification of the extent of transmural fibrosis, it is difficult to exclude the possibility that reductions in flow, function and metabolism represent chronically stunned myocardium coexisting with nontransmural infarction. Although the latter circumstance would not be completely consistent with normalization of function following revascularization, most studies examining function have shown improvement that falls short of complete recovery.

Finally, while experimental stunning is associated with normal flow and depressed function, restoration of perfusion following an episode of ischemia occurs through a residual stenosis. Although episodes of demand-induced ischemia during daily life seem unlikely to produce prolonged regional dysfunction unless produced by maximal or prolonged exercise (7), the presence of a residual stenosis may amplify the effects of stunning (5). At present, however, there is still no experimental evidence that chronic stunning per se has any benefit to the myocyte unless accompanied by concomitant reductions in energy utilization. In fact, chronic stunning would represent an effect of repetitive ischemia and not an intrinsic adaptation that sustains myocyte viability during recurrent episodes of ischemia. To address this will require better animal models in which these phenomena can be correlated with mechanisms at the cellular and molecular level.

References

1. Arani DT, Greene DG, Bunnell IL, Smith GL, Klocke FJ (1984) Reductions in coronary flow under resting conditions in collateral-dependent myocardium of patients with complete occlusion of the left anterior descending coronary artery. J Am Coll Cardiol 3: 668–674
2. Bolli R (1992) Myocardial stunning in man. Circulation 86 (6): 1671–1691
3. Canty JM Jr, Klocke FJ (1987) Reductions in regional myocardial function at rest in conscious dogs with chronically reduced regional coronary artery pressure. Circ Res 61 (5) Suppl II: 107–116
4. Canty JM Jr, Giglia J, Kandath D (1990) Effect of tachycardia on regional function and transmural myocardial perfusion during graded coronary pressure reduction in conscious dogs. Circulation 82: 1815–1825
5. Farber NE, Pieper GM, Gross GJ (1988) Postischemic recovery in the stunned myocardium after reperfusion in the presence or absence of a flow-limiting coronary artery stenosis. Am Heart J 116: 407–420
6. Frass O, Sharma HS, Knöll R, Duncker DJ, McFalls EO, Verdouw PD, Schaper W (1993) Enhanced gene expression of calcium regulatory proteins in stunned porcine myocardium. Cardiovasc Res 27: 2037–2043
7. Homans DC, Laxson DD, Sublett E, Pavek T, Crampton M (1991) Effect of exercise intensity and duration on regional function during and after exercise-induced ischemia. Circulation 83: 2029–2037
8. Mills I, Fallon JT, Wrenn D, Sasken H, Gray W, Bier J, Levine D, Berman S, Gilson M, Gewirtz H (1994) Adaptive responses of coronary circulation and myocardium to chronic reduction in perfusion pressure and flow. Am J Physiol 266 (Heart Circ Physiol 35): H447–H457
9. Ross J Jr (1991) Myocardial perfusion-contraction matching. Implications for coronary heart disease and hibernation. Circulation 83 (3): 1076–1083
10. Vanoverschelde J-L J, Wijns W, Depré C, Essamri B, Heyndrickx GR, Borgers M, Bol A, Melin JA (1993) Mechanisms of chronic regional postischemic dysfunction in humans: New insights from the study of noninfarcted collateral-dependent myocardium. Circulation 87: 1513–1523

10–12
© Steinkopff Verlag 1996

S. E. Downing

Myocardial hibernation: relationship to a model for segmental dyskinesis

Key words Myocardial ischemia – hibernation – perfusion-contraction matching – myocardial dyskinesis – isolated heart systems – K^+ channels

A close quantitative relationship between coronary flow and cardiac mechanical function has been recognized for more than 40 years (1). Similarly, in skeletal muscle oxygen consumption is a function of O_2 availability over a broad range (10). Thus, in both systems organ perfusion, substrate availability, metabolic activity, and mechanical function appear to be tightly linked variables. Because the phenomena resemble some characteristics of the hibernating mammal (6), this term was suggested to collectively define events in experimental low flow cardiac ischemia (2). The same term had been used previously to describe apparently similar events in selected patients with ischemic heart disease (9). The clinical implications of these observations in the context of ischemic heart disease seem intuitively obvious. In both settings the critical issue is that the linkage between low flow and down-regulation of function be sustained over a prolonged time base, that the integrity of the ischemic segment or organ be maintained, and that substantial recovery of function occur when flow is reconstituted.

In the experimental isolated piglet heart model, it has been amply demonstrated that severe normothermic ischemia (coronary flow, 10 % of control) is associated with sharply reduced function which remains stable for at least 2 h. Changes in myocardial high energy phosphate concentrations are minimal, and glycogen concentrations do not differ from time-matched non-ischemic control hearts (2). The latter finding is consistent with the recent observation that glycogen synthase activity is sharply increased (7). Reperfusion of these hearts by incrementally increasing flow over a 15-min time base results in return of mechanical function to about 80 % of pre-ischemic values (3). High energy phosphate concentrations are not significantly reduced. ATP averaged 23 μmol/g, and CP averaged 45 μmol/g dry weight. This may be compared with control hearts not subjected to ischemia in which ATP averaged 28 μmol/g and CP, 50 umol/g (3). The modest reduction in function is fully reversed by giving calcium.

Isolated heart systems differ in fundamental respects from *in vivo* circumstances. Major differences include absence of autonomic control, removal of circulating hormonal signals, absence of mechanical stresses associated with maintaining the systemic circulation, and frequently the use of crystalloid solutions as perfusate. Thus, caution should be exercised when findings in these models are extrapolated to the intact organism, and certainly to the patient with segmental ischemia. Models that use crystalloid typically have coronary flow rates of 12–20 times normal. Flow rates five times normal may be taken to represent "ischemia", although a more accurate term would be tissue "hypoxia". We chose to use red-cell-enhanced perfusate to provide more physiological conditions of flow and O_2 delivery (2).

An important question was whether these hearts would continue to manifest the same tight perfusion-contraction coupling and stable hibernation in the presence of enhanced adrenergic stimulation, as would be expected to occur *in vivo* during stress. Hearts were studied following the addition of norepinephrine (NE, 40 ng/ml) to the per-

S. Evans Downing, M. D. (✉)
Department of Pathology
Yale University School of Medicine
310 Cedar Street
P.O. Box 208023
New Haven, Connecticut 06520-8023, USA

fusate, and compared with saline controls (4). This concentration of NE increased the pressure-rate product by about 50 % prior to ischemia. Regardless, when flow was reduced to 10 %, mechanical performance fell to the same level as in controls not exposed to NE, and stable hibernation continued for the full 2 h studied. The hibernation mechanism completely overrode beta agonist stimulation by this high concentration of catecholamine (4).

Considering the demonstrated potency of the perfusion-contraction matching and acute hibernation phenomena, identification of a mechanistic basis has aroused considerable interest. Some have attributed it to mechanical events associated with arterial distention or collapse. However, this seems inconsistent with the fact that in crystalloid perfused preparations reduction of flow volume to values which are normal for blood perfused preparations is associated with marked reductions in contractile function. This suggests that the "erectile" mechanism is inordinately amplified in the high flow preparations. Most would take the view that other factors are involved, and probably of greater importance. Opening of ATP-gated potassium channels consequent to adenosine A1 receptor stimulation seemed a likely candidate in view of the demonstrated involvement of these channels in reducing infarct size and "stunning". The same piglet model described above, as well as a crystalloid perfused rabbit model, were used to address this issue (8). Addition of aprikalim, a K-ATP channel opener, caused marked coronary vasodilatation; glibenclamide had the opposite effect. However, both agents were without effect on perfusion-contraction coupling, acute hibernation, or the degree of metabolic or functional recovery following reperfusion in either species. Hence, these channels substantially modulate vascular smooth muscle, but not cardiac muscle. Other ion channels could be important, but have not been identified. The regulatory signal(s) remains elusive.

There is considerable uncertainty regarding the relationship of these physiological phenomena to segmental ischemia *in vivo,* particularly as they may apply to the human with coronary artery obstruction (9). Two hours of normothermic ischemia with a 90 % reduction in coronary flow would most certainly cause substantial irreversible myocyte injury. Hence, the effectiveness of the hibernation phenomenon in a dyskinetic segment may be quite different than in the quiescent isolated heart. This question was approached by exploring the consequences of passive stretch, as occurs in the dyskinetic segment *in vivo,* in our isolated rabbit heart model (5). After reduction of coronary flow to 10 %, and induction of acute hibernation, intraventricular pressure was elevated to systemic levels to mimic systolic stresses. Recovery of function after 90 min was markedly less than in ischemic hearts not subjected to elevated intraventricular pressures. Myocardial ATP and glycogen concentrations were also sharply lower (5). Depression of recovery correlated with the level and duration of passive stretching.

In preliminary studies with the rabbit model, similar findings were observed using pulsatile stretching to more closely model *in vivo* dyskinesis. This approach was extended to our piglet model for more detailed study (Offstad et al., manuscript in preparation). Recovery of systolic function after 2 h of ischemia and repetitive stretching was half that found in ischemic hearts not subjected to stretching. ATP concentrations were similarly reduced. Electron microscopy indicated structural changes consistent with ischemia, but no mechanical disruption was identified. Excess energy demands most likely explain the findings in this model for segmental dyskinesis. Thus, the acute hibernation mechanism could be much less effective in the *in vivo* dyskinetic segment as well. Variables such as severity and duration of ischemia, mechanical stresses, and metabolic state are likely to enter the equation as critical determinants of the effectiveness of the hibernation mechanism, and ultimately of tissue viability.

References

1. Case RB, Berglund E, Sarnoff SJ (1954) Ventricular function: II. Quantitative relationship between coronary flow and ventricular function with observations on unilateral failure. Circ Res 2: 319–325
2. Downing SE, Chen V (1990) Myocardial hibernation in the ischemic neonatal heart. Circ Res 66: 763–772
3. Downing SE, Chen V (1992) Acute hibernation and reperfusion of the ischemic heart. Circulation 82: 699–707
4. Downing SE, Chen V (1992) Effects of catecholamine stimulation on myocardial hibernation. Am Heart J 124: 589–596
5. Downing SE (1993) Wall tension and myocardial dysfunction after ischemia and reperfusion. Am J Physiol 264: H386–H393
6. Hochachka P, Guppy M (1987) Metabolic Arrest and the Control of Biological Time. Cambridge, Mass, Harvard University Press, pp 57–100

7. McNulty PH, Valenti JA, Shi CQ-X, Young LH, Sinusas AS (1994) Low flow myocardial ischemia induces persistent regional activation of glycogen synthase: a potential mechanism for increasing myocardial glucose storage (Abstract). Circulation 90: I209 (1120)
8. Offstad J, Kirkeboen KA, Ilebekk A, Downing SE (1994) ATP gated potassium channels in acute myocardial hibernation and reperfusion. Cardiovasc Res 28: 872–880
9. Rahimtoola SH, Griffith GC (1989) The hibernating myocardium. Am Heart J 117: 211–221
10. Whalen WJ, Buerk D, Thuning CA (1973) Blood flow-limited oxygen consumption in resting cat skeletal muscle. Am J Physiol 224: 763–768

13–16
© Steinkopff Verlag 1996

K. P. Gallagher

Myocardial hibernation in terms of the flow-function relationship

Key words Hibernation – stunning – myocardial ischemia – perfusion-contraction-matching

In the northern part of the United States, hibernation is a very real phenomenon. It refers, of course, to the dormant condition in which some types of animals pass through the trying conditions of winter. In fact, the Latin word from which the word derives is hibernus which refers to wintry conditions. In contrast to various woodland creatures who can sleep through the winter largely oblivious to its rigors, the human inhabitants of the North have to stay awake through winter no matter how much they would like to hibernate for several months. With our usual penchant for giving simple, catchy nicknames to very complicated concepts, the cardiovascular research community has adopted the word hibernation to describe the myocardium's response to coronary inflow restriction that is not severe enough to compromise viability. Faced with the "wintry" circumstances posed by inappropriately low oxygen availability, the idea is that the myocardium "hibernates" to protect itself against the consequences of prolonged supply/demand imbalance.

This appealing concept was popularized and defined by Rahimtoola as "...a state of persistently impaired myocardial and left ventricular function at rest due to reduced coronary blood flow that can be partially or completely restored to normal if the myocardial oxygen/demand relationship is favorably altered, either by improving blood flow and/or by reducing demand" (12). The concept of myocardial hibernation developed from clinical and experimental observations. Clinically, surgical revascularization was documented to improve regional cardiac function in portions of the left ventricle that had been characterized by significant preoperative dysfunction. The finding that preoperative dysfunction was sometimes reversible implied that the myocardium was viable and not merely scar tissue from an old infarct (11). Experimentally, studies demonstrated that a close relationship existed between local blood flow and contraction (5, 6). This suggested that low preoperative function in viable myocardium could have been due to chronically restricted coronary blood flow. Faced with reduced oxygen delivery, the amount of mechanical work performed by the myocardium decreased. The idea is that the myocardium tries to keep the supply/demand ratio evenly matched. If the numerator (perfusion) decreases, the denominator (contraction) can respond by decreasing, as well, to keep the ratio normal or nearly normal (13).

The supply/demand ratio is a difficult thing to measure directly. A surrogate means of evaluating the regional supply/demand ratio in the myocardium is to use the regional flow-function relationship. As depicted in Figure 1, systolic function, a major determinant of myocardial oxygen demand, is plotted on the y-axis. Blood flow, a main determinant of oxygen delivery given the high extraction ratio across the heart, is plotted on the x-axis. An idealized linear relationship is presented in the figure for the sake of simplicity but it must be acknowledged that a modestly curvilinear relationship has been reported by many investigators. The flow-function relationship was derived from experiments in which different degrees of severe coronary stenosis were produced while monitoring changes in regional function in anesthetized or conscious experimental animals, primarily dogs. In general, parameters of regional mechanical performance have been normalized as

K. P. Gallagher, Ph.D. (✉)
Parke-Davis Pharmaceutical Research Division
2800 Plymouth Road
Ann Arbor, MI 48105, USA

percentages of the baseline value. Blood flow values in the flow restricted zone have been most often normalized as percentages of simultaneously measured blood flow in the nonischemic area. When normalized in this manner, the flow-function relationship is virtually identical when evaluated at rest or when hemodynamic conditions are greatly altered, as in exercise (6). Blood flow values have also been normalized for heart rate, resulting in comparably similar relationships under different conditions (13). When myocardial blood flow is reduced, regional function correlates best with changes in subendocardial perfusion indicating that alterations in the deep layers of the left ventricle are preeminent in determining the degree of mechanical dysfunction produced by coronary inflow restriction. The relationship between perfusion and function in the outer layers is less straightforward and may be influenced by the phenomenon of nonischemic dysfunction due to tethering. For the sake of simplicity and to concentrate on the relationship that appears to be the least influenced by tethering, the position and slope of the line in Figure 1 approximates that derived for the relationship between changes in subendocardial blood flow and a widely used parameter of regional function, systolic wall thickening (5).

The point labeled H, in the middle of the idealized flow-function relationship, represents a potential operating point for myocardium that is hibernating. It could be argued that any point on the line represents a potential operating point for hibernation but at low levels of perfusion, recovery of function will be markedly impaired and at very low levels of perfusion, viability will be compromised. Therefore, a lower limit of perfusion probably exists to define hibernating myocardium but what that limit is and how it may vary under different circumstances has not been established.

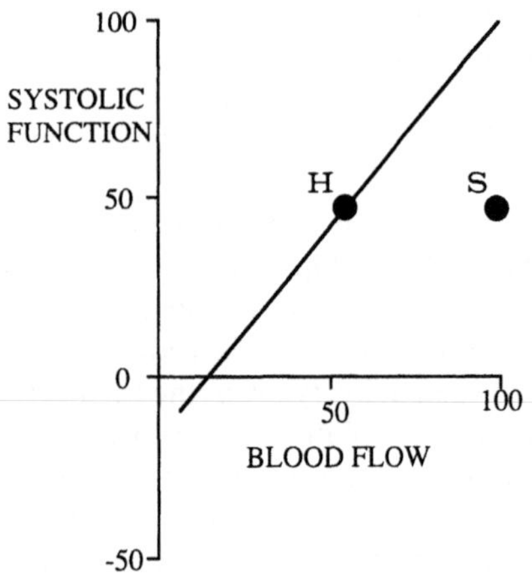

Fig. 1 Idealized (linear) flow-function relationship between regional systolic function and blood flow. The position and slope of the line corresponds approximately to the relationship between subendocardial blood flow and systolic wall thickening (5, 6). Function and flow are normalized as percentages of baseline values and percentages of simultaneously measured nonischemic zone flows, respectively. The point labeled H represents a potential operating point for hibernating myocardium. The point labeled S exemplifies stunned myocardium. Hibernating myocardium is characterized by proportionate changes in blood flow and function; stunned myocardium displays levels of dysfunction that are not in proportion to blood flow.

The studies describing the linear (or nearly linear) regional flow-function relationship were acute in nature. The various levels of steady dysfunction lasted for 5–10 minutes, only enough time to inject microspheres and satisfy the investigators that steady hemodynamic conditions prevailed. Myocardial hibernation, however, implies that chronic reductions in flow occur, leading to chronic regional hypofunction. Experimental studies have demonstrated that steady levels of inflow restriction over an hour or more can be sustained and are associated with reduced levels of contraction (9, 10, 14). Performing similar studies in experiments that extend over several days is more difficult but there are data indicating that "chronic" hibernation can be produced experimentally (3, 4).

One of the consistent features of experimental hibernation is that creatine pho phate and lactate gradually return to normal levels despite persistence of coronary inflow restriction (10, 14). Since they are markers of the metabolic milieu, their restoration to nearly normal levels has been interpreted to support the idea that the supply/demand ratio in hibernating myocardium is evenly matched. These results have also complicated elucidation of the mechanism by which perfusion and mechanical function are closely linked. The restoration of creatine phosphate and lactate to nearly normal levels means that some of the potential "error" signals have disappeared, despite persistence of inflow restriction and mechanical hypofunction. Regional contraction may be at an appropriately reduced level given the (lower) availability of oxygen when it is hibernating, but how does the myocardium "know" what is appropriate? Although a few solid hypotheses have been presented to answer this question (7, 15), it remains to be answered conclusively.

Whether or not chronic inflow restriction and mechanical hibernation are common events in human patients is a controversial issue. Impaired regional function can be associated with conditions other than hibernation, such as scarring after myocardial infarction or myocardial stunning. In noninfarcted myocardium, the contention of many investigators is that impaired regional function is more often the result of myocardial stunning (rather than chronic inflow restriction) after episodic bouts of coronary occlusion due to cyclical platelet aggregation or vasospasm. Given the lability of myocardial oxygen requirements, stunning could also be evident after demand induced ischemia if coronary inflow is restricted by severe narrowing of the coronaries.

In terms of the flow-function relationship, points located to the right of the standard flow-function curve indicate the condition of stunning because a given level of flow is associated with a disproportionately high degree of dysfunction as exemplified with the point labeled S in Figure 1. For reasons that are not entirely clear, administration of positive inotropic agents improves regional systolic function in stunned myocardium and this maneuver has become an experimental "rule of thumb" to aid in defining stunned myocardium. On a flow-function plot, for examples, positive inotropic stimulation would tend to move point S from the right of the standard curve up to a more normal operating position on the curve.

In hibernating myocardium, on the other hand, positive inotropic stimulation can lead to further decreases in regional contraction. Although there is evidence that hibernating myocardium does have contractile reserve (14), sustained positive inotropic stimulation is detrimental. Hibernating myocardium can be thought of as being restricted to operation on the flow-function curve. If positive inotropic stimulation reduced normalized flow on the x-axis, for example, point H would move down and left on the flow-function relation to a lower value of systolic function. If myocardial oxygen requirements were reduced by administering a negative inotropic agent, normalized perfusion may increase and regional function could improve. Thus, hibernating myocardium operates up or down (and stays on) the standard flow-function relationship, in contrast to stunned myocardium.

Thinking of hibernation and stunning in terms of the flow-function relationship enables a clear distinction to be made between the two concepts. Unfortunately, it is also an oversimplified way to approach the problem of distinguishing the two concepts in a human patient for a number of reasons. First, the flow-function relationship was largely derived as the instantaneous relationship between regional perfusion and mechanical function. As indicated by the disproportion between flow and function evident during stunning, the flow-function relationship is strongly influenced by history or the events preceding the measurement. Experimental evidence indicates that the intensity of ischemia during coronary occlusion is largely responsible for determining the extent and duration of mechanical stunning after blood flow is restored (2).

Second, the manner in which blood flow tends to be distributed in flow-restricted myocardium is nonuniform. Deeper myocardial layers will have less blood flow than the outer layers. Consequently, flow restriction severe enough to produce stunning may occur in the subendocardium at the same time less severe flow restriction (and no consequent stunning) is evident in the subepicardium (1, 13). Some investigators prefer a definition of hibernation which includes the proviso that true hibernation is confirmed only if function returns completely to normal after increasing blood flow or reducing demand. I think the emphasis should be on sustained viability and that hibernating myocardium can include "about to be stunned" elements. As long as there is enough blood flow to sustain viability, all of the myocardial layers can be considered as hibernating during flow restriction despite differential rates of functional recovery after perfusion is restored to nomal levels.

Third, distinguishing hibernation from stunning in human patients is constrained by the measurements that can be made clinically. Estimates of perfusion and regional function cannot always be made coincidentally, at appropriate times, or with solid information on preceding events. Likewise, the temporal and spatial resolutions of clinical measurements are more limited than those which can be made in experimental animals. Consequently, it may not be possible to differentiate regional stunning from hibernation in humans, at least in terms of flow and function. Potentially more promising may be the use of metabolic imaging techniques (8) that may generate new "rules of thumb" for characterizing the condition of the myocardium.

In conclusion, the flow-function relationship can aid in defining how hibernation and stunning differ from one another. Unfortunately the practical problem of distinguishing if one condition or the other, or both, exist in a particular human patient remains to be solved. Likewise, the mechanisms by which myocardial perfusion and mechanical function are linked so closely under some circumstances (eg., hibernation) and not in others (eg., stunning) remain to be determined conclusively.

References

1. Bolli R, Patel BS, Hartley CJ, Thornby JI, Jeroudi MO, Roberts R (1989) Nonuniform transmural recovery of contractile function in stunned myocardium. Am J Physiol 257 (Heart Circ Physiol 26): H375–H385
2. Bolli R, Zhu W-X, Thornby JI, O'Neill PG, Roberts R (1988) Time course and determinants of recovery of function after reversible ischemia in conscious dogs. Am J Physiol 254 (Heart Circ Physiol 23): H102–H114
3. Bolukoglu H, Liedtke AJ, Nellis SH, Eggleston AM, Subramanian R, Renstrom B (1992) An animal model of chronic coronary stenosis resulting in hibernating myocardium. Am J Physiol 263 (Heart Circ Physiol 32): H20–H29
4. Canty JM, Klocke FJ (1987) Reduction in regional myocardial function at rest in conscious dogs with chronically reduced regional coronary artery pressure. Circ Res 61: II-107–II-116
5. Gallagher KP, Matsuzaki M, Koziol JA, Kemper WS, Ross J Jr (1984) Regional myocardial perfusion and wall thickening during ischemia in conscious dogs. Am J Physiol 247 (Heart Circ Physiol 16): H727–H738
6. Gallagher KP, Matsuzaki M, Osakada G, Kemper WS, Ross J Jr (1983) Effect of exercise on the relationship between myocardial blood flow and systolic wall thickening in dogs with acute coronary stenosis. Circ Res 50: 716–729
7. Marban E (1991) Myocardial stunning and hibernation. The physiology behind the colloquialisms. Circulation 83: 681–688
8. Marwick TH, MacIntyre WJ, Lafont A, Nemec JJ, Salcedo EE (1992) Metabolic response of hibernating and infarcted myocardium to revascularization: a follow-up study of regional perfusion, function, and metabolism. Circulation 85: 1347–1353
9. Matsuzaki M, Gallagher KP, Kemper WS, White F, Ross J Jr (1983) Sustained regional dysfunction during prolonged partial coronary stenosis: Gradual recovery of function after reperfusion. Circulation 68: 170–182
10. Pantely GA, Malone SA, Rhen WS, Anselone CG, Arai A, Bristow JD (1990) Regeneration of myocardial phosphocreatine in pigs despite continued moderate ischemia. Circ Res 67: 1481–1493
11. Rahimtoola SH (1985) A perspective on the three large multicenter randomized clinical trials of coronary bypass surgery for chronic stable angina. Circulation 72: V123–V125
12. Rahimtoola SH (1989) The hibernating myocardium. Am Heart J 117: 211–219
13. Ross J Jr (1991) Myocardial perfusion contraction matching: Implications for coronary heart disease and hibernation. Circulation 83: 1076–1086
14. Schulz R, Guth BD, Pieper K, Martin C, Heusch G (1992) Recruitment of an inotropic reserve in moderately ischemic myocardium at the expense of metabolic recovery: a model of short-term hibernation. Circ Res 70: 1282–1295
15. Tubau JF, Rahimtoola SH (1992) Hibernating myocardium: A historical perspective. Cardiovasc Drugs Therap 6: 267–271

17–19
© Steinkopff Verlag 1996

A. Ilebekk
J. Offstad
K. Lande
K. A. Kirkebøen

Contractile pattern in acutely hibernating myocardium

Key words Coronary blood flow – hibernation – low-flow ischemia – myocardial metabolism – segment length – stunning

In the hibernating myocardium contractile function and energy consumption are downregulated in response to reduced coronary blood flow (2, 4, 7 – 9). Thus, the myocardium may survive prolonged periods of reduced blood flow without overt signs of ischemia, and it may regain normal contractile function when blood flow restrictions are terminated. The mechanism for this phenomenon is presently unknown, but to get insight into the mechanism involved, it is important to characterize all aspects of it as closely as possibly. Since a direct comparison of regional contractile pattern in acutely hibernating and stunned myocardium has not been reported, we here present such a comparison. We also relate changes in the regional contractile pattern to alterations in local myocardial oxygen consumption ($M\dot{V}O_2$).

In seven open-chest pigs, anesthetized with sodium pentobarbital, we reduced mid-LAD flow by about 30 % for 1 h using a hydraulic occluder. Thereafter, we allowed a recovery period of 2 h with unrestricted coronary blood flow. Segment lengths were recorded by ultrasound technique in the region to be made ischemic, and in a remote, control region (6). In four of these and four other pigs we sampled arterial and regional venous blood for determination of blood gases and pH and for analysis of regional lactate release and oxygen consumption.

Changes in contractile pattern through a cardiac cycle in normal, hibernating, and stunned myocardium are presented in the figure. Contractile pattern after 5 – 10 and approximately 55 min of low-flow ischemia were not different, and the latter is presented in Fig. 1. Contractile pattern in stunned myocardium was recorded after approximately 1 h of free flow, when stunning was close to maximum and reactive hyperemia was no longer present. Systolic segment length shortening decreased by 40 ± 5 and 40 ± 6 % (mean ± SEM) in hibernating and stunned myocardium, respectively. In both hibernating and stunned myocardium end-diastolic segment length rose, and early systolic bulging as well as early diastolic shortening developed (see Fig. 1). The increments in end-diastolic segment length (5.0 ± 0.9 and 3.6 ± 1.3 %), in early systolic bulging (1.4 ± 0.4 and 1.3 ± 0.4 % of end-diastolic segment length) and in end-systolic segment length (17.9 ± 2.1 and 16.0 ± 2.3 %), in hibernating and stunned myocardium, respectively, were not statistically different. However, early diastolic shortening amounted to 7.7 ± 0.8 % in hibernating myocardium, compared to 5.5 ± 0.6 % in stunned myocardium (difference: $p < 0.05$).

Schulz and coworkers (9) have previously described early diastolic wall thickening (equivalent to early diastolic segment length shortening) in hibernating myocardium, and regard it as a prognostic sign of viability. The contractile pattern of stunned myocardium has also previously been reported, although after brief periods of total ischemia (1). The similarity of contractile patterns in hibernating and stunned myocardium implies that it appears difficult or impossible to discriminate between these two altered myocardial states by a detailed analysis of the contractile patterns.

The significance of a greater early diastolic shortening in hibernating than in stunned myocardium is uncertain.

Prof. Dr. med. A. Ilebekk (✉) · J. Offstad · K. Lande
K. A. Kirkebøen
Institute for Experimental Medical Research
University of Oslo
Ulleval Hospital
0407 Oslo, Norway

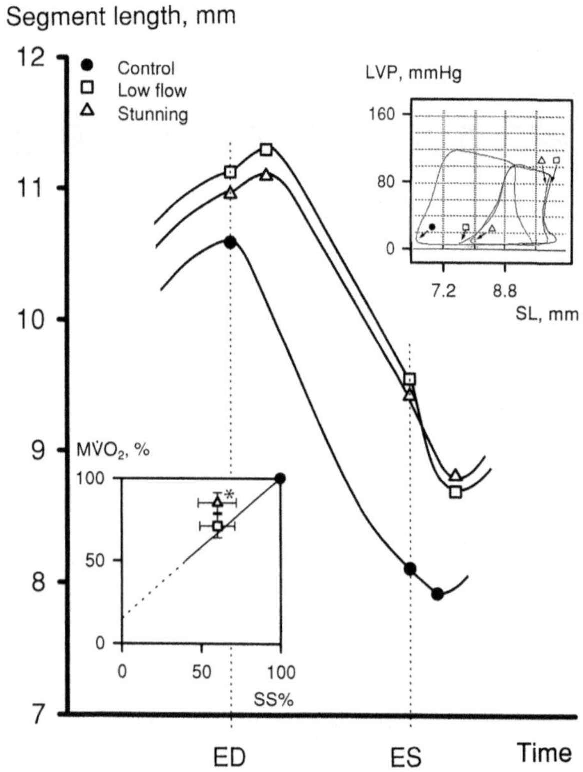

Fig. 1 Illustration of segment length changes before (control), after approximately 55 min of reduced blood flow (low-flow), and after approximately 1 h of unrestricted flow (stunning). Data represent mean values and SEM (when indicated). Early systolic bulging was not significantly different and amounted to 0.17 ± 0.05 and 0.14 ± 0.05 mm in acutely hibernating (low flow) and stunned myocardium, respectively, whereas early diastolic shortening was greater (0.86 ± 0.10 mm) in acutely hibernating myocardium than in stunned myocardium (0.60 ± 0.13 mm) (difference; $p < 0.05$) (crossing lines in main figure). *The upper, right insert* shows segment length – left ventricular pressure loops at control, low flow, and stunning in one experiment. Note the most pronounced early diastolic shortening during low flow (lower, left corner of the loop). *The lower left insert* shows that $\dot{M}VO_2$ in stunned myocardium was significantly greater than in acutely hibernating myocardium (*; $p < 0.05$) despite a similar reduction in systolic segment length shortening (SS %). The proposed line of identity crosses the $\dot{M}VO_2$-axis to indicate the magnitude of basal metabolism.
ED and ES; end-diastole and end-systole, LVP; left ventricular pressure, SL; segment length.

Our data cannot discriminate between passive elastic recoil, stretching by adjacent non-ischemic fibers, and diastolic contraction due to delayed actin-myosin disengagement. However, the correlation between early diastolic shortening and postischemic recovery of function both after total ischemia (10) and acute hibernation (9), suggests that diastolic segment length shortening reflects active tension development. We found that control $M\dot{V}O_2$ fell from 330 ± 15 μmol/min · 100 g to a reduced, but stable value throughout the low-flow period. Despite similar systolic segment length shortening, but longer early diastolic shortening in hibernating than stunned myocardium, $M\dot{V}O_2$ was significantly higher and amounted to 290 ± 24 μmol/min · 100 g in stunned-, compared to 240 ± 10 μmol/min · 100 g in hibernating myocardium (see Fig. 1). Thus, the disproportionately higher $M\dot{V}O_2$ in stunned than hibernating myocardium cannot be explained by differences in either systolic- or early diastolic contractile patterns. Our data obtained in the acutely hibernating myocardium, support the proposed close correlation between local myocardial contractile function and local coronary blood flow (5). We also show that this relation is lost in stunned myocardium, as has been shown during pharmacologically induced myocardial dysfunction (3).

Despite unchanged regional contractile function and $M\dot{V}O_2$ throughout the period with reduced coronary blood flow, lactate release and local venous pH and pCO_2 showed a biphasic response. Lactate release peaked after 5 min with a release of 27 ± 9 μmol/min · 100 g, compared to a consumption of 40 ± 8 μmol/min · 100 g in the control period (difference: $p < 0.01$). After 20 min of low flow, lactate release stabilized close to zero. At 5 min of low flow, local venous pCO_2 rose to 9.3 ± 0.5 kPa ($p < 0.01$) (control $pCO_2 = 7.9 \pm 0.4$ kPa) and local pH fell to 7.28 ± 0.01 ($p < 0.01$) (control 7.34 ± 0.01). Both local venous pCO_2 and pH stabilized at less extreme values during the last 30 – 40 min of the low flow period: pCO_2 at about 8.9 ± 0.4 kPa ($p < 0.05$ versus control) and pH at 7.30 ± 0.03 (ns versus control). Such biphasic changes in blood gases and myocardial lactate balance as well as a rebuilding of creatine phosphate during ongoing flow reductions have previously been recognized (2, 7, 9) and apparently represent a key feature of the hibernating myocardium. We think that the degree and velocity of early contractile downregulation in response to ischemia markedly modulate the subsequent signs of ischemia and also the degree and velocity of subsequent metabolic adaptation.

In conclusion, three key features of acute hibernation can be separated. The first one is an acute downregulation of contractile function in response to an ischemic insult, allowing maintenance of ionic balance and structure provided sufficient restflow. The second one is a metabolic adaptation demonstrated by the disappearance of lactate release and almost normalization of blood gases and pH during ongoing flow-reductions. The third feature of the acutely hibernating myocardium is the potential for restoration of normal contractile function when coronary blood flow is no longer restricted. A transient phase with myocardial stunning may, however, be expected before normal contractile function is reestablished.

References

1. Aksnes G, Kirkebøen KA, Christensen G, Ilebekk A (1992) Characteristics and development of myocardial stunning in the pig. Am J Physiol 263: H544–H551
2. Arai AE, Pantely GA, Anselone CG, Bristow J, Bristow JD (1991) Active downregulation of myocardial energy requirements during prolonged moderate ischemia in swine. Circ Res 69: 1458–1469
3. Buffington CW, Strum DP, Watanabe S (1994) Regional oxygen consumption persists in dyskinetic canine myocardium. J Cardiovasc Pharmacol 24: 37–44
4. Downing SE, Chen V (1990) Myocardial hibernation in the ischemic neonatal heart. Circ Res 66: 763–772
5. Gallagher KP, Matsuzaki M, Koziol JA, Kemper WS, Ross J Jr (1984) Regional myocardial perfusion and wall thickening during ischemia in conscious dogs. Am J Physiol 16: H727–H738
6. Offstad J, Kirkebøen KA, Lande K, Ilebekk A (1993) Cardiac adaption to one hour of mild regional low flow ischemia in the pig. Cardiovasc Res 27: 2248–2253
7. Pantely GA, Malone SA, Rhen WS, Anselone CG, Arai A, Bristow J, Bristow JD (1990) Regeneration of myocardial phosphocreatine in pigs despite continued moderate ischemia. Circ Res 67: 1481–1493
8. Ross J Jr (1991) Myocardial perfusion-contraction matching: implications for coronary heart disease and hibernation. Circulation 83: 1076–1083
9. Schulz R, Guth BD, Pieper K, Martin C, Heusch G (1992) Recruitment of an inotropic reserve in moderately ischemic myocardium at the expense of metabolic recovery. A model of short-term hibernation. Circ Res 70: 1282–1295
10. Takayama M, Norris RM, Brown MA, Armiger LC, Rivers JT, White HD (1988) Postischemic shortening of acutely ischemic myocardium predicts early and late recovery of function after coronary artery reperfusion. Circulation 78: 994–1007

E. Marban

Excitation-contraction coupling in hibernating myocardium

Key words Intracellular calcium – contraction – ischemia – NMR spectroscopy

The new sophistication in revascularization therapy for coronary artery disease has heightened our awareness of the diverse effects of perfusion on cardiac function. Total ischemia leads to a prompt cessation of contraction (1) by mechanisms that include a decrease in myocardial turgor, metabolite accumulation, and eventual inexcitability (2). A more subtle form of contractile failure is myocardial "hibernation" (3, 4), defined as the reversible contractile depression that occurs during a mild to moderate decrease in coronary perfusion. Considerable evidence favors the notion that force can respond to changes in flow even in the absence of ischemia ("Gregg's phenomenon"), but the mechanism remains unclear (5).

In the present article I briefly review our very incomplete understanding of excitation-contraction (E-C) coupling in the hibernating myocardium. We used a highly restrictive definition of hibernation in which we demanded that the changes in contractility during low flow be rapidly reversible and in which we excluded from consideration any dysfunction accompanied by frank ischemia, as judged by metabolite accumulation and net lactate production. The reader is referred elsewhere for comprehensive discussions of E-C coupling in health and in a variety of disease states (6, 7), and to the other articles in this issue for discussion of alternative (and clinically more realistic) models of hibernation.

Supported by N.I.H. R01 44065

E. Marban, M.D., Ph. D. (✉)
Division of Cardiology
Department of Medicine
Ross 844
The Johns Hopkins University School of Medicine
Baltimore, MD 21205, USA

Energy metabolism in an acute model of hibernation

To simulate myocardial hibernation, Kitakaze and I (8) used Langendorff-perfused isovolumically contracting ferret hearts probed with NMR spectroscopy. We first determined the range of coronary pressures over which force could be changed without concomitant metabolic evidence of ischemia. Figure 1 shows pooled data from 5 hearts obtained with an experimental protocol in which coronary perfusion pressure was stepped from 80 mm Hg to various other levels. We measured lactate efflux (A), pH_i and Pi (B), and developed pressure (C) to define precisely the coronary pressure at which ischemia first becomes apparent. Over the range of coronary pressures above 60 mm Hg, pressure development by the left ventricle varies more than two-fold (panel C, $P < 0.001$) despite the absence of significant changes in lactate production (A), pH_i (B), or [Pi] (B) over this range ($P \geq 0.1$ by ANOVA). The dashed vertical line thus demarcates coronary pressures above 60 mm Hg, where energy metabolism is comparable to control, from those of $\leq$ 55 mm Hg where significant differences begin to occur. The range above 60 mm Hg may be where pure acute "hibernation" occurs, given the paucity of metabolic evidence of ischemia and the complete reversibility of the contractile changes at these pressures.

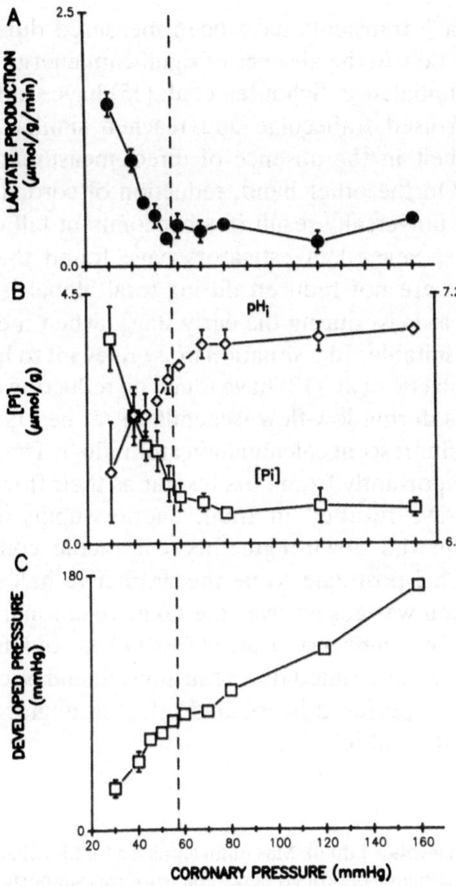

Fig. 1 Effects of coronary pressure on lactate production (A), Pi and pH_i (B), and developed pressure during twitch contractions in 2 mM $[Ca]_0$ (means ± SE from 5 hearts not loaded with either Ca^{2+} indicator). The coronary pressure began at 80 mm Hg and was returned to that value after each experimental determination. Developed pressure at 80 mm Hg remained stable (± 5 %) during the course of each experiment. [Reproduced from Kitakaze and Marban (8), by permission].

Calcium transients in acutely hibernating myocardium

The central abnormality of E-C coupling in hibernating myocardium is revealed in Fig. 2. Ca^{2+} transients were measured using NMR and 5F-BAPTA as described previously. Column A shows left ventricular developed pressure (DP), the Ca^{2+} transient, and a ^{31}P NMR spectrum obtained under control conditions (80 mm Hg perfusion pressure). During each cardiac cycle, $[Ca^{2+}]_i$ rises from about 150 nM in diastole to 1.7 μM at peak systole, consistent with estimates from aequorin in papillary muscles (9). The ^{31}P NMR spectrum is typical of well-oxygenated myocardium and shows a (very small) Pi peak at 4 – 5 ppm, a prominent phosphocreatine (PCr) resonance at 0 ppm, and the three ATP peaks. The shift between Pi and PCr reports a pH_i of 7.11. Coronary pressure was then decreased to 60 mm Hg, and the corresponding records in column B were obtained when developed pressure had reached a new steady state at slightly less than 50 % of the control value (compare A & B, top panels). Interestingly, another Ca^{2+} transient acquired at this time reveals a marked decrease in amplitude: diastolic $[Ca^{2+}]_i$ was little changed, but $[Ca^{2+}]_i$ now reaches only ~ 500 nM in systole. On the other hand, the ^{31}P spectrum changes very little; at 60 mm Hg, prominent PCr and ATP signals persist, and the Pi resonance increases only slightly. The striking decrease in $[Ca^{2+}]_i$ is thus not associated with clear-cut metabolic evidence of ischemia. The decrease in the amplitude of Ca^{2+} transients suffices to explain the negative inotropic effect (9, 10); no changes in myofilament responsiveness need be postulated. The fall in force was quickly reversible (C, upper panel), as was that in systolic $[Ca^{2+}]_i$ (C, lower panel); this intervention thus satisfies the criteria described above for hibernating myocardium. Such changes in Ca^{2+} transients occurred consistently and were statistically significant (8).

The results indicate that a decrease in Ca^{2+} transients underlies the contractile dysfunction of myocardial hibernation. The stunned myocardium is characterized by a decrease in myofilament responsiveness; there is no decrease in Ca^{2+} transients (6). Given the major differences in the factors that trigger stunning on one hand and hibernation on the other, a fundamental discrepancy in the E-C coupling abnormality in the two conditions should not come as a surprise.

Interpretation and caveats

With moderate decreases in perfusion pressure, as in Fig. 2, the paucity of changes in the ^{31}P NMR spectra contrast with the clear-cut effect of coronary pressure on Ca^{2+} transients. Such perfusion-induced changes in $[Ca^{2+}]_i$ are striking, but their mechanism is not yet clear. Whereas changes in Pi, pH_i and ATP certainly contribute to contractile failure when ischemia is prolonged and severe (11), such factors cannot explain the modulation of contractile force by less extreme alterations of coronary perfusion. Notably, force can actually increase when perfusion pressure is raised above ordinary control levels (5, 12), suggesting that factors other than ischemia must be operative. An alternative mechanism which has attracted considerable attention is the "garden hose effect": distension of the intracardiac coronary arteries is proposed to stretch the myocardial cells surrounding the vessels, resulting in increased contractile force via a Frank-Starling mechanism (13). This idea is supported by histologic examination of arrested hearts, which exhibit a modest increase in sarcomere length at supra-normal coronary pressures (14). In contrast, Kitakaze and I (8) found that an increase in perfusion pressure leads to a rise in force even in hearts in which the end-diastolic length has already been stretched to optimal levels. This observation argues against changes in sarcomere length as the sole cause of the changes in the force of contraction and in $[Ca^{2+}]_i$. A thorough re-examination of the biochemical basis of vascularly-induced alterations in cardiac contraction is clearly warranted. The demonstration that perfusion pressure modulates the amplitude of Ca^{2+} transients should further motivate the ongoing search for specific mediators of E-C coupling elaborated by endothelial cells, smooth muscle or myocardial cells in response to changes in coronary perfusion.

The data reviewed here are the only ones available in which Ca^{2+} transients have been measured during low coronary flow in the absence of significant energy supply-demand imbalance. Schouten et al. (15) have studied isolated perfused trabeculae and reached similar conclusions, albeit in the absence of direct measurements of $[Ca^{2+}]_i$. On the other hand, reduction of coronary flow does not universally result in a concomitant fall of Ca^{2+} transients. Several investigators have found that Ca^{2+} transients are not reduced during total global ischemia (16, 17), at least during the early stages when the hearts remain excitable. In a situation more relevant to hibernation, Camacho et al. (18) have found no reduction of Ca^{2+} transients during low-flow ischemia in rat hearts loaded with the fluorescent calcium indicator indo-1. Their study differs importantly from ours insofar as their flow reductions always resulted in frank energy supply-demand imbalance; the down-regulatory contractile compensation which I postulate to be the distinctive hallmark of hibernation was absent over the range of coronary flows explored by Camacho et al. Nevertheless, our findings with fully-compensated flow reductions should be checked using blood-perfused hearts and other strategies for the quantification of $[Ca^{2+}]_i$.

Acknowledgements I thank Masafumi Kitakaze for his collaboration on the experiments described here. The work was supported by the National Institutes of Health (R01 HL44065).

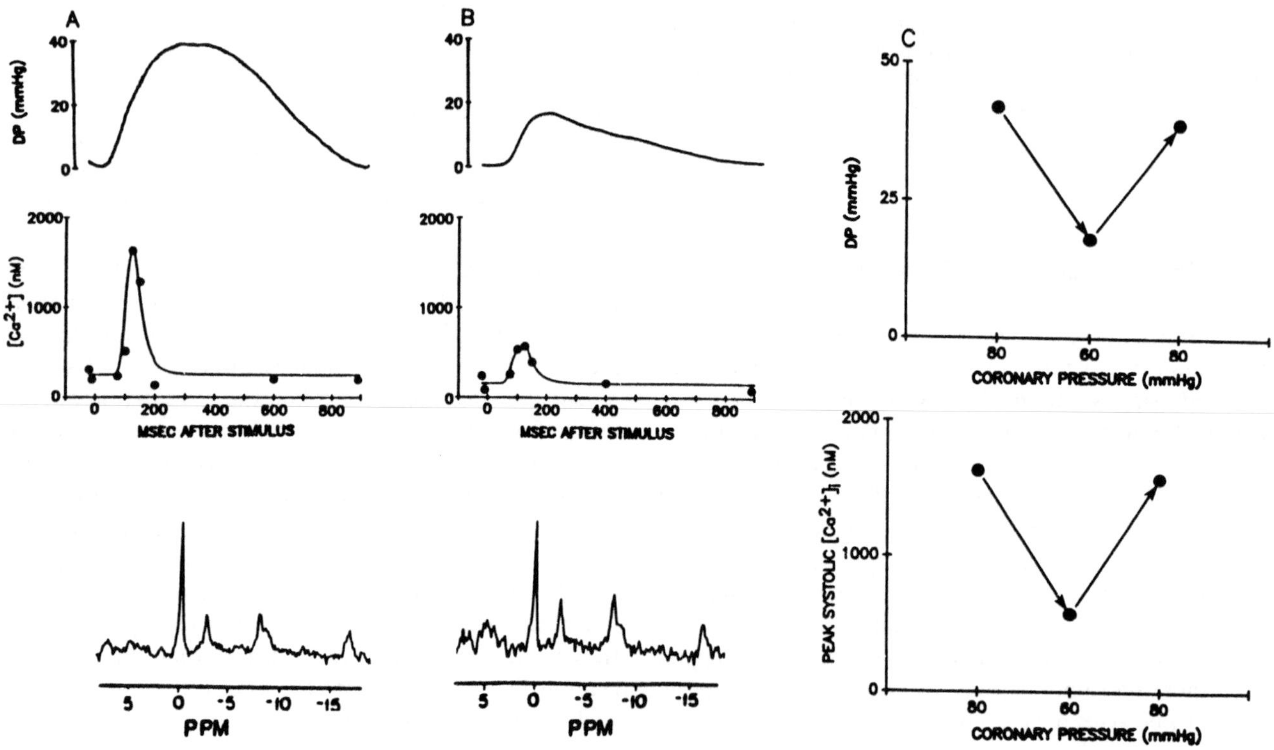

Fig. 2 Measurements of $[Ca^{2+}]_i$ in a perfused heart with 5F-BAPTA at two different perfusion pressures. A: Contractile pressure, Ca^{2+} transient and ^{31}P spectrum during control perfusion (80 mm Hg coronary pressure, 8 mM $[Ca]_0$). B: "Hibernating" myocardium induced by lowering coronary pressure to 60 mm Hg. Note the decrease in force and in systolic $[Ca^{2+}]_i$, with little change in energy metabolism as gauged by the ^{31}P spectrum. C: Developed pressure (top) and peak-systolic $[Ca^{2+}]_i$ (bottom) in the two stages of the experiment shown in A & B, and after returning to a coronary pressure of 80 mm Hg. [Adapted from Kitakaze and Marban (8), by permission].

References

1. Tennant R, Wiggers CJ (1935) The effect of coronary occlusion on myocardiol contraction. Am J Physiol 112: 351–361
2. Koretsune Y, Corretti M, Kusuoka H, Marban E (1991) Mechanism of ischemic contractile failure: inexcitability, metabolite accumulation, or vascular collapse? Circ Res 68: 255–262
3. Braunwald E, Rutherford JD (1986) Reversible ischemic left ventricular dysfunction: Evidence for the "hibernating myocardium". J Am Coll Cardiol 8: 1467–1470
4. Rahimtoola SH, Griffith GC (1989) The hibernating myocardium. Am Heart J 117: 211–221
5. Feigl EO (1983) Coronary physiology. Physiol Rev 63: 1–205
6. Marban E (1991) Myocardial stunning and hibernation: the physiology behind the colloquialisms. Circulation 83: 681–688
7. Atar D, Gao WD, Marban E (1995) Alterations of excitation-contraction coupling in stunned myocardium and in failing myocardium. J Mol Cell Cardiol, in press
8. Kitakaze M, Marban E (1989) Cellular mechanism of the modulation of contractile function by coronary perfusion pressure in ferret hearts. J Physiol (Lond) 414: 455–472
9. Wier WG, Yue DT (1986) Intracellular $[Ca^{2+}]$ transients underlying the short-term force-interval relationship in ferret ventricular myocardium. J Physiol (Lond) 376: 507–530
10. Marban E, Kitakaze M, Chacko VP, Pike MM (1988) Ca^{2+} transients in perfused hearts revealed by gated ^{19}F NMR spectroscopy. Circ Res 63: 673–678
11. Allen DG, Orchard CH (1986) Myocardial contractile function during ischemia and hypoxia. Circ Res 60: 153–168
12. Opie LH (1965) Coronary flow rate and perfusion pressure as determinants of mechanical function and oxidative metabolism of isolated perfused rat heart. J Physiol 180: 529–541
13. Arnold G, Kosche F, Miessner E, Neitzert A, Lochner W (1968) The importance of the perfusion pressure in the coronary arteries for the contractility and the oxygen consumption of the heart. Pflügers Archiv 299: 339–356
14. Poche R, Arnold G, Gahlen D (1971) The influence of coronary perfusion pressure on metabolism and ultrastructure of the myocardium of the arrested aerobically perfused isolated guinea-pig heart. Virchows Archiv 8: 252–266
15. Schouten VJ, Allart CP, Westerhof N (1992) Effect of perfusion pressure on force of contraction in thin papillary muscles and trabeculae from rat heart. J Physiol (Lond) 491: 585–604
16. Lee HC, Mohabir R, Smith N, Franz MR, Clusin WT (1988) Effect of ischemia on calcium-dependent fluorescence transients in rabbit hearts containing Indo 1. Circulation 78: 1047–1059
17. Kihara Y, Grossman W, Morgan JP (1989) Direct measurement of changes in intracellular calcium transients during hypoxia, ischemia, and reperfusion of the intact mammalian heart. Circ Res 65: 1029–1044
18. Camacho SA, Figueredo VM, Brandes R, Weiner MW (1993) Ca^{2+}-dependent fluorescence transients and phosphate metabolism during low-flow ischemia in rat hearts. Am J Physiol 256: H114–H122

24–26

G. A. Pantely
J. D. Bristow

Hibernating myocardium: a hypometabolic state for energy conservation

Key words Myocardial ischemia – myocardial metabolism

Introduction

Two phenomena can explain prolonged, yet reversible, myocardial contractile dysfunction. The first, myocardial stunning, is a reperfusion-induced abnormality. The second, which is the topic of this discussion, is myocardial hibernation. As originally proposed by Rahimtoola (1), hibernating myocardium is defined by 3 components. It is a hypocontractile region of the left ventricle in which

1. function is decreased to match reduced flow,
2. metabolic balance is present despite reduced flow,
3. cells remain viable, resuming normal contractile function after flow is restored.

The data supporting components 1 and 3 have been summarized in an excellent review article (2). The metabolic state has been a more difficult issue. Rahimtoola felt that while the hypoperfused region was initially ischemic, it did not remain chronically ischemic "in the strict sense". The vagueness of the terminology and lack of evidence that hypoperfused myocardium was not ischemic were obstacles in establishing the concept of hibernating myocardium. This present discussion focuses on the metabolic state of hypoperfused myocardium.

G. A. Pantely, M.D. ✉ · J. D. Bristow M.D.
Division of Cardiology, L 462
Oregon Health Sciences University
3181 S.W. Sam Jackson Park Road
Portland, Oregon 97201, USA

Potential metabolic responses to moderate hypoperfusion

A reduction in myocardial flow leads to an abrupt decrease in high energy phosphate (HEP) production, resulting in energy imbalance (HEP use > production). A reduction in intracellular HEP stores and increased ATP production by anaerobic metabolism are signs that HEP use exceeds production. To ensure cell viability, energy balance must be restored before intracellular energy sources are severely reduced. Potential metabolic responses to maintain systolic function and cell viability during persistent hypoperfusion include:

1. HEP use is reduced to match production. Intracellular HEP stores are not replenished during the continued hypoperfusion. This persistent abnormal energy state indicates a passive response to the energy imbalance.
2. HEP use is reduced to match production. However, HEP stores are replenished despite the continued hypoperfusion. This implies active regulation of these processes.

In the first alternative, cell viability is possible if intracellular HEP sources are not severely reduced. Systolic function is determined solely by oxygen availability. In the second alternative, reduced intracellular HEP levels are gradually corrected. The metabolic state of the cell returns to or near normal despite reduced energy production, as Rahimtoola speculated. This is an active, regulated response, one that represents a "hypometabolic state for energy conservation" (3). Experimental evidence is available that moderately hypoperfused myocardium can achieve something close to this interesting metabolic response. This will be outlined in the next section. Although this discussion emphasizes our work, other groups have significantly contributed to the understanding of metabolic adaptations in hypoperfused myocardium.

Experimental evidence supporting the concept of hibernating myocardium

Experiments were performed in anesthetized pigs. Within 10 minutes after the onset of moderate regional ischemia (47 % reduction in left anterior descending coronary artery flow), myocardial oxygen consumption falls by 44 % and systolic wall thickening by 75 %. Subendocardial phosphocreatine (PCr) falls by 61 %, ATP by 46 %, and anaerobic metabolism is present with lactate production and high tissue lactate levels (Figure 1) (4 – 6). However, remarkable metabolic changes evolve as the reduction in flow continues (4 – 8). Over the next 60 minutes, anaerobic metabolism ceases and HEP repletion is initiated with PCr content returning to normal. ATP content remains reduced but stable. These metabolic changes are not due to pathologic abnormalities such as depletion of substrate for anaerobic metabolism or inability to convert PCr to ATP (5, 7, 8). However, this state is easily upset by increasing energy use with pacing (5) or a positive inotropic agent (7, 8), resulting in the reappearance of anaerobic metabolism and a fall in PCr.

The lack of anaerobic metabolism and regeneration of PCr despite continued hypoperfusion are important findings. They indicate that HEP use is slightly below that of production (5, 6). Since PCr is only produced from ATP, it costs one ATP molecule to produce one PCr molecule. It is not certain why hypoperfused cells with diminished ATP content so quickly restore PCr to normal. However, PCr content may be a sensitive measure of how successfully the cell compensates for reduced energy production.

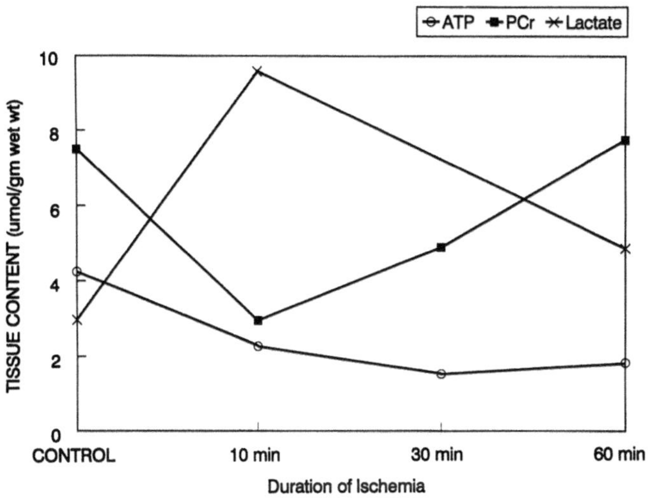

Fig. 1 Changes in subendocardial tissue content of ATP (–O–), phosphocreatine (–■–), and lactate (–X–) during a 47 % reduction in transmural left anterior descending coronary artery flow for 60 minutes. Data are adapted from references 4 and 5.

Complete conservation of energy requires restoration of ATP stores which still did not occur after 5 hours of moderate hypoperfusion (9). ATP content could possibly return to normal, but this may require more time. ADP and AMP, precursors of ATP, are rapidly depleted in cells during ischemia. With these substrate deficiencies, ATP repletion occurs by slower de novo synthetic pathways.

In these models of controlled ischemia, hibernating myocardium occurs when the hypoperfusion is of moderate severity, of relatively brief duration (hours) and oxygen demand is stable (4 – 8). However, this is a delicate state that can easily be upset, exceeding the ability of the hypoperfused myocardium to maintain viability.

These results make it difficult to know whether "ischemia" is present despite reduced function or reduced flow. Ischemia is present in hypofunctioning myocardium when flow is reduced in relation to baseline, and anaerobic metabolism plus reduced intracellular HEP levels are also present. However, when a hypofunctioning region with reduced flow has aerobic metabolism and normal or near normal PCr and lactate levels, it may best be defined as hibernating, rather than ischemic, myocardium.

Human myocardium is probably capable of metabolic adaptations similar to those observed during hypoperfusion in animals. The situation in humans, however, is more complex with frequent changes in myocardial oxygen demand or supply occurring during a day. It is unlikely that a hibernating state similar to the animal model exists for prolonged periods in chronically hypofunctioning myocardium in humans (10).

Now that the concept of hibernating myocardium is more convincingly established, the mechanisms of hibernation need to be defined. Understanding these mechanisms could have broad theoretical and practical implications.

Conclusions

Moderately hypoperfused myocardium in animals initiates an active process that transiently reduces regional energy consumption below that required by the reduced flow. This eliminates most metabolic abnormalities of ischemia despite ongoing hypoperfusion. These interesting early metabolic adaptations help to confirm the concept of hibernating myocardium, a hypometabolic state for energy conservation. A similar metabolic response probably can occur in human myocardium. However, the complexities of coronary disease may make it difficult to demonstrate these metabolic adaptations in chronically hypofunctioning myocardium in humans.

References

1. Rahimtoola SH (1985) A perspective on the three large multicenter randomized clinical trials of coronary bypass surgery for chronic stable angina. Circulation 72 (suppl V): V-123–V-135
2. Ross J Jr (1991) Myocardial perfusion-contraction matching. Implications for coronary heart disease and hibernation. Circulation 83: 1076–1083
3. Hochachka PW (1986) Defense strategies against hypoxia and hypothermia. Science 231: 234–241
4. Pantely GA, Malone SA, Rhen WS, Anselone CG, Arai A, Bristow J, Bristow JD (1990) Regeneration of myocardial phosphocreatine in pigs despite continued moderate ischemia. Circ Res 67: 1481–1493
5. Arai AE, Pantely GA, Anselone CG, Bristow J, Bristow JD (1991) Active downregulation of myocardial energy requirements during prolonged moderate ischemia in swine. Circ Res 69: 1458–1469
6. Bristow JD, Arai AE, Anselone CG, Pantely GA (1991) Response to myocardial ischemia as a regulated process. Circulation 84: 2580–2587
7. Schulz R, Guth BD, Pieper K, Martin C, Heusch G (1992) Recruitment of an inotropic reserve in moderately ischemic myocardium at the expense of metabolic recovery. A model of short-term hibernation. Circ Res 70: 1282–1295
8. Schulz R, Rose J, Martin C, Brodde OE, Heusch G (1993) Development of short-term myocardial hibernation. Its limitation by the severity of ischemia and inotropic stimulation. Circulation 88: 684–695
9. Neill WA, Ingwall JS, Andrews E, Gopal MA, Klein K, Kramer M, Oxendine JM, Piotrowski ZH, Reis I (1986) Stabilization of a derangement in adenosine triphosphate metabolism during sustained, partial ischemia in the dog heart. J Am Coll Cardiol 8: 894–900
10. Vanoverschelde JJ, Wijns W, Depré C, Essamri B, Heyndrickx GR, Borgers M, Bol A, Melin JA (1993) Mechanisms of chronic regional postischemic dysfunction in humans. New insights from the study of noninfarcted collateral-dependent myocardium. Circulation 87: 1513–1523

27–29

J. D. Schipke

Myocardial hibernation

Key words Myocardium – hibernation – downregulation – ischemia – perfusion-contraction matching

Introduction

Hibernation is induced via the photoperiod and is a humorally controlled form used by some homeothermic animals to survive the adverse conditions of the winter. During winter sleep, body temperature is decreased to ambient temperature. Heart rate, metabolism and other physiologic functions exhibit corresponding decreases. Spontaneous or provoked return to baseline is possible at any time (6).

It is now almost ten years since the term myocardial hibernation was used to describe myocardial ischemia (11). Usage of this term seems inappropriate since the definition as used in zoology is not easily transferable into medicine and therefore the paradigm of myocardial hibernation is frequently imprecisely used in the literature. Not only to facilitate communication but also because of its high clinical significance, this particular ischemic condition deserves meticulous definition.

Hibernating myocardium

The condition of reduced oxygen supply due to reduced perfusion has been termed ischemia. Traditionally, it reflects a mismatch between oxygen consumption and oxygen supply so that its persistence will induce cell death. After pathological studies revealed that postoperatively recovered asynergic myocardium contained little or no fibrotic tissue (2), it became conceivable that myocardial function could recover even after long-lasting ischemia.

In 1984, Rahimtoola introduced the term myocardial hibernation to describe a chronic ischemia with dyskinetic myocardial segments and reduced perfusion but with active metabolism. Later, myocardial hibernation was described as an act of self preservation which becomes effective within a limited range of oxygen supply reductions (11) to protect myocardium from irreversible damage (3, 8). The interval needed for hibernating myocardium to recover upon reperfusion is not known. However, some studies suggest quick functional recovery (9, 11).

Because hibernating myocardium can benefit from reperfusion, it must be differentiated from other dyskinetic myocardium. Seemingly, more patients than assumed can expect improvement of myocardial function (4), and more and more patients have already benefitted from revascularization (5, 9). The improved function is generally understood to result from increased oxygen supply and improved metabolism (5). Interestingly, solely restoring physiologic pressures in the coronary arteries (= garden hose effect) was made responsible for the improved function (9).

Mechanisms

Various candidates were suspected to initiate myocardial hibernation. During moderate ischemia, deranged high energy phosphates could induce reduced function. In our study on isolated, blood-perfused canine hearts we systematically reduced the coronary arterial pressure (CAP)

PD Dr. J. D. Schipke (✉)
Institut für Experimentelle Chirurgie
Universität Düsseldorf
Moorenstraße 5
40225 Düsseldorf

from control to different low values. At a critical functional CAP (35 mmHg), left ventricular peak pressure (LVSP) was decreased to a steady level, but PCr- or ATP-concentrations did not decrease. This stability persisted until CAP was lowered to 14 mmHg, the critical metabolic CAP, where LVSP kept decreasing and marked metabolic changes were noted by decreased PCr- and increased Pi-concentrations, suggesting an unstable and ischemic heart (Fig. 1). Returning CAP to normal from the zone between these two critical CAPs resulted in complete recovery of function (12). Since stable, although sometimes decreased, ATP- and PCr-concentrations were also reported from others (10, 16), the concentrations of high energy phosphates are not very likely responsible for hibernation. In turn, reduced turnover of high energy phosphates in hypoxic myocardium and not their concentrations were made responsible for the reduced ventricular function (1).

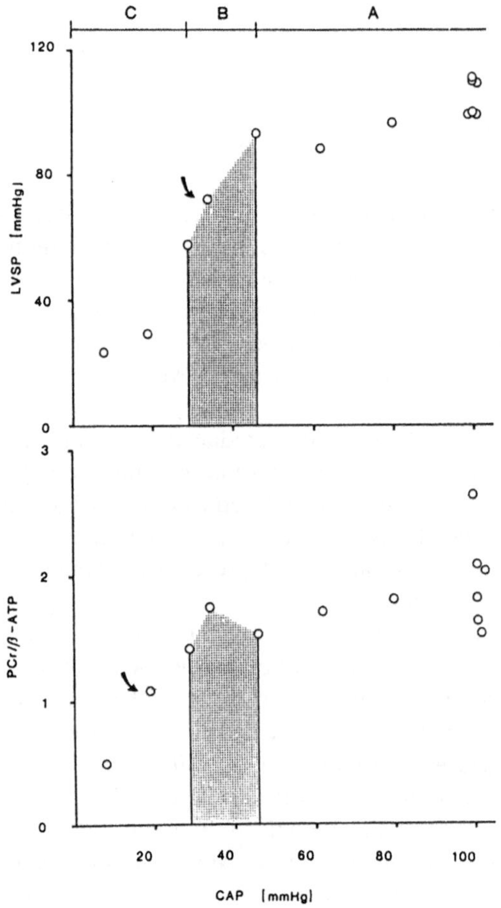

Fig. 1 Effects of reductions in coronary arterial pressure (CAP) on ventricular function (left ventricular peak systolic pressure: LVSP; top) and the ratio between PCr and β-ATP-concentrations (PCr/β-ATP; bottom). Reductions in perfusion pressure were not associated with impaired ventricular function as long as they took place within the autoregulatory pressure range (A). Additional reductions in perfusion pressure that induced moderate reductions in coronary blood flow resulted in a particular ischemia with reduced but stable function (B: shaded area): perfusion and contraction matched: the myocardium was hibernating. The function of such myocardium recovered after institution of physiologic perfusion. Additional reductions in perfusion pressure and oxygen supply below the hibernating range produced ischemia in the more classical sense: oxygen supply and oxygen demand did no longer match (C). Function was furthermore impaired and progressively decreased, and concentration of high energy phosphates was decreased compared to ranges A and B.

The search for candidates continues and from one study, the reduced amplitude of Ca^{++}-transients in the ischemic myocardium (8) was included, whereas from preliminary studies both adenosine (13) and ATP-dependent potassium channels (14) were excluded from being involved in the development of myocardial hibernation. Other preliminary studies on isolated cells in turn, lead to the conclusion that endothelial cells sense hypoxia releasing a novel factor(s) which directly inhibits crossbridge cycling and thus, myocyte contraction and in doing so match cardiac contraction to oxygen supply (15).

It is well established that reductions in myocardial oxygen supply result in a decrease in contractile function. Little evidence exists, however, as to whether the reduction in energy demand is in proportion to the reduction in function. Employing the MVO_2/pressure-volume relation, we observed at moderately reduced coronary arterial pressures (from 90 to 60 mmHg) an increase in the contractile efficiency, i.e. the contractile apparatus converted the reduced oxygen more economically to energy. This finding was independent from whether glucose, glucose and lactate, or glucose und palmitate was provided. However, if only palmitate was provided as substrate, contractile efficiency was not increased during moderate ischemia (7). Thus, the increased O_2-utilisation during moderate ischemia can be attributed – at least in part – to the fact that the myocardium can switch towards the energetically more favourable substrate.

Summary

From available results, the following schematic can be drawn: Reductions in perfusion pressure are not associated with impaired ventricular function as long as they take place within the autoregulatory range. Additional reductions in perfusion pressure that moderately diminish coronary blood flow will result in a particular ischemia with decreased but stable function: perfusion and contraction match, the myocardium hibernates. The process responsible for this new equilibrium could be termed down regulation of function.

The trigger inducing hibernation is so far unknown. The strategy, however, is similar to that used by hibernating animals. Likewise, myocardial hibernation is a protective mechanism. As hibernators recover initial function after unfavourable periods are terminated, hibernating myocardium recovers after institution of physiologic perfusion. It is under debate, whether function quickly recovers or remains temporarily depressed. As hibernating animals might finally even die, if unfavourable periods last too long, myocardium might become irreversibly injured due to ischemia lasting too long.

Additional reductions in perfusion pressure and oxygen supply below the hibernating range produce ischemia in the more classical sense, because oxygen supply and demand no longer match. Damage will become irreversible in case the situation persists longer than about 20 min. After onset of reperfusion, the myocardial function would remain depressed, however, for a considerable period: myocardial stunning.

Considering the regional heterogeneities of myocardial blood flow, distinct differentiation between moderate and severe ischemia is difficult. Ischemia will induce more articulate damage in subendocardial than in subepicardial layers. Similarly, damage in the ischemic core will be more pronounced than in the border zone. Presence or absence of collaterals will make prognosis of the outcome of ischemia even more difficult. Myocardium can hibernate or become necrotic, in parallel; its function can quickly or slowly recover upon reperfusion. The existence of such mixed forms could explain much of the dissent about the phenomenon of myocardial hibernation. On the other hand, actively employing the (unknown) underlying mechanisms of down regulation of function and myocardial hibernation could possibly shift jeopardized myocardium from severe to moderate ischemia and thus preserve it from becoming necrotic. Independent from the therapeutic aspect, hibernating myocardium deserves appropriate diagnosis and revascularization to avoid it from unnecessarily hibernating beyond winter.

Acknowledgement Reading and correcting of the manuscript by Ms. N. Palomero-Gallagher (M. Sc. Bio) is greatly appreciated.

References

1. Bittl JA, Balschi JA, Ingwall JS (1987) Contractile failure and high-energy phosphate turnover during hypoxia: 31P-NMR surface coil studies in living rat. Circ Res 60: 871–878
2. Bodenheimer MM, Banka VS, Hermann GA, Trout RG, Pasdar H, Helfant RH (1976) Reversible Asynergy. Circulation 5: 792–796
3. Braunwald E, Rutherford JD (1986) Reversible ischemic left ventricular dysfunction: evidence for the "hibernating myocardium". J Am Coll Cardiol 8: 1467–1470
4. Broderick T, Sawada S, Armstrong WF, Ryan T, Dillon JC, Bourdillon PDV, Feigenbaum H (1990) Improvement in rest and exercise-induced wall motion abnormalities after coronary angioplasty: an exercise echocardiographic study. J Am Coll Cardiol 15 (3): 591–599
5. Cohen M, Charney R, Hershman R, Fuster V, Gorlin R (1988) Reversal of chronic ischemic myocardial dysfunction after transluminal coronary angioplasty. J Am Coll Cardiol 12: 1193–1198
6. Hoffmann RA (1964) Terrestrial animals in cold: hibernators. In: Dill DB, Adolph EF, Wilber CG (eds) Handbook of Physiology, section 4, Adaption to the environment; American Physiological Society, Washington, pp 379–403
7. Krenz M, Sunderdiek V, Schwanke U, Arnold G, Schipke JD (1995) Hibernierendes Myokard-Einfluß von Substratangebot und Schwere der Minderperfusion auf Änderungen des kontraktilen Wirkungsgrades. Z Kardiol 84 Suppl: 31 (Abstract)
8. Marban E (1991) Myocardial stunning and hibernation. Circulation 83: 681–688
9. Melchior J, Doriot PA, Chatelani P, Meier B, Urban P, Finci L, Rutishauser W (1987) Improvement of left ventricular contraction and relaxation synchronism after recanalization of chronic total coronary occlusion by angioplasty. J Am Coll Cardiol 9 (4): 763–768
10. Pantely GA, Malone SA, Rhen WS, Anselone CG, Arai A, Bristow J, Bristow JD (1990) Regeneration of myocardial phosphocreatine in pigs despite continued moderate ischemia. Circ Res 67: 1481–1493
11. Rahimtoola SH (1989) The hibernating myocardium. Am Heart J 117:111–121
12. Schipke JD, Harasawa Y, Chacko VP, Burkhoff D, Sagawa K, Jacobus WE (1989) Critical perfusion pressures for functional and metabolic derangements in the hibernating, isolated blood-perfused canine heart. Faseb J 3: A249 (Abstract)
13. Schulz R, Rose J, Heusch G (1994) Endogenous adenosine is not involved in the development of short-term myocardial hibernation. J Mol Cell Cardiol 26: 65 (Abstract)
14. Schulz R, Rose J, Martin C, Heusch G (1994) ATP-dependent potassium channels are not involved in the development of short-term myocardial hibernation. Eur Heart J 14 (suppl): 220 (Abstract)
15. Shah AM, Mebazza A, Cuda G et al. (1994) Hypoxic endothelial cells inhibit myocardial crossbridge cycling and contraction: the mechanism underlying myocardial contraction? Eur Heart J 15 Suppl: 115 (Abstract)
16. Sunderdiek U, Bergfeld I, Schwenen M, Arnold G, Schipke JD (1992) Myocardial function and energy balance during reduced myocardial perfusion. Eur Heart J 13: 438 (Abstract)

30 – 32

R. Schulz
G. Heusch

Acute adaptation to ischemia: Short-term hibernating myocardium

Key words Myocardial ischemia – perfusion-contraction-matching – inotropic reserve

The term "hibernation" – a paradigm borrowed from zoology – implies a regulatory reduction of energy expenditure in adaptation to reduced energy supply, thereby allowing survival. In the heart, the situation of reduced contractile function (reflecting energy expenditure) during persistent reduction in blood flow (reflecting energy supply) was termed „myocardial hibernation"; by definition, the myocardium remains viable and contractile function recovers upon restoration of blood flow (4). While the initial period of adaptation to ischemia lasting for up to several hours, i.e., short-term myocardial hibernation, is well characterized in animal models, long-term myocardial hibernation lasting over weeks or months can only be inferred from clinical observations (4).

Transition from an initial ischemic supply-demand imbalance to short-term myocardial hibernation

Within the first few seconds following an acute reduction of myocardial blood flow, energy demand of the hypoperfused myocardium clearly exceeds the reduced energy supply. However, this imbalance between energy supply and demand is an inherently unstable condition since contractile function and thus energy demand rapidly decreases following the onset of ischemia. In the subsequent steady-state condition, the amount of contractile dysfunction is in proportion to the reduction of myocardial blood flow, i.e., a state of perfusion-contraction-matching exists (5).

R. Schulz · Prof. Dr. G. Heusch (✉)
Abteilung für Pathophysiologie
Universitätsklinikum Essen
Hufelandstraße 55, 45147 Essen

Metabolism of short-term hibernating myocardium

Within the first 5 min of ischemia, myocardial creatine phosphate content is reduced and lactate consumption is reversed to net lactate production. When ischemia is prolonged to 60 – 90 min, however, myocardial creatine phosphate content recovers to near control values (1, 3, 6), and lactate production is attenuated (2, 6), whereas regional contractile dysfunction remains reduced (2, 3, 6). Apparently, the reduction in regional contractile function during moderate ischemia permits the partial recovery of ischemia-induced alterations in metabolism.

Recruitment of an inotropic reserve at the expense of metabolic recovery in short-term hibernating myocardium

Although basal contractile function is depressed, the hypoperfused myocardium retains its responsiveness to an inotropic challenge (Fig. 1) (6). When, after 85 min of ischemia, dobutamine is infused selectively into the ischemic myocardium of anesthetized pigs, contractile function increases, although regional blood flow remains reduced. Thus, energy is available in the ischemic myocardium which is not used to support baseline function, but permits the increase in contractile function upon an inotropic challenge. However, the increase in contractile function during inotropic stimulation once more decreases myocardial creatine phosphate content and increases lactate production (Fig. 1), indicating a renewed supply-demand imbalance.

Limitations of short-term hibernation

The development of such delicate balance between regional myocardial blood flow and function during early ischemia is disturbed by unfavorable alterations in supply and demand. When after 5 min of ischemia, at a blood flow reduction compatible with the development of short-term myocardial hibernation over 90 min, energy supply is further reduced by a further reduction of myocardial blood flow, necroses develop. Likewise, increasing energy demand by continuous inotropic stimulation with dobutamine induces necroses (8). Thus, both the further reduction in energy supply by an increasing severity of ischemia and an enhanced energy expenditure by continuous inotropic stimulation impair the development of short-term myocardial hibernation and precipitate myocardial infarction.

Open questions

1) How long can the ischemic myocardium maintain its metabolic integrity? It is possible that the metabolic status of short-term hibernating myocardium once again deteriorates over time. On the other hand, it is possible that the successfully adapted myocardium can maintain such a state indefinitely and will proceed into long-term hibernation. Long-term myocardial hibernation therefore may or may not develop from short-term myocardial hibernation.
2) What are the mechanisms responsible for the transition from an initial supply/demand imbalance to a state of perfusion-contraction matching? Alterations in the β-adrenoceptor density or affinity as the underlying mechanism for the development of short-term myocardial hibernation have been excluded (8). Also, the increased adenosine release during ischemia is not involved in the development of short-term myocardial hibernation as increased catabolism of endogenous adenosine by infusion of adenosine deaminase does not interfere with baseline contractile function, metabolic recovery, the recruitment of inotropic reserve by dobutamine and myocardial viability (7).

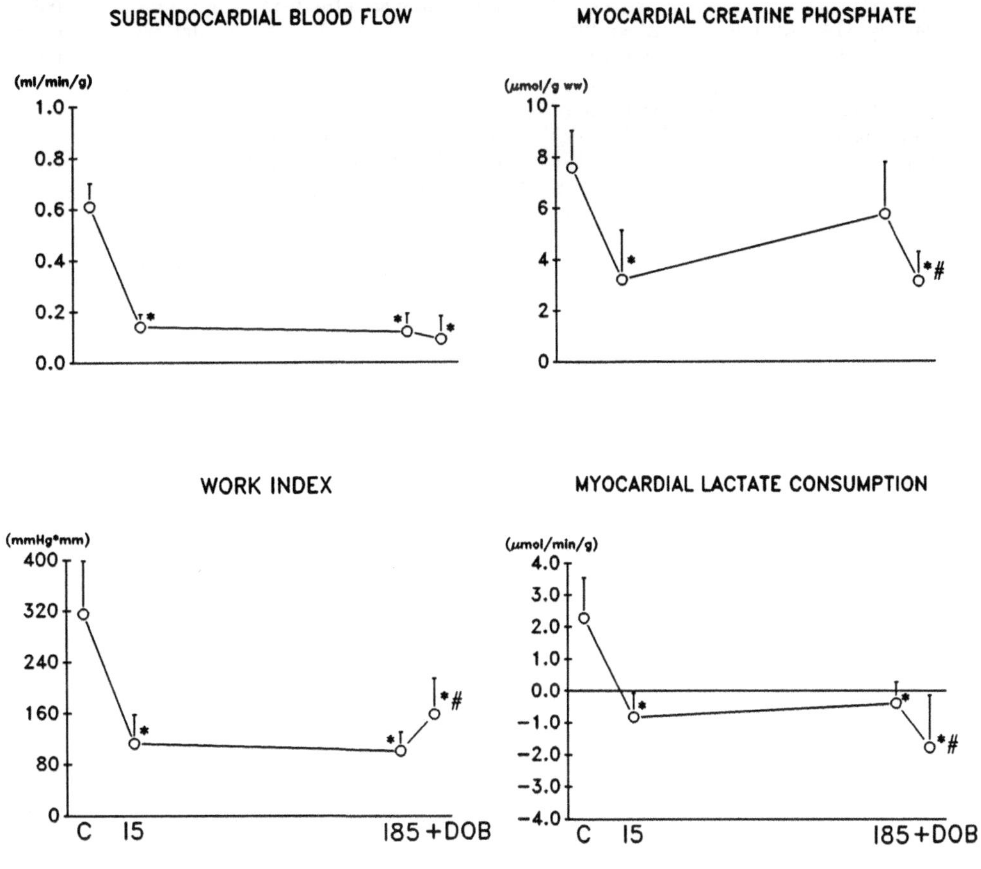

Fig. 1 The reduction in subendocardial blood flow of the anterior myocardium at 5 min ischemia (I5) is associated with decreased regional contractile function. Creatine phosphate falls and lactate consumption is reversed to net lactate production. With the extension of ischemia to 85 min (I85) at a constant subendocardial blood flow, there is a tendency for a further decrease in regional contractile function. In contrast, lactate production is attenuated and creatine phosphate recovers to a value no longer significantly different from control. Infusion of dobutamine (+DOB) after 85 min of ischemia increases regional contractile function at an unchanged subendocardial blood flow. This increase in contractile function, however, is associated once more with a decreased creatine phosphate content and increased lactate production. From (6)

Also, none of these features is affected by blockade of ATP-dependent potassium channels with glibenclamide, ruling out that activation of ATP-dependent potassium channels is involved in the development of short-term myocardial hibernation (9).

3) How long can the ischemic myocardium respond to an inotropic stimulation? In contrast to dysfunctional, irreversibly damaged myocardium, the hibernating myocardium retains an inotropic reserve. The recruitment of such inotropic reserve, which is at the expense of metabolic recovery, can be used to identify hibernating myocardium. A progressive loss of myofibrils in ischemic myocardium, however, may result in a reduction and finally loss of response to an inotropic challenge, despite persistent viability.

4) Does chronic contractile dysfunction in patients reflect true hibernation, i.e. a situation of chronic contractile dysfunction during persistent ischemia, or repetitive episodes of ischemia and reperfusion, i.e. repetitive stunning?

5) Can myocardial hibernation be induced or reinforced? This is a challenging therapeutic goal, as it would extend the time frame for reperfusion interventions in patients with acute ischemic syndromes. In that respect, short-term myocardial hibernation, i.e. endogenous cardioprotective mechanisms during acute ischemic syndromes, may be a much more common and important phenomenon than long-term myocardial hibernation.

References

1. Downing SE, Chen V (1990) Myocardial hibernation in the ischemic neonatal heart. Circ Res 66: 763–772
2. Fedele FA, Gewirtz H, Capone RJ, Sharaf B, Most AS (1988) Metabolic response to prolonged reduction of myocardial blood flow distal to a severe coronary artery stenosis. Circulation 78: 729–735
3. Pantely GA, Malone SA, Rhen WS, Anselone CG, Arai A, Bristow J, Bristow JD (1990) Regeneration of myocardial phosphocreatine in pigs despite continued moderate ischemia. Circ Res 67: 1481–1493
4. Rahimtoola SH (1985) A perspective on the three large multicenter randomized clinical trials of coronary bypass surgery for chronic stable angina. Circulation 72 Suppl V: V-123–V-135
5. Ross Jr J (1991) Myocardial perfusion-contraction matching. Implications for coronary heart disease and hibernation. Circulation 83: 1076–1083
6. Schulz R, Guth BD, Pieper K, Martin C, Heusch G (1992) Recruitment of an inotropic reserve in moderately ischemic myocardium at the expense of metabolic recovery: a model of short-term hibernation. Circ Res 70: 1282–1295
7. Schulz R, Rose J, Heusch G (1994) Endogenous adenosine is not involved in the development of short-term myocardial hibernation. J Moll Cell Cardiol 26: 234 (abstr)
8. Schulz R, Rose J, Martin C, Brodde OE, Heusch G (1993) Development of short-term myocardial hibernation: its limitation by the severity of ischemia and inotropic stimulation. Circulation 88: 684–695
9. Schulz R, Rose J, Martin C, Heusch G (1993) Activation of ATP-dependent potassium channels is not involved in the development of short-term myocardial hibernation in swine. Circulation 88: I-632 (abstr)

33–35
© Steinkopff Verlag 1996

H. Gewirtz

Myocardial hibernation: unresolved physiological and clinical issues

Key words Myocardial blood flow – myocardial oxygen consumption – myocardial contraction

Introduction

It is impossible to discuss myocardial hibernation without consideration of myocardial stunning. Further, to understand either process it is imperative that their definitions be kept firmly in mind. An essential feature common both to hibernation and stunning is reversibly impaired contractile function of the myocardium (1, 2). Myocardial stunning, however, is associated with "normal" levels of myocardial blood flow and oxygen consumption (3, 4). Since myocardial systolic function by definition is depressed, "normal" levels of myocardial oxygen consumption in stunning must be regarded as excessive relative to the level of mechanical work performed. In contrast, myocardial oxygen consumption, blood flow, and systolic function all are proportionately reduced in hibernation (5, 6). Thus, from a conceptual point-of-view myocardial hibernation can and should be distinguished from stunning based on the prevailing level of regional myocardial blood flow and oxygen consumption. Balanced reduction of myocardial blood flow, function and oxygen comsumption should be considered hibernation while "normal" myocardial blood flow and oxygen comsumption with impaired systolic function should be considered stunning.

H. Gewirtz, M.D.
Nuclear Cardiology
Vincent Burnham 3
Massachusetts General Hospital
32 Fruit Street
Boston, Massachusetts 02114, USA

Controversies: unresolved physiological and clinical issues

Employing the above definitions, one can address several related questions. For instance, can repeated episodes of stunning result in hibernation? Can hibernating myocardium undergo stunning? Is it possible for the same region of the heart to exhibit both hibernation and stunning at the same time?

A preliminary report with a porcine model of external coronary artery stenosis indicates that repeated episodes of coronary occlusion/reperfusion can occur over a period of a month without myocardial infarction and may result in persistent impairment of left ventricular systolic function (7). Since regional myocardial blood flow in the stenosis zone in this study (7) was only modestly reduced, if at all, the authors concluded chronic LV dysfunction was caused by stunning not hibernation. The data presented, however, do not rule out a role for hibernation as a primary cause of chronically impaired systolic function.

A recent human study (8) described a group of patients in whom regional left ventricular function was impaired in face of resting myocardial blood flow (and oxygen consumption) which was ~ 20 % lower than that of the reference region of the same heart. Myocardial blood flow in collateral dependent zones with dysfunction, however, was similar to that of the reference area of hearts from another group of patients in which wall motion in collateral dependent regions was normal and flow in the collateral dependent zone equal to that of the reference area (8). Since basal regional myocardial blood flow was "nearly normal" and flow reserve reduced in a limited number of individuals studied, the authors concluded that repeated episodes of myocardial ischemia (i.e. "stunning") caused chronic impairment of systolic function and that chronic hypoperfusion (i.e. "hibernation") was less likely to be responsible. Evidence demonstrating intermittent coronary artery occlusion/reperfusion or demand-induced ischemia, however, was not presented. Further, proper classification of the physiological status of these patients depends on the reference region chosen. If, as is customary, a region of the same heart with normal function and flow is selected, then the collateral dependent segments should be classed as hibernating since regional myocardial blood flow, function and oxygen consumption all were reduced. The extent of the reduction (~ 20 %) is quite consistent with data obtained in a chronic porcine model of myocardial hibernation (5) as well as other observations made in humans (9).

The above considerations should not be taken to mean that chronic, repeated episodes of stunning cannot give way to chronic hibernation. However, since stunning by definition refers to a state of post-ischemic mechanical dysfunction in face or "normal" resting blood flow, one must propose at some point that basal myocardial blood flow declines and remains reduced in response to impaired mechanical function to complete the transition from chronic impairment of contractile function initiated by stunning to chronic impairment maintained by hibernation. The decline in resting myocardial blood flow in these circumstances may reflect recovery of microvessels from stunning with resultant return of metabolic regulatory function. Thus myocardial hibernation may be reached by more than one pathway. In some cases progressive proximal stenosis of the coronary circulation eventually could result in a steady decline in resting flow and equal reduction in function and myocardial oxygen consumption (5). Alternatively, episodic occlusion/reperfusion with both myocardial and vascular stunning could eventually revert to a state of persistent low flow, function and oxygen consumption if microvascular stunning resolved and metabolic flow control was restored.

The degree to which myocardial oxygen consumption is matched to mechanical function and blood flow is of considerable interest in evaluation of myocardial stunning and hibernation. Unfortunately, a major determinant of myocardial oxygen consumption, namely myocardial contractility, is difficult to measure and therefore has not been considered in most discussions of myocardial hibernation and stunning. Without this information, it is difficult to say just how much "function" (usually considered in terms of regional wall motion) is impaired and, therefore, how closely matched or mis-matched myocardial blood flow and oxygen consumption are relative to it.

The issue of contractile state also is relevant to discussion of the possibility of stunning superimposed on hibernation and even the simultaneous existence of the two states in the same segment of myocardium (10). If we recall the common clinical and experimental observation that myocardial ischemia can be ameliorated by drugs which reduce myocardial contractility, then it is not clear that a reduction in blood flow from a chronically reduced baseline will have the same effect on myocardial function as a comparable reduction from a "normal" level of flow. Likewise, an increase in myocardial oxygen demand may not necessarily result in acute ischemia. Accordingly, the notion proposed in recent reviews (10, 11) that collateral dependent myocardium with impaired vasodilator reserve is vulnerable to repeated episodes of ischemia, possibly "silent," simply because myocardial blood flow and flow reserve may be reduced at rest, ignores the fact – despite reduced resting blood flow – that 1) flow reserve is not exhausted (5); 2) regional function can improve in response to inotropic stimulation, and 3) the myocardium may adapt in a fashion which renders it less not more vulnerable to acute ischemia. Thus, while it is logical to propose that acute on chronic reduction in myocardial perfusion (or acute increase in oxygen demand) could lead to "stunning" superimposed on hibernation, additional studies are required to test this hypothesis. Finally, chronic, reversible impairment of myocardial systolic function, like jaundice, should be considered a physiological entity having multiple potential etiologies. In some cases stunning may be the primary cause or could represent an intermediary state in transition to hibernation. In others chronic hibernation may be present from the outset. Animal models (5, 7) and human observations (8, 9) exist which support both mechanisms.

References

1. Kloner RA, Przyklenk K (1992) Hibernation and stunning of the myocardium. (Editorial). New Engl J Med 325: 1877–1879
2. Rahimtoola SH (1989) The hibernating myocardium. Am Heart J 117: 211–221
3. Heyndrickx G, Wijns W, Vogelaers D, Degrieck Y, Bol A, Vandeplassche G, Melin JA (1993) Recovery of regional contractile function and oxidative metabolism in stunned myocardium induced by 1-hour circumflex coronary artery stenosis in chronically instrumented dogs. Circ Res 72: 901–913
4. Bergmann SR, Weinheimer CJ, Brown MA, Perez JE (1994) Enhancement of regional myocardial efficiency and persistence of perfusion, oxidative, and functional reserve with paired pacing of stunned myocardium. Circulation 89: 2290–2296

5. Mills I, Fallon JT, Wrenn D, Sasken HF, Gray W, Bier J, Levine D, Berman S, Gilson M, Gewirtz H (1994) Adaptive responses of the coronary circulation and myocardium to chronic reduction in perfusion pressure and flow. Am J Physiol 266: (Heart Circ Physiol 35); H447–457
6. Schulz R, Guth BD, Pieper K, Martin C, Heusch G (1992) Recruitment of an inotropic reserve in moderately ischemic myocardium at the expense of metabolic recovery. A model of short term hibernation. Circ Res 70: 1282–1295
7. Shen YT, Hasebe N, Zhang H, Vatner SF (1993) Impaired regional myocardial function during ameroid induced chronic coronary artery stenosis in conscious pigs: Hibernation or stunning? (Abstract). Circulation 88 (Suppl I): I-188
8. Vanoverschelde JLJ, Wijns W, Depre C, Essamri B, Heyndrickx GR, Borgers M, Bo IA, Melin JA (1993) Mechanisms of chronic regional postischemic dysfunction in humans: New insights from the study of noninfarcted collateral-dependent myocardium. Circulation 87: 1513–1523
9. Gewirtz H, Fischman AJ, Abraham SA, Gilson M, Strauss HW, Alpert NM (1994) Positron emission tomographic measurements of absolute regional myocardial blood flow permits identification of nonviable myocardium in patients with chronic myocardial infarction. J Am Coll Cardiol 23: 851–859
10. Bolli R (1992) Myocardial "stunning" in man. (Review). Circulation 86: 1671–1691
11. Buxton DB (1993) Dysfunction in collateral-dependent myocardium: Hibernation or stunning. (Editorial). Circulation 87: 1756–1757

36–38

G. R. Heyndrickx

Hibernating myocardium

Key words Hibernation – stunning – chronic ischemia

The concept of hibernating myocardium was introduced in 1984 by Rahimtoola when he hypothezised that chronic regional myocardial dysfunction could be viewed as a self protective adaptive process of down regulation of contractile function and metabolism in response to chronic hypoperfusion (1). This new steady state of flow-function match could eventually remain stable for a prolonged period of time and be reversed upon myocardial revascularization.

While this hypothesis of functional and metabolic down regulation in response to chronic hypoperfusion remains mostly unproven there is no doubt that chronic dysfunctioning myocardial segments may regain function after revascularization.

The facts:

1. Chronic left ventricular segmental dysfunction is frequently observed in the absence of signs of ongoing ischemia – no ST/T-changes, no enzyme leakage, no evidence for previous myocardial infarction – and may bear a considerable burden on the overall left ventricular function.
2. It is true that during the early hours after the onset of ischemia, the occurrence of a number of adaptive changes such as the progressive return to normal of myocardial creatine phosphate content and the progressive attenuation of the ischemia-induced net lactate production suggests down regulation of cellular function. It is also true that prolonged inotropic stimulation in these conditions may increase further the severity of ischemia and enhance energy expenditure and precipitate myocardial infarction (2). There is no evidence that this condition, called short term hibernation, is the mechanism that leads to chronic reversible dysfunction.
3. Myocardial biopsies taken from chronic dysfunctioning segments at the time of surgery contain a variable amount of myocytes which display rather typical electron microscopic abnormalities. These cells, the so called hibernating cells, are characterized by the loss of sarcomeres and the accumulation of intracellular glycogen. This observation precludes the notion of immediate normalisation of function after reperfusion (3).
4. PET studies have demonstrated that, in most instances, basal regional myocardial perfusion in these segments is near normal or only moderately reduced. The reduction in flow is, however, out of proportion to the severe depression in regional function, evidencing a flow-function mismatch (4).
5. Recent studies have shown that these abnormally contracting segments have a greatly reduced coronary flow reserve despite near normal basal flow (4).
6. Despite reduced flow reserve a certain amount of contractile reserve can be recruited during appropriate inotropic stimulation as demonstrated by dobutamine echo tests (5). This contractile response is only temporary, reflecting the lack of normal coronary flow reserve.
7. While complete or partial recovery of regional function upon revascularisation can be observed, it is of interest to note that akinetic segments with low myocardial flow do not recover as often as akinetic seg-

G. R. Heyndrickx, M.D., Ph.D., FACC, FESC (✉)
Cardiovascular Center
Onze Lieve Vrouw Ziekenhuis
Moorselbaan 164
9300 Aalst, Belgium

Fig. 1

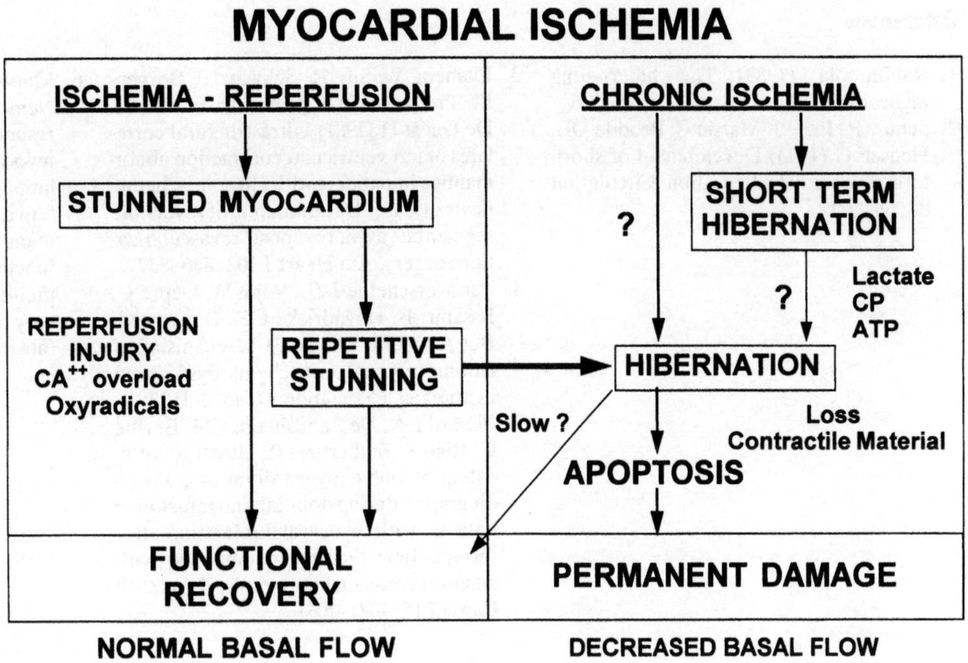

ments in which flow is only moderately reduced or near normal. In addition, segments displaying the largest concentration of hibernating cells which therefore should benefit theoretically the most from revascularization, are the least to recover regional function (6, 7).

These findings may suggest that after all, hibernating myocardium is not such a stable condition as previously acknowledged, but may evolve slowly towards permanent myocardial damage. One possible mechanism is a chronic loss of myocytes through a process known as apoptosis, in which fragmentation of nuclear DNA precedes phagocytosis by surrounding myocytes.

Mechanisms

In the absence of any experimental model of chronically hibernating myocardium, proposals to explain the underlying pathophysiological mechanisms have to be derived from clinical studies. In most clinical studies in which quantitative measurements of regional flow were performed a normal or slightly decreased basal perfusion is observed in chronic dysfunctioning segments which did improve after revascularisation, whereas segments with severe decreases in regional flow rarely recover function upon reperfusion. The presence of near normal basal flow together with the significantly reduced coronary flow reserve suggests a more plausible cause to describe this phenomenon of hibernating myocardium i.e.: the occurrence of multiple and repetitive bouts of myocardial stunning. It is easily conceivable that segments, not-withstanding normal basal perfusion, may be subjected to multiple episodes of high – demand ischemia during daily life as a result of the limited coronary flow reserve. These repetitive episodes of reversible high – demand ischemia would prevent recovery of function in between the episodes and result in an accumulation of functional deficit, first without cellular abnormalities (myocardial stunning) and finally with pathological consequences and the progressive loss of contractile material (hibernating myocardium); (Fig. 1).

References

1. Rahimtoola (1989) The hibernating myocardium. Am Heart J 117: 216–226
2. Schulz R, Rose J, Martin C, Brodde OE, Heusch G (1993) Development of short-term myocardial hibernation. Circulation 88: 684–695
3. Flameng W, Suy R, Schwarz F, Borgers M, Piessens J, Thone F, Van Ermen H, De Geest H (1981) Ultrastructural correlates of left ventricular contraction abnormalities in patients with chronic ischemic heart disease: Determinants of reversible segmental asynergy post revascularization surgery. Am Heart J 102: 846–857
4. Vanoverschelde J-JL, Wijns W, Depré C, Essamri B, Heyndrickx GR, Borgers M, Bol A, Melin JA (1993) Mechanisms of chronic regional postischemic dysfunction in humans. Circulation 87: 1512–1523
5. Pierard LA, De Landsheere CM, Berthe C, Rigo P, Kulbertus HE (1990) Identification of viable myocardium by echocardiography during dobutamine infusion in patients with myocardial infarction after thrombolytic therapy: comparison with positron emission tomography. J Am Coll Cardiol 15: 1021–1031
6. Marwick TH, MacIntyre WJ, Lafont A, Nemec JJ, Salcedo EE (1992) Metabolic responses of hibernating and infarcted myocardium to revascularization. Circulation 85: 1347–1353
7. Shivalkar B, Borgers M, Maes A, Mortelmans L, Flameng W (1994) Low regional function assessment with high metabolism predicts functional recovery after coronary bypass surgery. Circulation 90: I-251 (abstract)

39–41

S. H. Rahimtoola

Hibernating myocardium: a brief article

Key words Myocardial ischemia – reperfusion – ventricular function – myocardial infarction

Hibernating myocardium is a state of persistently impaired myocardial and left ventricular (LV) function at rest due to reduced coronary blood flow that can be partially or completely restored to normal if the myocardial oxygen supply/demand relationship is favorably altered, either by improving blood flow and/or by reducing demand. In a preliminary report, Conversano and co-workers have confirmed that in man there is a reduction of myocardial blood flow in hibernating myocardium when compared to normals (40 ± 5 vs 113 ± 33 ml/min/100 g).

Hibernating myocardium is a result of downgrading of cardiac function so that blood flow and function are once again in equilibrium, and as a result, neither myocardial necrosis nor ischemic symptoms are present. Obviously, if the myocardial oxygen supply/demand balance is subsequently altered unfavorably, either temporarily or permanently, then symptoms and signs of ischemia and/or of necrosis again occur.

Hibernating myocardium may be a unique pathophysiological myocardial state which at the present time we may not be able to characterize or define perfectly; more research and data are needed. Hearse's suggestion that it may be more appropriately viewed as an example of an "exquisitively regulated tissue successfully adapting its activity to prevailing circumstance" may be most apt. Hibernating myocardium has provided a thrust for a lot of investigative work, both basic and clinical, and for the more complete diagnosis and appropriate management of patients with LV dysfunction at rest.

Many articles in this special series will deal with the basic aspects of myocardial hibernation; therefore, in this brief article, I will concentrate on the clinical aspects.

Prof. S. H. Rahimtoola (✉)
University of Southern California
2025 Zonal Avenue
Los Angeles, California 90033, USA

Clinical syndromes with myocardial hibernation

Hibernating myocardium has so far been demonstrated to occur in the clinical syndromes of unstable angina, chronic stable angina, with myocardial infarction and in LV dysfunction and/or heart failure.

Unstable and stable angina

A large number of studies has demonstrated that LV dysfunction at rest improves with revascularization. The best predictor of improvement of global LV function (e.g., LV ejection fraction) is the number of viable but dysfunctional myocardial segments. The exact frequency of occurrence of hibernating myocardium in these two clinical syndromes is not precisely known, one study showed it to be almost three times more common in unstable angina than in stable angina (75 % vs 28 %). We have presented data to show that 10-year survival after coronary bypass surgery was significantly better in patients with unstable angina and preoperative LV dysfunction than in those with stable angina and preoperative LV dysfunction. In fact, up to 6 years after surgery, in patients with unstable angina and preoperative LV dysfunction, the survival was similar to that of patients with unstable and stable angina who had normal preoperative LV function.

Acute myocardial infarction

Myocardial hibernation is known to occur in a region of LV wall at a distance from the area of infarction and in the LV wall in the area of infarction or presumed infarction. A randomized trial of PTCA in patients with singlevessel disease and myocardial infarction showed that patients randomized to PTCA had greater improvements of various measurements including LV ejection fraction than those randomized to no PTCA. Another study has shown that after myocardial infarction patients who had hibernating myocardium demonstrated by positron emission tomography had a 33 % incidence of a subsequent cardiac event compared to 3 % of patients who had no hibernating myocardium. One study has demonstrated that 20 % of LV segments in 20 patients with old Q-wave infarction had hibernating myocardium.

LV dysfunction and/or heart failure

Several case reports have documented that patients who presented with heart failure had hibernating myocardium. Revascularization of hibernating myocardium resulted in marked improvement of heart failure, functional class, and in LV ejection fraction.

One study has shown that 11 % of patients referred for cardiac transplantation because of presumed irreversible myocardial damage and chronic resistant heart failure had hibernating myocardium. These patients were revascularized and their 3.5 year survival was 72 %.

Three studies have shown that in patients with severe LV dysfunction/heart failure, those who had hibernating myocardium (demonstrated by positron emission tomography) and were revascularized on follow-up had a mortality of 4 % (vs 14 to 33 % in those who were not revascularized), death or myocardial infarction of 4 % (vs 50 to 62 % in those who were not revascularized). In one of these studies, the 2-year survival in those who were revascularized was 88 % vs 50 % (p = 0.03) in those who were not revascularized.

Recovery of hibernating myocardium

The rate of recovery of resting LV dysfunction after revascularization and study of the morphological changes in the dysfunctional myocardium has allowed to describe hibernating myocardium as acute, subacute or chronic (Fig. 1).

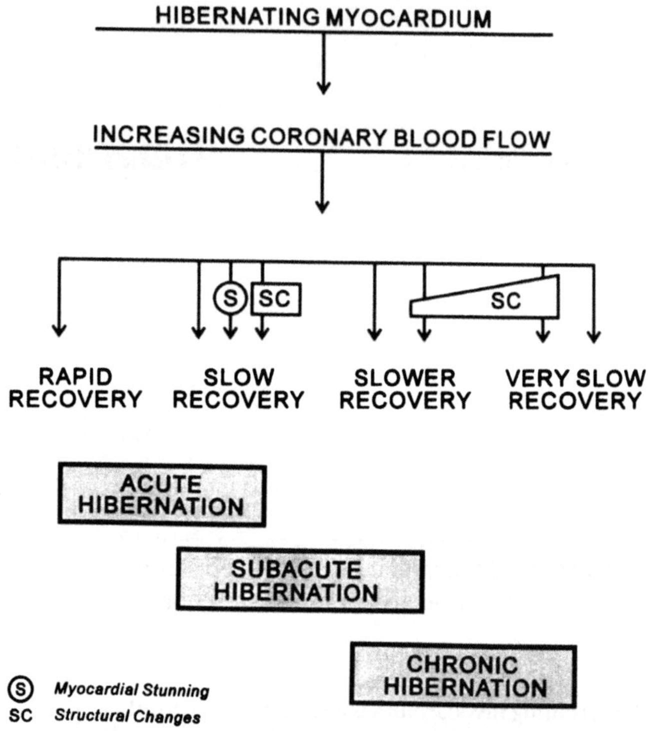

Fig. 1 Rates of recovery (rapid to very slow) of left ventricular function after increasing coronary blood in hibernating myocardium. The role of stunned myocardium and of structural changes in the myocardium is shown. The possible range of acute, subacute and chronic myocardial hibernation based on rate of recovery of left ventricular function is illustrated.

Table 1 Hibernating myocardium

Experimental	short term	chronic
Clinical	acute/subacute	subacute/chronic
Hibernating myocardium	normal some structural changes	near normal some structural changes marked structural changes[†]
Adjacent myocardium	infarcted fibrotic normal	infarcted fibrotic normal
Prior to hibernation	acute ischemic episode(s) gradual reduction of blood flow? stunning?	acute ischemic episode(s) gradual reduction of blood flow? stunning?
Recovery from hibernation	rapid/slow stunning may occur LV function: normal less abnormal	rapid/slow/very slow stunning? LV function: normal less abnormal

[†] "Dedifferentiation" or "diffuse atrophy/wasting from reduced function"

Acute

Hibernating myocardium that recovers "immediately" or very rapidly after myocardial revascularization is presumptive evidence of normal or almost normal myocardium; this has been confirmed by electron microscopic studies of myocardial biopsies. Experimental studies of acute hibernation provide additional confirmation.

Chronic

Hibernating myocardium may take a long time (up to 1 year in one patient) to recover completely. Electron microscopic studies of myocardial biopsies have demonstrated marked abnormalities which can be expected to take a long time to recover.

Subacute

In one acute experimental study, hibernating myocardium took time to recover which suggests that hibernation was followed by stunning. In three different reports, hibernation which was presumably present for some time recovered slowly after revascularization. In these patients, some structural changes could have been present which took time to recover or hibernation was followed by a period of stunning or both.

Some aspects of myocardial hibernation are summarized in Table 1.

References

1. Borgers M, Thone F, Wonters L, Ausina J, Shivalkar B, Flameng W (1993) Structural correlates of regional myocardial dysfunction in patients with critical coronary artery stenosis: Chronic hibernation? Cardiovasc Path 2: 237–245
2. Braunwald E, Rutherford JD (1986) Reversible ischemic left ventricular dysfunction: Evidence for the "hibernating myocardium". J Am Coll Cardiol 8: 1467–1470
3. Bristow JD, Arai AE, Anselone CG, Pantely GA (1991) Response to myocardial ischemia as a regulated process. Circulation 84: 2580–2587
4. Flameng W, Vanhaecke J, Van Belle H, Borgers M, DeBeer L, Minten J (1987) Relation between coronary artery stenosis and myocardial purine metabolism, histology and regional function in humans. J Am Coll Cardiol 9: 1235–1242
5. Galli M, Marcassa C, Bolli R, Giannezzi P, Temporelli PL, Imparato A, Silva Orrego PL, Giubbini R, Giordano A, Tavazzil L (1994) Spontaneous delayed recovery of perfusion and contraction after the first 5 weeks after anterior infarction: Evidence for the presence of hibernating myocardium in the infarcted area. Circulation 90: 1386–1397
6. Hearse D (1994) Myocardial ischaemia: Can we agree on a definition for the 21st Century? Editorial. Cardiovasc Res 28: 1737–1744
7. Rahimtoola SH (1982) Coronary bypass surgery for chronic angina – 1981: A perspective. Circulation 65: 225–241
8. Rahimtoola SH (1982) Postoperative exercise response in the evaluation of the physiological status after coronary bypass surgery. Circulation 65 (Suppl II): II-106–II-114
9. Rahimtoola SH (1985) A perspective on three large multicenter randomized clinical trial of coronary bypass surgery for chronic stable angina. Circulation 72 (Suppl V): 123–5
10. Rahimtoola SH (1989) The hibernating myocardium. Am Heart J 177: 211–21
11. Ross J Jr (1991) Myocardial perfusion-contraction matching: Implications for coronary heart disease and hibernation. Circulation 83: 1076–1082
12. Schulz R, Guth BD, Pieper K, Martin C, Heusch G (1992) Recruitment of an inotropic reserve in moderately ischemic myocardium at the expense of metabolic recovery. A model of short-term hibernation. Circ Res 70: 1282–1295

42–44

J. Ross, Jr.

Myocardial hibernation, stunning, or both?

Key words Ischemia – myocardial function – coronary blood flow – reperfusion

Myocardial "hibernation" is a term first used by Rahimtoola (10) for a condition of sustained abnormal contraction presumed due to chronic underperfusion in patients with coronary heart disease, in whom revascularization could lead to recovery of global or regional ventricular function. Braunwald and Rutherford (3) suggested that hibernating myocardium results from months or years of ischemia, and that ventricular dysfunction persists until blood flow is restored.

This postulated condition may bear a relation to the phenomenon of low-flow "perfusion-contraction matching" that we have described in several settings of acute and sustained experimental ischemia (12). In this context, reduced myocardial blood flow particularly to the subendocardium leads to reduction of myocardial contraction; the decreased level of contraction and altered substrate utilization (impaired oxidative metabolism and increased glycolytic metabolism), in turn, may bring energy supply and demand back into balance. The appropriateness of this "matching" between energy supply and contraction during the ischemic period will determine whether prolonged ischemic contractile dysfunction will be reversible, or whether it will result in tissue necrosis (12). On the other hand, the complete absence of residual perfusion during ischemia will result in progressive myocardial damage which begins at about 20 min and is complete in 60 – 90 min (11).

We have demonstrated experimentally that low-flow perfusion-contraction matching can be substained over an intermediate period of 5 h (8). When ischemia, characterized by reduction of subendocardial flow alone by about 50 % associated with reduced regional contraction, was maintained for this period in conscious dogs, function did not return early after reperfusion, but it recovered completely at 1 week without necrosis of the left ventricular free wall (8). An undefined metabolic adaptation could have occurred during this 5 h period to help maintain cardiac muscle viability, or the reduction of contraction *per se* reduced the metabolic requirements sufficiently so that diminished aerobic metabolism coupled with increased anaerobic glycolysis were sufficient to protect the myocardium at this moderate level of ischemia. The term myocardial stunning (2) has been applied to describe a phenomenon first reported in 1978 by Hendrickx et al. in experimental animals as transient contractile dysfunction, sometimes prolonged, which followed a 15-min period of coronary occlusion when coronary blood flow was restored (6). Stunning was undoubtedly present during the recovery period after our 5 h period of flow reduction, since myocardial blood flow became normal while dysfunction persisted without tissue damage (8); thus, depending upon when regional function was measured during the course of this experiment, either low-flow perfusion-contraction matching (which might be characterized as a form of hibernation) or stunning was

Supported in part by a Coronary Heart Disease SCOR Grant HL 17682 awarded by the National Heart, Lung and Blood Institute, and by an endowed chair awarded by the San Diego County Chapter of the American Heart Assocation.

Dr. J. Ross, Jr. (✉)
Department of Medicine (M-013B)
University of California, San Diego
School of Medicine
La Jolla, California 92093, USA

present. Recently, more prolonged reduction of blood flow for 7 days in swine associated with persistent contractile dysfunction also was found to be compatible with lack of tissue necrosis (1).

In some experimental studies the term hibernation has been used broadly, such as a period of severe global underperfusion for 2 h causing reduced contraction with persistent metabolic evidence of ischemia (5), or a 1-h period of mild ischemia in which abnormalities of high-energy phosphate stores were initially present but resolved with continued underperfusion (9).

In chronic coronary heart disease in the clinical setting, hibernation and stunning could occur separately or together as a cause of substained contractile dysfunction, either as sustained low coronary flow at rest, or as periods of low flow alternating with reflow followed by prolonged stunning (12). The potential therapeutic significance of long-term perfusion-contraction matching, or chronic hibernation, lies primarily in the setting of chronic coronary heart disease associated with significant left ventricular dysfunction, particularly when there is little or no clinical evidence of ongoing ischemia (angina pectoris or ECG changes) at the time the patient is evaluated, when the question arises as to whether or not a revascularization procedure will beneficially affect cardiac function. Thus, if the myocardium is viable, successful revascularization of one or more such regions of dysfunction can be expected to improve global left ventricular function. Proof of such a chronic hibernation syndrome, either experimentally or clinically, would require that repeated measurements show both reduced regional blood flow and impaired function at rest over a sustained period prior to revascularization.

Vanoverschelde et al. (14) recently studied patients with coronary artery occlusion without myocardial infarction in whom collateral development was evident. In some patients, severe regional myocardial dysfunction was present at rest, coronary vasodilator reserve was usually reduced, but the average resting coronary blood flow by ^{13}N-ammonia using PET imaging in the involved region was not significantly different from that in patients with similar coronary anatomy who had no resting myocardial dysfunction. In a subgroup of patients in whom flow reserve was measured, an inverse correlation was found between the resting wall motion score and coronary blood flow reserve, but no correlation was reported between resting wall motion score and resting coronary blood flow. Also, in patients with resting wall motion abnormalities there was often evidence of metabolic and ultrastructural abnormalities in the dysfunctional region. In a number of the patients studied, improvement in regional function after myocardial revascularization was shown. The authors concluded from these findings that impaired function was likely the result of repeated ischemic episodes with persistent stunning, and that the observed functional, metabolic and structural alterations, in fact, describe "chronic myocardial hibernation" (14).

However, several individual patients in their study clearly show reduced resting coronary blood flow associated with markedly impaired wall motion (14). Moreover, subendocardial flow, which is the best predictor of regional wall motion during ischemia (12), could not be measured in that study. In addition, others have described low basal coronary blood flow associated with impaired regional contraction in the clinical setting of severe coronary stenosis (4, 7, 13). In the study by Tillisch et al. (13) one subgroup of patients studied by PET with ^{13}N-ammonia to assess blood flow showed reduced resting coronary flow with increased glucose uptake, and this subgroup showed improved contractile function following revascularization. Therefore, the valuable study by Vanoverschelde et al. (14) does not settle the issue of whether hibernation (defined herein and by most others as a condition of low coronary flow), repeated ischemia with stunning, or both, were responsible for impaired wall motion reversible by revascularization.

It can be concluded that there is a subgroup of patients who have reduced resting coronary perfusion, often with evidence of abnormal metabolism, in whom prolonged perfusion-contraction matching or chronic hibernation may be postulated to exist, but serial studies will be needed in such patients to document the persistence of chronic underperfusion. In the absence of angina pectoris or signs of ischemia, if such a condition exists additional adaptations may occur which prevent significant ischemia but do not restore function (12). In other patients who have reversible contraction abnormalities, but normal resting perfusion and impaired coronary flow reserve, the existence of prolonged stunning associated with repeated episodes of stress-induced ischemia seems a more logical explanation than myocardial hibernation.

Clear-cut evidence for chronic hibernation in the clinical setting seems likely to remain elusive because of the nature of the studies needed to document it. However, current evidence supports the view that either chronic hibernation, stunning, or their coexistence can be responsible for regional myocardial contractile dysfunction that is reversible by revascularization.

References

1. Bolukoglu H, Liedtke J, Nellis S, Eggleston A, Subramanian R, Renstrom B (1992) An animal model of chronic coronary stenosis resulting in hibernating myocardium. Am J Physiol 263: H20–H29
2. Braunwald E, Kloner RA (1982) The stunned myocardium: prolonged, postischemic ventricular dysfunction. Circulation 66: 1146–1149
3. Braunwald E, Rutherford JD (1986) Reversible ischemic left ventricular dysfunction: Evidence for the "hibernating myocardium". J Am Coll Cardiol 8: 1467–1470
4. Brunken R, Tillisch J, Schwaiger M, Child JS, Marshall R, Mandelkern M, Phelps ME, Schelbert HR (1986) Regional perfusion, glucose metabolism, and wall motion in patients with chronic electrocardiographic Q wave infarctions: evidence for persistence of viable tissue in some infarct regions by positron emission tomography. Circulation 73: 951–963
5. Downing SE, Chen V (1990) Myocardial hibernation in the ischemic neonatal heart. Circ Res 66: 763–772
6. Heyndrickx GR, Baig H, Nelkins P, Leusen K, Fishbein MC, Vatner SF (1978) Depression of regional blood flow and wall thickening after brief coronary occlusions. Am J Physiol 234: H653–H659
7. Marshall RC, Tillisch JH, Phelps ME, Huang S-C, Carson R, Henze E, Schelbert HR (1983) Identification and differentiation of resting myocardial ischemia and infarction in man with positron computed tomography, ^{18}F-labeled fluorodeoxyglucose and N-13 ammonia. Circulation 67: 766–778
8. Matsuzaki M, Gallagher KP, Kemper WS, White F, Ross J Jr (1983) Sustained regional dysfunction, produced by prolonged coronary stenosis: Gradual recovery after reperfusion. Circulation 68: 170–182
9. Pantely GA, Malone SA, Rhen WS, Anselone CG, Arai A, Bristow J, Bristow JD (1990) Regeneration of myocardial phosphocreatine in pigs despite continued moderate ischemia. Clin Res 67: 1481–1493
10. Rahimtoola SH (1985) A perspective on the three large multicenter randomized clinical trials of coronary bypass surgery for chronic stable angina. Circulation 72 (suppl V): V-123–V-135
11. Ross J Jr (1991) Mechanical consequences of regional myocardial ischemia. In: Fozzard HA, Haber A, Jennings RB, Katz AM, Morgan HE (eds) The heart and cardiovascular system: scientific foundations. Vol II. Raven Press, New York, 2nd Ed, pp 1997–2020
12. Ross J Jr (1991) Myocardial perfusion-contraction matching. Implications for coronary heart disease and hibernation. Circulation 83: 1076–1083
13. Tillisch J, Brunken R, Marshall R, Schwaiger M, Mandelkern M, Phelps M, Schelbert H (1986) Reversibility of cardiac wall-motion abnormalities predicted by positron-tomography. N Engl J Med 314: 884–888
14. Vanoverschelde J-LJ, Wihns W, Depré C, Essamri B, Heyndrickx GR, Borgers M, Bol A, Melin JA (1993) Mechanisms of chronic regional postischemic dysfunction in humans. New insights from the study of noninfarcted collateral-dependent myocardium. Circulation 87: 1513–1523

45–47
© Steinkopff Verlag 1996

M. Borgers
J. Ausma

Structural aspects of the chronic hibernating myocardium in man

Key words Dedifferentiation – structural remodeling – chronic hibernation

Functional outcome after revascularization of chronic hibernating left ventricular segments is less predictable than initially thought. The earlier proposed criterium of the hibernating state – that functional recovery occurs immediately after revascularization – has been called into question. The time-course and the degree of functional recovery after revascularization are two of the unresolved issues. The morphologic changes in the myocardium of hypocontractile segments, especially the possible structural counterparts underlying chronic ischemia, are not well documented. In recent studies (1, 4, 6, 10) light and electron microscopy was performed on myocardial tissue removed from the anterior wall of the left ventricle during coronary artery bypass grafting.

The patients included in these studies fulfilled the following criteria:
- severe stenosis of the coronary artery
- abnormal anterior wall motion
- no signs of infarction on ECG
- preoperative flow-metabolic mismatch as documented by PET
- postoperative (3–6 months) recovery of regional contractile function
- return to flow-metabolic match as documented by PET.

The main change in cardiomyocytes from hypo/akinetic non-infarcted myocardium consists of a loss of contractile material (sarcomeres) (Fig. 1). The depletion of sarcomeres is initially seen at the center of the cell (perinuclear

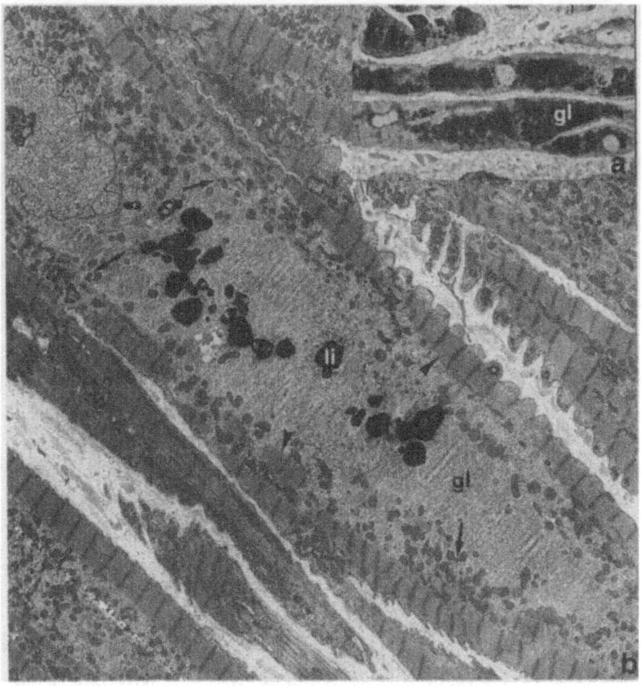

Fig. 1 Light (a) and electron microscopic (b) pictures showing subcellular changes in cardiomyocytes of chronic hibernating myocardium: depletion of sarcomeres (present only at the cell periphery [arrowhead]), accumulation of glycogen (gl), and the presence of numerous small mitochondria (arrows). li: lipofuscin (a: x 350; b: x 3.250).

M. Borgers · J. Ausma
Department of Molecular Cell Biology & Genetics
Cardiovascular Research
Institute of Maastricht
University of Limburg
Maastricht, The Netherlands

Prof. Dr. M. Borgers (✉)
Department of Morphology, Life Sciences
Janssen Research Foundation
Turnhoutseweg 30
2340 Beerse, Belgium

region) and may extend towards the periphery, involving the whole cytoplasm. This change, however, is distinct from atrophy since the space left by the dissoluted sarcomeres is occupied by glycogen (Fig. 1). Another characteristic change is the presence of numerous small donut-like mitochondria in the areas adjacent to the glycogen-rich perinuclear zones. A third change concerns the nuclei, in which the heterochromatin is evenly distributed over the nucleoplasm. Finally, there is a loss of the sarcoplasmic reticulum. Organized sarcoplasmic reticulum is virtually absent; instead, a network of disorganized profiles of reticular membranes is present in the myolytic areas. Fragments of rough endoplasmic reticulum are frequently found. In addition, the sarcolemma no longer presents protrusions (T-tubules) into the cytoplasm. These morphologic aspects are reminiscent of embryonic/fetal cells. Remarkably, typical degenerative changes, such as cytoplasmic vacuolization, cytosolic edema, mitochondrial swelling, membrane disruption, accumulation of secondary lysosomes, membrane whorls, and lipid droplets are virtually absent. The substructures present in the cells of such affected segments appear globally to be perfectly healthy. However, in segments in which microinfarcts (probably not severe enough to be picked up by ECG) were detected histologically, the cardiomyocytes bordering such infarcts have characteristics of the hibernating cells but also present signs of degenerative atrophy, a finding which others have made (7). Among the possible causes of the structural alterations in chronic hibernating myocardium, we propose contractile unloading of the myocytes (quiescence giving rise to increased breakdown and decreased synthesis of contractile proteins) (8), in combination with a metabolic substrate switch (glucose being preferred over fatty acid in the presence of lowered oxygen availability. Accumulation of glycogen may represent an excess of glucose uptake/utilization). In addition, an increased wall stress (stretch) might contribute to the above structural remodeling. In view of the morphological observations (the accumulation of glycogen, the paucity of contractile material, the occurrence of rough endoplasmic reticulum and the redistribution of heterochromatin), which suggest dedifferentiation, we looked at the expression – and organization patterns – of some markers of cardiomyocyte differentiation. Alpha-smooth muscle actin, cardiotin and titin were found to be expressed and distributed in patterns resembling those of the embryonic phenotype, which led us to hypothesize that cardiomyocytes in chronic hibernating myocardium have acquired aspects of dedifferentiation (2).

The question that needs to be answered now is whether such cells redifferentiate after blood flow is restored. Identification of factors that trigger myolysis and/or myofibrillogenesis is crucially important with reference to the potential reversibility of the change. Evidence has been presented that cardiomyocytes, at different stages of differentiation, are capable of adaptively remodeling the contractile system and that they have significant structural plasticity (5). The question of reversibility however, will remain unanswered until an animal model becomes available in which these structural changes can be reproduced. Interestingly, we recently showed structural changes in atrial cardiomyocytes after chronic atrial fibrillation in the goat (3) that corresponded to the changes seen in chronic hibernating myocardium in man. Again, contractile unloading and stretch of the myocardium are considered to be causally involved in this model.

Apart from changes to cardiomyocytes, an increase in extracellular matrix components such as collagen (types I and III) and fibronectin surrounding the cardiomyocytes is often seen in hibernating segments. It has been proposed recently that there is a close relationship between the ability to recover function and the amount of connective tissue (9).

Although it is not known to what extent cardiomyocyte alterations and connective tissue remodeling contribute to the abnormal wall motion of hibernating segments, these factors are believed to play a major role in the determination of the speed and degree of functional recovery after revascularization. Segments in which these structural changes predominate will most likely show a delayed recovery since structural remodeling to regain a normal amount of contractile material requires time. The ultimate limiting factor for recovery, however, may be the presence of increased amounts of connective tissue.

References

1. Ausma J, Ramaekers F, Flameng W, Borgers M (1994) Cellular Adaptation in Hibernating Myocardium in Man. Cardiac Adaptation and Failure. In: Hori M, Maruyama Y, Reneman RS (eds). Springer-Verlag, Tokyo, in press
2. Ausma J, Schaart G, Thoné F, Shivalkar B, Flameng W, Depré C, Vanoverschelde JL, Ramaekers F, Borgers M (1995) Chronic ischemic viable myocardium in man: aspects of dedifferentiation. Cardiovasc Pathol, in press
3. Borgers M, Ausma J, Wijffels M, Allessie M (1994) Atrial fibrillation in the goat: a model for chronic hibernating myocardium. Circulation 90: I-467

4. Borgers M, Thoné F, Wouters L, Ausma J, Shivalkar B, Flameng W (1993) Structural correlates of regional myocardial dysfunction in patients with critically coronary artery stenosis: chronic hibernation? Cardiovasc Pathol 2: 237–245
5. Borisov AB (1991) Myofibrilogenesis and reversible disassembly of myofibrils as adaptive reactions of cardiac muscle cells. Acta Physiol Scand S599: 71–80
6. Maes A, Shivalkar B, Flameng W, Nuyts J, Borgers M, Ausma J, Bormans G, Schiepers C, De Roo M, Mortelmans L (1994) Histological alterations in chronically hypoperfused myocardium: correlation with PET findings. Circulation 90: 735–745
7. Schwarz ER, Schaper J, vom Dahl J, Altehoefer C, Buell U, Schoendube F, Messmer BJ, Sheehan FH (1994) Myocardial hibernation is not sufficient to prevent morphological disarrangements with ischemic cell alterations and increased fibrosis. Circulation 90: I-378
8. Sharp WW, Terracio L, Borg TK, Samarel AM (1993) Contractile activity modulates actin synthesis and turnover in cultured neonatal rat heart cells. Circ Res 73: 172–183
9. Shivalkar B, Borgers M, Maes A, Mortelmans L, Flameng W (1994) Low regional function associated with high metabolism predicts functional recovery after coronary bypass surgery. Circulation 90: I-251
10. Vanoverschelde J-LJ, Wijns W, Depré C, Essamri B, Heyndricks GR, Borgers M, Bol A, Melin J (1993) Mechanisms of chronic regional postischemic dysfunction in humans: new insights from the study of non-infarcted collateral dependent myocardium. Circulation 87: 1513–1523

48–49
© Steinkopff Verlag 1996

A. Elsässer
Jutta Schaper

Hibernating myocardium: adaptation or degeneration?

Key words Hibernation – morphology – cardiac function

The definition of hibernating myocardium (HM) implies that due to chronic underperfusion, the function of the myocardial area afflicted is reduced. It is claimed that the tissue survives at a new level of reduced oxygen supply and demand. After restoration of adequate perfusion, cardiac function will recover (Rahimtoola S. H.: The hibernating myocardium, Am Heart J. 117, 211–220, 1989).

Among the various possibilities to test this hypothesis the morphological investigation of biopsies, removed during coronary bypass surgery from well-defined myocardial regions, offers one of the most direct approaches for the evaluation of the integrity of the tissue under the conditions of hibernating. We used electron microscopy as well as immunohistochemistry for an extensive study of this problem. Prior to surgery, the patients underwent cardiological routine examination completed by dobutamine echocardiography and thallium scintigraphy. Only patients with moderate to severe regional wall motion disturbances were included in this study.

Basically, three different structural alterations are observed in hibernating myocardium:
1) changes of size and shape of the myocytes
2) intracellular degenerative changes of the myocytes
3) extracellular alterations of the myocardium.

Dr. A. Elsässer (✉) · J. Schaper
Max-Planck-Institut
für Physiologische und Klinische Forschung
Abteilung Experimentelle Kardiologie
Benekestraße 2
61231 Bad Nauheim

Ad 1) Many myocytes are of normal size, but others are either hypertrophied or show atrophy of different degrees. Usually, the hibernating myocardium shows a mixture of all three different cellular appearances in one particular viewing field in the microscope.

Ad 2) Intracellular alterations include loss of the myofilaments and the occurrence of nonspecified cytoplasm, an accumulation of numerous small mitochondria showing different stages of degeneration, changes of size and shape of the nuclei, and disorganization of the cytoskeleton. The contractile proteins myosin, the thin filament complex, titin, and α-actinin were reduced to a similar extent. The cytoskeleton, consisting of desmin, tubulin and the associated protein vinculin showed a significant disorganization and accumulation, usually in the same cells that exhibited a lack of contractile filaments. These morphological changes are indicative of a loss of both, contractile function as well as of cellular integrity; the latter normally ensured by the cytoskeleton.

By electron microscopy, sequestration of cellular particles from the myocytes into the extracellular space is observed. This is interpreted as a selfprotective mechanism of the cells, because a myocyte of decreased size needs less energy. This mechanism will most probably, in addition to the loss of myofilaments and therefore of contractile function, enable the cells to survive for a longer period of time. Another sign of an alteration of the energetic situation is an abundant intracellular storage of glycogen.

These intracellular changes exist in variable combinations and are present in a great number of myocytes but not in all of these, i.e., comparable to the variation of cell size there exists also an inhomogeneity in the distribution of cellular degeneration.

Ad 3) The extracellular space is enlarged and shows an increase in all extracellular matrix components, i.e., of adhesive and structural proteins as well as of fibroblasts and macrophages. The macrophages are numerous and apparently activated and induced to phagocytosis by sequestrated cell particles. A certain heterogeneous distribution of the occurrence of fibrosis was likewise observed. It may finally replace myocytes in larger areas of the myocardium so that after a longer duration of hibernation the entire area afflicted may exclusively consist of fibrotic material.

In some regions of the hibernating myocardium an increased capillary density can be observed. Most probably, this is a regional protective factor for the tissue.

The intracellular and extracellular changes are often of the same severity, however, there is also the possibility of a dominance of intra- or extracellular degeneration.

Summary of morphological changes in hibernating myocardium

– myocyte size	– existence of normal, hypertrophic, atrophic cells
– intracellular	– loss of myofilaments
	– accumulation of mitochondria with different stages of degeneration
	– occurrence of non-specified cytoplasm and vacuoles
	– disorganization of the cytoskeleton
	– sequestration of cellular particles into the extracellular space
– extracellular	– increase of extracellular matrix components: adhesive and structural proteins
	– increase of extracellular cells, i.e., macrophages and fibroblasts
	– change of capillary density
	– alteration of the capillary endothelial cells

The changes demonstrated here are regarded as an adaptation to the reduced perfusion situation. This adaptation, however, consists of a degeneration of the myocytes and an increase in the components of the extracellular space.

Up to a certain degree of severity the alterations are reversible. When, however, the disorganization of the cytoskeleton and the loss of myofilaments as well as the increase in collagen are far progressed, a recovery of function after restoration of an adequate perfusion is not possible. The final stage of degeneration is cell death and synthesis of scar tissue.

In addition, not only the degree of the degenerative alterations is important, but the number of cells afflicted by it is decisive for the recovery of function after restoration of perfusion.

Based on the morphological findings presented here we believe that repetitive ischemic episodes produce cellular degeneration and final cell death leading to scar formation in the non-contracting "hibernating" cardiac region. The adaptive, cell preserving mechanism as proposed for hibernating myocardium, if it exists at all, is incapable to preserve the structural integrity and cannot prevent further deterioration of the tissue.

50–52

R. O. Bonow

The hibernating myocardium: identification of viable myocardium in patients with coronary artery disease and chronic left ventricular dysfunction

Key words Myocardial ischemia – hibernation – ventricular dysfunction – PET – scintigraphy

In a large subset of patients with coronary artery disease (CAD) and left ventricular (LV) dysfunction, LV performance is reduced on the basis of regionally ischemic or hibernating myocardium rather than irreversibly infarcted myocardium. The detection of reversibly dysfunctional myocardium is clinically relevant, as regional and global LV function in such patients may improve substantially after revascularization. Noninvasive imaging methods to assess myocardial metabolic activity, membrane integrity, and inotropic reserve are ideally suited for this assessment.

Positron emission tomography

Positron emission tomography (PET) has emerged as a promising method for demonstrating viable myocardium in patients with compromised LV function (1, 2). Myocardial viability by PET is identified on the basis of intact metabolic activity in regions of severely underperfused and dysfunctional myocardium. The most extensive experience thus far has been achieved using ^{18}F-fluorodeoxyglucose (FDG) as a marker of regional exogenous glucose utilization in such hypoperfused regions. In particular, a pattern of enhanced FDG uptake in regions with reduced perfusion (termed the FDG: blood flow "mismatch") indicates viable tissue that has preferentially shifted its metabolic substrate toward glucose rather than fatty acids or lactate. The finding of preserved metabolic activity in myocardial regions with reduced blood flow has been demonstrated in several studies to be an accurate clinical marker with which to distinguish viable myocardium from myocardial fibrosis, with positive and negative predictive accuracies in the range of 85 % for identifying regions that will manifest improved function after revascularization (1, 2). Thus, PET appears to yield excellent viability information.

Robert O. Bonow, M.D. (✉)
Division of Cardiology
Northwestern University Medical School
250 East Superior Street, Suite 524
Chicago, Illinois 60611, USA

Thallium-201 imaging

The requirements for cellular viability include intact sarcolemmal function to maintain electrochemical gradients across the cell membrane, as well as preserved metabolic activity to generate high energy phosphates. These processes also require adequate myocardial blood flow to deliver substrates and wash out the metabolites of the metabolic processes. As the retention of thallium-201 is an active process that is a function of cell viability and cell membrane activity, as well as blood flow, thallium-201 should in theory be taken up and retained by myocardial regions that also retain FDG and other metabolic tracers. However, many regions of severely ischemic or hibernating myocardium appear to have irreversible thallium defects on standard exercise-redistribution imaging. It has been shown that up to 50 % of regions with "irreversible" thallium defects will improve in function after revascularization. Thus, standard thallium scintigraphy may not provide satisfactory precision in differentiating between LV dysfunction arising from infarcted versus hibernating myocardium (3, 4).

These relatively poor results with exercise-redistribution imaging may be overcome using other imaging protocols. These include 1) late (24–72 h) redistribution imaging, 2) thallium reinjection imaging, in which imaging is repeated after a small additional dose of thallium is injected at rest after a period of redistribution following stress imaging, or 3) thallium imaging without exercise using a rest-redistribution protocol. These imaging protocols improve the accuracy of thallium imaging in identifying viable myocardium and, in some series, these results approach those obtained with PET imaging (3–5).

Technetium-99m sestamibi imaging

Unlike thallium-201, Tc-99m sestamibi does not redistribute appreciably after an injection during exercise or at rest. Thus, sestamibi may have inherent disadvantages relative to thallium for viability assessment. This concept is supported by studies demonstrating that rest-exercise sestamibi imaging underestimates viable myocardium in patients with chronic CAD and LV dysfunction compared to exercise-redistribution-reinjection thallium imaging, although recent data suggest that quantitative analyses may increase sestamibi's accuracy for identify viable tissue (5, 6). Until more definitive data are available, sestamibi remains an investigational rather than a preferred agent for clinical myocardial viability assessment.

Dobutamine echocardiography

Previously ischemic, stunned myocardium can be identified following administration of inotropic agents such as dopamine, isoproterenol, and dobutamine, as well as by postextrasystolic potentiation. Experimental studies in dogs have demonstrated that postischemic dysfunctional myocardium bears considerable contractile reserve that may be recruited after moderate inotropic stimulation without causing detrimental effects. Recently, low-dose dobutamine infusion to enhance regional systolic wall thickening during echocardiography have been proposed and applied successfully to patients after thrombolytic therapy for acute myocardial infarction and in patients with chronic LV dysfunction. The results of these studies, thus far in small numbers of patients, suggest that this method provides data as accurate as that achieved using scintigraphic methods (4, 7, 8).

Clinical implications

The identification of viable myocardium has become an area of intense interest for several reasons. Among these is the rather unique potential of nuclear cardiology techniques to distinguish viable regions on the basis of perfusion, cell membrane integrity, and metabolic activity and the ability of dobutamine echocardiography to assess regional inotropic reserve. Although the available data imply that each of these methods has similar diagnostic accuracy (1, 2, 4, 6, 7, 8), larger scale studies comparing PET, thallium-201, and dobutamine echocardiography are required in patients undergoing revascularization to determine the relative efficacies of these methods in identifying viable myocardium.

The evolving PET data indicate that the identification of viable myocardial tissue in patients with CAD and LV dysfunction has several important, clinically relevant implications. First, the augmentation in regional systolic function after revascularization, as predicted by FDG:blood flow mismatch, results in a significant and predictable increase in global LV ejection fraction (1, 2). This increase in LV ejection fraction after revascularization in patients with FDG:blood flow mismatch appears to translate into an improvement in prognosis (1, 2, 9, 10). Recently published data suggest that survival is improved by myocardial revascularization in patients with FDG:blood flow mismatch compared to the survival results during medical therapy (9, 10). Finally, the improvement in LV function after revascularization, as predicted by FDG:blood flow mismatch, is also associated with a significant improvement in symptoms of congestive heart failure (10). Although more definitive data are required before full conclusions can be drawn, these data suggest that patients with impaired left ventricular function and FDG:blood flow mismatch are a subgroup of patients who may have substantial improvement in outcome if identified and treated with myocardial revascularization. These patients appear to have the potential for improved left ventricular function, improved symptoms, and improved survival. Whether these clinical outcome data derived from PET studies can be generalized to viability markers obtained from thallium imaging or dobutamine echocardiography awaits further study.

References

1. Schelbert H (1994) Metabolic imaging to assess myocardial viability. J Nucl Med 35 (suppl): 8S–14S
2. Maddahi J, Schelbert H, Brunken R, Di Carli M (1994) Role of thallium-201 and PET imaging in evaluation of myocardial viability and management of patients with coronary artery disease and left ventricular dysfunction. J Nucl Med 35: 707–715
3. Bonow RO, Dilsizian V (1992) Assessing viable myocardium with thallium-201. Am J Cardiol 70: 10E–17E
4. Dilsizian V, Bonow RO (1993) Current diagnostic techniques of assessing myocardial viability in hibernating and stunned myocardium. Circulation 87: 1–20
5. Dilsizian V, Arrighi JA, Diodati JG, Quyyumi AA, Bacharach SL, Marin-Neto JA, Uddin S, Bonow RO (1994) Myocardial viability in patients with chronic ischemic left ventricular dysfunction: Comparison of ^{99m}Tc-sestamibi, ^{201}thallium, and ^{18}F-fluorodeoxyglucose. Circulation 89: 578–587
6. Udelson JE, Coleman PS, Matherall JA, Pandian NG, Gomes AR, Griffith JL, Shea NL, Oates E, Konstam MA (1994) Predicting recovery of severe regional ventricular dysfunction: Comparison of resting scintigraphy with thallium-201 and technetium-99m sestamibi. Circulation 89: 2552–2561
7. Cigarroa CG, de Filippi CR, Brickner E, Alvarez LG, Wait MA, Grayburn PA (1993) Dobutamine stress echocardiography identifies hibernating myocardium and predicts recovery of left ventricular function after coronary revascularization. Circulation 88: 430–436
8. Bonow RO (1995) The hibernating myocardium: Implications for management of congestive heart failure. Am J Cardiol (in press)
9. Eitzman D, Al-Aouar Z, Kanter HL, vom Dahl J, Kirsh M, Deeb GM, Schwaiger M (1992) Clinical outcome of patients with advanced coronary artery disease after viability studies with positron emission tomography. J Am Coll Cardiol 20: 559–565
10. Di Carli MF, Davidson M, Little R, Khanna S, Mody FV, Brunken RC, Czernin J, Rokhsar S, Stevenson LW, Laks H, Hawkins R, Schelbert HR, Phelps ME, Maddahi J (1994) Value of metabolic imaging with positron emission tomography for evaluating prognosis in patients with coronary artery disease and left ventricular. Am J Cardiol 73: 527–533

53–55

R. Ferrari

Commentary on hibernating myocardium and its clinical relevance

Key words Hibernating myocardium – myocardial ischaemia – heart failure – myocardial viability – ischaemic cardiomyopathy

Introduction

Differentiation of viable myocardium from non-viable myocardium in patients with coronary artery disease and left ventricular dysfunction is an issue of clinical relevance in this age of myocardial revascularization.

Impaired left ventricular function may occur transiently during an attack of angina and is usually reversible. It may persist over hours or even days in patients after an episode of ischaemia followed by reperfusion, leading to the so-called condition of "stunning". In patients with persistent limitation of coronary flow, left ventricular dysfunction may be present over months or years, or indefinitely in subjects with fibrosis, scar formation and remodelling after myocardial infarction, leading to the syndrome of heart failure. Chronic left ventricular dysfunction does not necessarily mean permanent or irreversible cell damage. Hypoperfused myocytes can remain viable but akinetic. This type of dysfunction has been called "hibernating myocardium" (1).

The diagnosis of hibernation is clinically relevant because it has therapeutic implications, as regional and global left ventricular function due to hibernation will improve after revascularization and it is associated with improved survival (2).

The true clinical gold standard for hibernation is the improvement in systolic function of dysfunctional myocardial segments after revascularization. Such a retrospective standard is, however, insufficient. An accurate prospective diagnosis of patients with potentially reversible left ventricular dysfunction is essential for the identification of ideal candidates for revascularization procedures. Thus, the hibernating myocardium poses a series of clinical issue. The three fundamental questions are: 1) how and with what accuracy this entity can be recognized?; 2) how should it be best treated? and 3) can reperfusion of hibernating myocardium be considered an alternative to transplantation?

How hibernating myocardium can be recognized

A number of methods are available to assess viability and contractile reserve in regions with hypokinetic or akinetic wall motion. They include cardiac imaging techniques that evaluate myocardial viability on the basis of myocardial perfusion, cell membrane integrity and metabolic activity and the infusion of a low-dose positive inotropic agent during echocardiography to evaluate contractile reserve (3).

Positron emission tomography (PET) provides the capacity to quantitate noninvasively regional blood flow and to assess regional metabolic activity independent of flow. In addition it provides enhanced image resolution and routine correction for body attenuation. In this way it overcomes the two major limitations of thallium imaging: poor resolution and photon attenuation. Recently, 18-F-flurodeoxyglucose (FDG) has emerged as a marker of regional exogenous glucose utilization in hypoperfused

Prof. R. Ferrari (✉)
Cattedra di Cardiologia and Fundazione Clinica del Lavoro,
Centro di Fisiopatologia Cardiovascolare "S. Maugeri"
Universita' degli Studi di Brescia c/o Spedali Civili
P. le Spedali Civili, 1
25123 Brescia, Italy

regions. FDG is a glucose analogue that undergoes the same transport and phosphorylation of glucose but does not enter glycolysis or glycogen synthesis. An increase of FDG uptake in regions with reduced perfusion, the so-called FDG-blood flow mismatch, provides a metabolic signal for identifying viable myocardium (3). The technique, however, is expensive and not readly available.

Thallium myocardial imaging is an established method to assess perfusion and sarcolemmal integrity and hence to detect myocardial viability. Regional thallium activity on redistribution images acquired either early (3 – 4 hours) or late (8 – 72 hours) after stress is commonly used to demonstrate the distribution of viable myocardial cells and the extent of myocardial fibrosis. Rest-redistribution is also successfully used to distinguish viable from non-viable myocardium. Thallium reinjection after stress-redistribution imaging has also been proposed. All these protocols have advantages and disadvantages (3). Different opinions exist on which protocol should be used for the detection of hibernating myocardium. This, depends on the underlying clinical question and on the meaning of the term hibernation. In our experience, the clinical question in a patient with left ventricular dysfunction possibly due to hibernation is one of viability and not of inducible ischaemia. Therefore, we use rest-redistribution thallium imaging (4).

Echocardiography during low-dose dobutamine infusion has been successfully used to identify viable versus necrotic myocardium after successful thrombolysis. The administration of a positive inotropic agent in the setting of reduced coronary flow reserve (like in hibernation) has been hampered by the risk of increasing myocardial demand, thereby producing myocardial ischaemia and persistent regional dysfunction. Despite this limitation, recent data suggest that low-dose dobutamine echocardiography is a safe and accurate method for assessing hibernating myocardium (5). We have evaluated its role in identifying hibernation in 33 CAD patients with positive thallium rest-redistribution test and persistent left ventricular dysfunction (6). Reversible dysfunction was identified by functional improvement of akinetic areas immediately after surgical revascularization, detected by intraoperative epicardial echocardiography and both 2 weeks and 3 months later, by means of transthoracic echocardiography. Infusion of dobutamine predicted reversible dysfunction with a sensitivity of 86.8 % specificity of 81.6 %. In our study dobutamine echocardiography predicted the immediate functional recovery after revascularization with higher accuracy than thallium rest-redistribution. On the contrary, scintigraphic imaging was better correlated than dobutamine echocardiography with long-term recovery of function (4). This discrepancy stresses that the two tests have different clinical significance as they explore two different aspects of the same issue: viability and contractile reserve of the akinetic myocytes. We believe that demonstration of viability provides the ultimate rationale for revascularization. Presence of contractile reserve provides information on the overall operative risk, thus overriding the additional concept that global systolic ejection fraction is a crucial determinant of surgical risk (7). Global ejection fraction, in fact, can be related to different physiopathological mechanisms.

How should it best be treated?

It is clear that hibernation myocardium should be reperfused.

It is our conviction, however, that, in a decision-making process, several steps should be fullfilled before recommending myocardial revascularization. 1. the symptomatic status of the patient is important. This should not be limited to the presence of angina pectoris or of inducible ischaemia, but also to the presence of signs of heart failure in absence of other symptoms. 2. coronary anatomy has to be suitable for revascularization either by open-heart surgery or angioplasty. 3. the extension and severity of the ventricular dysfunction has to justify an interventional procedure, the risk of which is not negligible. 4. the demonstration of viable myocardium by one or more of the possible imaging modalites is essential, particularly to predict long-term recovery after revascularization. 5. the demonstration of a contractile reserve by low-dose dobutamine echocardiography is also important as it confirms viability and provides further information on the surgical risk.

No data exists regarding a possible pharmacological treatment. Theoretically drugs which improve coronary perfusion and protect the myocyte against ischaemia might be usefull.

Can reperfusion of hibernating myocardium be considered as an alternative to transplantation?

Revascularization of patients with end-stage ischaemic cardiomyopathy and clinical manifestation of congestive heart failure rather than angina may be considered an alternative to transplantation. Data regarding this possibility are few. In our study (6), one-third of patients had dyspnea as the only symptom, a severe reduction of ejection fraction and some of these patients were potential candidates for transplantation. Examining the existing literature on revascularization of severe ischaemic cardiomyopathies and pooling together the data, it seems that perioperative mortality rate is between 15 % and 20 %, with 72 % – 75 % survival at 3 years. There is a clear improvement of symptoms and of global ejection fraction. Demonstration of viability, however, is essential for a positive outcome (7).

However, we believe that to answer this fondamental question we need a proper clinical study in which CAD patients (with demonstration of large areas of hibernating myocardium and awaiting transplantation) will be randomized to revascularization or standard medical therapy.

Conclusion

The discovery by Rahimtoola that chronic left ventricular regional dysfunction due to prolonged hypoperfusion can recover after full reperfusion has radically changed the current physiopathological concept of myocardial ischaemia and the actual treatment of CAD patients. We need, however, proper studies aimed to evaluate the role of the different diagnostic metodologies for detection of myocardial hibernation and to assess the clinical efficacy of revascularization of hibernating myocardium in terms of reduction of morbidity and mortality. From the clinical point of view attention and resorces should be concentrated on those case with large extension of hibernating myocardium, in which the differentiation of viable from non-viable myocardium and the stratification of operative risk is the real overriding clinical concern. It is this subset of patients which will justify further investigation in this fascinating field and which hopefully, will improve our therapeutical possibility.

Acknowledgment This work was supported by the National Research Council (C.N.R) target project "Prevention and control disease factors" n. 91.00156 PF 41. The authors thank Miss Roberta Bonetti for secretarial assistance in preparing the manuscript.

References

1. Rahimtoola S (1989) The hibernating myocardium. Am Heart J 117: 211–221
2. Eitzman D, Al-Aouar Z, Kanter HL (1992) Clinical outcome of patients with advanced coronary artery disease after viability studies with positron emission tomography. J Am Coll Cardiol 20: 559–565
3. Dilsizian V, Bonow R (1993) Current diagnostic techniques of assessing myocardial viability in patients with hibernating and stunned myocardium. Circulation 87: 1–20
4. Giubbini R, Alfieri O, Ferrari R, Milan E, Rossini P, Lorusso R, Berra P, La Canna G (1993) Thallium rest-redistribtion and echo-dobutamine tests to predict functional improvement after by pass surgery in patients with left ventricular dysfunction. Circulation 88 (4): 2883
5. Cigarroa CG, De Filippi CR, Brickner ME, Alvarez LG, Wait MA, Grayburn PA (1993) Dobutamine stress echocardiography identifies hibernating myocardium and predicts recovery of left ventricular function after coronary revascularization. Circulation 88: 430–436
6. La Canna G, Alfieri O, Giubbini R, Gargano M, Ferrari R, Visioli O (1994) Echocardiography during infusion of dobutamine for identification of reversible dysfunction in patients with chronic coronary artery disease. J Am Coll Cardiol 23: 617–626
7. Ferrari R, La Canna G, Giubbini R, Ceconi C, Pardini A, Coletti G, Berra P, Alfieri O (1994) Hibernating myocardium. In: Eds. M Yacoub, J Pepper (eds) Annual of Cardiac Surgery. pp 28–32

56–58

W. Flameng
B. Shivalkar

Hibernating myocardium, a clinical entity

Key words Chronic myocardial ischemia – hibernation – PET scanning

Before the term "hibernating myocardium" was introduced by Rahimtoola (1), it was shown by us that a subpopulation of patients could be defined who had a significant coronary artery stenosis and impaired wall motion in the absence of myocardial infarction (2). These patients could only be identified by a multivariate analysis using parameters related to preoperative regional wall motion, electrocardiogram, severity of coronary stenosis and viability of the myocardium. Data on myocardial viability were derived from histological examination of intraoperatively obtained biopsy material.

In another study (3), we could demonstrate that this subset of patients shows functional recovery of these regions after revascularization and that the patients showed a superior cardiac and total survival two years after bypass surgery, as compared to patients with postinfarction hypokinesis. If hibernating myocardium is defined as a hypocontractile, hypoperfused but viable region of the heart which regains contractility after revascularization, the subpopulation of patients we were able to identify, fulfils these criteria and can be classified as such.

Several questions arise when dealing with hibernation in the clinical setting. The major problem is diagnosis and identification of myocardial hibernation in patients suffering from coronary artery disease.

Prof. Dr. W. Flameng (✉) · B. Shivalkar
Cardiale Heelkunde
Universitair Ziekenhuis Gasthuisberg – Kuleuven
Herestraat 49
B-3000 Leuven, Belgium

This invariably involves identification of dysfunctional and hypoperfused myocardium which is viable. The presently available non-invasive tools such as positron emission tomography provide simultaneous information about perfusion and metabolism (viability). Viability assessment is an important issue, as the absolute proof of viability is direct histological examination of myocardial biopsy material obtained during surgery.

Another very pressing, and until now perhaps the most intriguing problem is why there is not always an immediate and unconditional recovery of the revascularized myocardium.

Assuming that hibernation involves adaptive mechanisms, cellular structural changes must be inevitable.

In the past decade we have concentrated on studying myocyte structural changes which might be subject to such a functional adaptation to chronic ischemia. Likewise, we also attempt to predict which patients might benefit from revascularization before taking that therapeutic option (ref 2–7).

Is the hibernating myocardium dedifferentiating?

From our earlier studies in patients undergoing coronary artery bypass surgery it became evident that although the hibernating myocardium is viable, the volume fraction of contractile material in hibernating myocytes is severely reduced and replaced by glycogen and small mitochondria. These findings made us suggest, for the first time during a symposium in "Left ventricular function in stunned and hibernating myocardium" at the XIII th Congress of the European Society of Cardiology in 1991 (8) that the hibernating myocardium is dedifferentiating. Since then, increasing evidence for such an adaptive mechanism is provided by Borgers and co-workers and will be elaborated in another article of this issue.

Anyway, full functional recovery after revascularization will depend upon the ability of the myocardium to "repair" the subcellular changes or to redifferentiate. If the loss of sarcomeres however is irreversible, recovery of function will depend upon the amount of structurally unaltered myocytes, which, in analogy with the stunned myocardium, regain contractility with ongoing reperfusion. We found that about 20 – 25 % of the myocytes in hibernating myocardium show some degree of myolysis. In a recent study we could identify a small subset of patients having up to 60 – 70 % of myolytic cells and these patients did not show functional recovery at 2 months after successful revascularization. We described these areas as "end stage hibernation".

Non-invasive identification of hibernating myocardium

The prerequisite for myocardial hibernation besides hypoperfusion and hypofunction, which show an improvement after revascularization, is viability of the myocardium. This viability however, is the most difficult to demonstrate in a non-invasive manner. A combined flow-metabolic study of the myocardium with PET permits the identification of viable tissue in chronically ischemic myocardium, which is indistinguishable from scar tissue on the basis of perfusion criteria alone (9). In a recent study (10) we correlated PET findings of blood flow and metabolism in chronically hypoperfused myocardium with histology. We studied 30 patients suffering from coronary artery disease. In each patient, myocardial blood flow and metabolism were measured with PET 1 or 2 days before revascularization. During surgery, 2 biopsies were taken from the left ventricular anterior wall. Ventriculography demonstrated wall motion abnormalities in 23 patients. Thirteen patients with a mismatch pattern i.e. preserved FDG uptake but decreased flow, in the biopsy region showed only 11 ± 6 vol% fibrosis but 21 ± 5 % cells

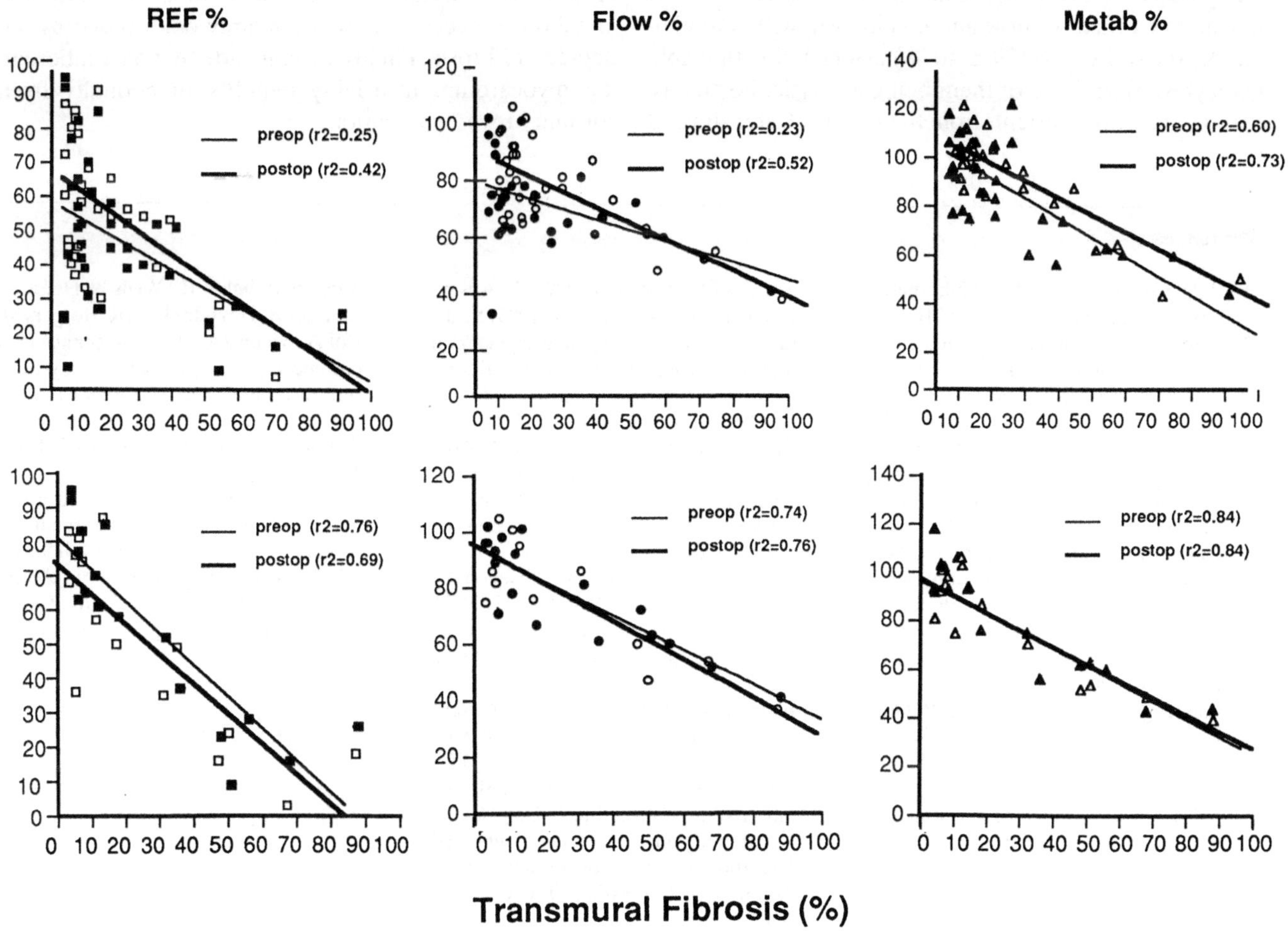

Fig. 1 *Top panel:* shows all patients with the pre- and postoperative data plotted against the transmural fibrosis. There is an improved correlation after revascularization. *Lower panel:* shows all patients except group 2 i.e. hibernating group. In these patients the transmural fibrosis appears to be an important predictor of the preoperative REF, flow and metabolism.

with reduced contractile material and increased glycogen content. Ten patients showed concordant flow / metabolism defects. The biopsies revealed extensive fibrosis (44 ± 16 %) and 23 ± 4 % of glycogen storing cells. There were 7 patients with normal anterior wall motion. Their biopsies showed only 7 ± 3 % fibrosis and 7 ± 4 % glycogen accumulating cells.

In another recent study, we performed pre- and 3 months postoperatively PET scanning and Equilibrium gated nuclear angiography (EGNA for regional ejection fraction = REF) in 36 coronary bypass surgery candidates. Histology was obtained from intra-operative biopsies as mentioned before. A principal component analysis was done using as variables the preoperative data, further a multivariate cluster analysis, divided the patients into 4 subpopulations: 1) a cluster of patients with normal function, flow, and metabolism, no fibrosis and viable myocytes ($n = 9$), 2) patients with low function, low flow but normal FDG-uptake, low fibrosis and viable myocytes including a moderate amount of myolytic cells (23 ± 10 %) ($n = 19$), 3) patients with low function, low flow and low metabolism, a high degree of fibrosis (62 ± 16 %) intermingled with viable cells resembling those in the second group ($n = 5$) and 4) a small group of patients ($n = 3$) having low function, flow and metabolism with a moderate degree of fibrosis (29 ± 10 %) associated with viable myocytes, 57 ± 23 % of them being myolytic. Postrevascularization, only patients from the second cluster showed significant improvement in function (REF from 39 ± 11 % to 50 ± 13 %, $p < 0.05$), identifying these areas as hibernating. A stepwise logistic regression showed a combination of low preoperative function and high FDG-uptake to be the best predictor of functional recovery ($p < 0.008$). A multivariate analysis showed that preoperative REF, flow and metabolism correlated significantly with fibrosis and that these correlations improved postoperatively ($p < 0.0001$), see figure 1.

Conclusions

From our previous and recent studies on the natural history of coronary artery disease, it becomes obvious that myocardial hibernation exists as a clinical entity and can be identified by the association of low function – high metabolism in terms of FDG-uptake. The hibernating myocardium is viable but shows definite subcellular alterations resembling those of dedifferentiated tissue. However, it remains to be proven if the hibernating myocardium is really dedifferentiating.

The non-hibernating myocardium remains unchanged after revascularization in terms of function, flow and metabolism because these are mainly determined by the degree of fibrosis. Finally we conclude that only hibernating myocardium invariably benefits functionally from coronary revascularization.

References

1. Rahimtoola SH (1989) The hibernating myocardium. Am Heart J 117: 211–221
2. Flameng W, Wouters L, Sergeant P, Lewi P, Borgers M, Thone F, Suy R (1984) Multivariate analysis of angiographic, histologic, and electrocardiographic data in patients with coronary heart disease. Circulation 70: 7–17
3. Flameng W, Suy R, Schwarz F, Borgers M, Piessens J, Thone F, Van Ermen H, De Geest H (1981) Ultrastructural correlates of left ventricular contraction abnormalities in patients with chronic ischemic heart disease: determinants of reversible segmental asynergy. Am Heart J 102: 846–857
4. Flameng W, Vanhaecke J, Van Belle H, Borgers M, De Beer L, Minten J (1987) Relation between coronary artery stenosis and myocardial purine metabolism, histology and regional functions in humans. J Am Coll Cardiol 9: 1235–1242
5. Borgers M, Thone F, Wouters L, Ausma J, Shivalkar B, Flameng W (1993) Structural correlates of regional myocardial dysfunction in patients with critical coronary artery stenosis: chronic hibernation? Cardiovasc Pathol 2: 237–245
6. Borgers M, De Nollin S, Thone F, Wouters L, Van Vaeck L, Flameng W (1993) Distribution of calcium in a subset of chronic hibernating myocardium in man. Histochem J 25: 312–318
7. Shivalkar B, Borgers W, Daenen W, Gewillig M, Flameng W (1994) ALCAPA Syndrome: An example of chronic myocardial hypoperfusion? J Am Coll Cardiol 23: 772–778
8. Flameng W, Shivalkar B (1991) Reversible myocardial dysfunction after coronary surgical revascularization. in: Left ventricular function in stunned and hibernating myocardium. Eds. Buller N, Henderson AH, Krayenbühl HP, Excerpta Medica, Amsterdam, Hong Kong, Princeton, Sydney, Tokyo, pp 99–109
9. Van Overschelde JL, Wyns W, Depré C, Essamri B, Heyndrickx GR, Borgers M, Bol A, Melin JA (1993) Mechanisms of chronic regional postischemic dysfunction in humans: new insights from the study of non-infarcted collateral-dependent myocardium. Circulation 87: 1513–1523
10. Maes A, Flameng W, Nuyts J, Borgers M, Shivalkar B, Ausma J, Bormans G, Schiepers C, De Roo M, Mortelmans L (1994) Histological alterations in chronically hypoperfused myocardium. Correlation with PET findings. Circulation 90: 735–745

59–61

M. Schwaiger

Identification of "hibernating myocardium" by imaging approaches

Key words Myocardial ischemia – hibernation – PET – scintigraphy

The terms "hibernating" and "stunned" myocardium have become widely accepted among experimentally or clinically oriented cardiologists. In contrast to "stunned" myocardium, which has been defined in the animal laboratory, the term "hibernating" myocardium is based on the clinical observation of functional recovery following surgical revascularization in patients with impaired LV-function (1).

The description of hibernating myocardium by Rahimtoola also included the presence of reduced myocardial perfusion (1). However, it was impossible, at the time of the clinical definition of "hibernating" myocardium, to accurately assess or predict regional myocardial perfusion in patients with coronary artery disease. Even today, the hypothesis of reduced myocardial perfusion and/or existence of "chronic ischemia" in hibernating myocardium remains controversial and awaits further improvement of techniques to measure blood flow in the human heart with high spatial resolution (2). The clinical presentations of coronary artery disease reflect the dynamic nature of coronary artery disease. The functional significance of a coronary artery stenosis varies depending on oxygen demand within the affected vascular bed. Even if regional myocardial blood flow could be measured with high accuracy, the measurement of relatively reduced myocardial blood flow in "hibernating" myocardium may represent the decreased oxygen demand of dysfunctioning myocardium and not the presence of "chronic ischemia". However, in the same patient, ischemia may occur during periods of physical activity, mental stress or sympathetic stimulation. Since the reversibility of dysfunction represents the most important clinical issue, the discussion of hypoperfusion or "chronic ischemia" in hibernating myocardium addresses primarily an academic question and does not directly affect the clinical decision making process.

M. Schwaiger, M.D. (✉)
Nuklearmedizinische Klinik
und Poliklinik der TU München
Klinikum rechts der Isar
Ismaninger Straße 22
81675 München, FRG

Due to the lack of accepted animal models, imaging procedures are challenged to provide new insights into the pathophysiology of hibernating human myocardium. However, in most patients dysfunctioning myocardium reflects a mixture of ischemic cell injury with coexistence of normal, hibernating, stunned, and scar tissue. Specific tissue characterization with high spatial resolution is necessary to study the regional interplay of physiologic parameters such as flow, metabolism and contractile reserve in the affected myocardium (3, 4). Currently available scintigraphic imaging approaches provide a spatial resolution of about 10–15 mm, yielding information limiting the pathophysiologic evaluation to large transmural segments. However, the unique specifity of tracer information provides separation of physiologic characteristics by contrast of the signal.

The scintigraphic techniques follow two general strategies. Firstly, the potassium analogues thallium-201 and Rubidium-82 have been used to probe the integrity of myocardial cell membranes as marker of tissue viability. Secondly, the use of metabolic tracers has been employed to study myocardial substrate retention as indicator for continuing metabolism in "hibernating" myocardium.

Thallium-201 scintigraphy has undergone various methodological variations based on the observation, that standard redistribution imaging has only limited sensitivity in detection of tissue viability. Resting thallium-201 scintigraphy, reinjection techniques and injection of thallium-201 together with administration of nitrates have been proposed to increase the sensitivity of this technique (5). Thallium-201 scintigraphy remains currently the most validated approach in assessing the extent of viable myocardium in patients with dysfunctioning myocardium. However, this scintigraphic assessment is limited by technical factors such as partial volume effect, attenuation artefacts and significant interobserver variability. More recently, semiquantitative analysis of tissue tracer retention has been shown to improve the separation of viable from nonviable myocardium (5).

Metabolic imaging requires in most instances positron emission tomography (PET). This technology offers improved image quality, attenuation correction and availability of short-lived radioisotopes for labelling of biologically active compounds. Using F-18 deoxyglucose as a marker of glucose metabolism, several studies have shown that reversibly dysfunctioning myocardium displays normal or even increased FDG-uptake. These data suggest that glucose metabolism is not only altered during ischemia, but also in "hibernating" myocardium. This clinically derived hypothesis is supported by increasing experimental evidence. First, ultrastructural and histological evaluation of tissue biopsies obtained from "hibernating" myocardial segments suggest degeneration of myocytes and increased glycogen storage, reflecting altered regulation of carbohydrate storage in these cells (6). Second, recent results evaluating the glucose transport proteins in "hibernating" human myocardium show an increased ratio of GLUT-1 to GLUT-4 transport proteins suggesting uncoupling of glucose transport from insulin stimulation in "hibernating" cells (7).

The comparison of tissue retention of blood flow markers and FDG by PET allows to identify segments with apparently reduced blood flow but maintained glucose metabolism (mismatch). This pattern of "mismatch" has become the hallmark of "hibernating" myocardium as defined by PET. This "mismatch" pattern is associated with a high likelihood of tissue recovery following revascularization (8). The extent of this abnormality has been also associated with the degree of global left ventricular functional recovery following revascularization. More recently, studies have indicated the important prognostic implication of this "mismatch" pattern. Retrospective analysis of patients undergoing PET studies revealed that patients with mismatch not undergoing revascularization suffered a significantly higher incidence of cardiovascular complication, as compared to those with the same scintigraphic pattern who underwent revascularization (9).

Newer PET imaging approaches include the use of C-11 acetate which is a marker of myocardial oxygen consumption. Although myocardial oxygen consumption may be slightly reduced in "hibernating" myocardium as assessed by C-11 acetate, it remains significantly higher than in scar tissue. Using such quantitative index of myocardial oxygen consumption provided by C-11 acetate, it appears to allow for separation of viable but dysfunctioning myocardium from scar tissue (10).

It is most important, that cardiologists and cardiovascular surgeons become aware of the high diagnostic accuracy of various new imaging approaches to identify hibernating myocardium. Recent investigations concentrating on clinical outcome, rather than functional recovery, indicate the prognostic potential of scintigraphic tissue characterization (9). More studies are necessary to define the impact of imaging approaches on the clinical selection of patients for revascularization and on clinical outcome. Such studies have to demonstrate that revascularization, based on presence of "hibernating myocardium", improves survival and, even more importantly, that the decision against revascularization in the absence of "hibernating myocardium" does not negatively affect outcome in patients with impaired LV-function and advanced CAD.

References

1. Rahimtoola SH (1989) The hibernating myocardium. Am Heart J 117: 211–221
2. Vanoverschelde J-LJ, Wijns W, Depré C, Essamri B, Heyndrickx GR, Borgers M, Bol A, Melin JA (1993) Mechanisms of chronic regional postischemic dysfunction in humans. New insights from the study of noninfarcted collateral-dependent myocardium. Circulation 87 (5): 1513–1523
3. Schulz R, Guth BD, Pieper K, Martin C, Heusch G (1992) Recruitment of an inotropic reserve in moderately ischemic myocardium at the expense of metabolic recovery. A model of short-term hibernation. Circulation Res 70: 1282–1295

4. Schelbert HR (1994) Metabolic imaging to assess myocardial viability. J Nucl Med 35 (4 Suppl): 8S–14S
5. Dilsizian V, Bonow RO (1993) Current diagnostic techniques of assessing myocardial viability in patients with hibernating and stunned myocardium. Circulation 87 (1): 1–20
6. Maes A, Flameng W, Nuyts J, Borgers M, Shivalkar B, Ausma J, Bormans G, Schiepers C, DeRoo M, Mortelmans L (1994) Histological alterations in chronically hypoperfused myocardium. Correlation with PET findings. Circulation 90 (2): 735–745
7. Schwaiger M, Sun D, Deeb N, Nguyen N, Haas F, Sebening F, Brosius F III (1994) Expression of myocardial glucose transporter (GLUT) mRNAs in patients with advanced coronary artery disease. Circulation 90 (4): I-113
8. Schwaiger M, Hicks R (1991) The clinical role of metabolic imaging of the heart by positron emission tomography. J Nucl Med 32: 565–578
9. Eitzman D, Al-Aouar Z, Kanter HL van Dahl J, Kirsh M, Deeb G, Schwaiger M (1992) Clinical outcome of patients with advanced coronary artery disease after viability studies with positron emission tomography. J Am Coll Cardiol 20: 559–565
10. Gropler R, Siegel B, Sampathkumaran K, Perez J, Sobel B, Bergmann S, Geltman E (1992) Dependence of recovery of contractile function on maintenance of oxidative metabolism after myocardial infarction. J Am Col Cardiol 19 (5): 989–997

Myocardial Stunning

65 – 68

S. F. Vatner
G. R. Heyndrickx

Ubiquity of myocardial stunning

Key words Stunning – hibernation – ischemia

We observed over two decades ago that myocardium rendered ischemic, but not irreversibly damaged, exhibited prolonged depression of regional myocardial function, long after the complete return of blood flow and resumption of a normal electrocardiographic pattern (3). At that time we did not appreciate the extent to which this characteristic of ischemic myocardium would be involved mechanistically in so many experimental and clinical settings. With the additional work of Kloner and Braunwald, the phenomenon of delayed recovery of postischemic tissue became known as "stunned myocardium" (2).

Classical myocardial stunning

The purpose of this brief review is to elucidate the ubiquity of myocardial stunning.

At first it was thought that myocardial stunning was elicited only following complete occlusion of a major coronary artery for less than 15 min. Characteristically on reperfusion, regional myocardial function would tend to resume rapidly during the reactive hyperemia phase and then, as reactive hyperemia subsided, would become depressed further to recover gradually over the subsequent 24-h period (Fig. 1). This is the classical picture of myocardial stunning. The clinical counterpart of this type of stunning is that which is observed after the brief coronary occlusion required for coronary angioplasty (10).

Myocardial stunning as a component of reperfusion injury

With the advent of thrombolytic therapy and the demonstration of the utility of coronary artery reperfusion to salvage ischemic myocardium, interest developed not only in recovery of tissue, but even more important, recovery of myocardial function. Controlled studies in animals studied serially over a month period of coronary artery reperfusion after coronary occlusion of 1 – 3 h duration, demonstrated gradual, prolonged recovery of regional myocardial function (7), (Fig. 2). This delayed recovery of function most likely included a component of myocardial stunning.

Myocardial stunning after ischemia resulting from an imbalance between O_2 supply and demand

In the presence of coronary artery disease

It is now apparent that myocardial stunning can result following a variety of etiologies causing myocardial ischemia, i.e., a complete occlusion of a major coronary artery is not a requisite. One such example occurs in patients and animal models with a fixed coronary artery stenosis. Under these conditions, with the increases of myocardial metabolic demand that occur with stress, e.g., with exercise, a regional imbalance between myocardial O_2 demand and supply occurs resulting in intense myocardial ischemia.

Supported in part by the U.S. Public Health Service Grants HL 33065, HL 38070-08, and HL 33107-11.

Dr. S. F. Vatner (✉) · G. R. Heyndrickx
New England Regional Primate Research Center
One Pine Hill Drive
P.O. Box 9102
Southborough, Massachusetts 01772-9102, U.S.A.
Cardiovascular Center
Aalst, Belgium

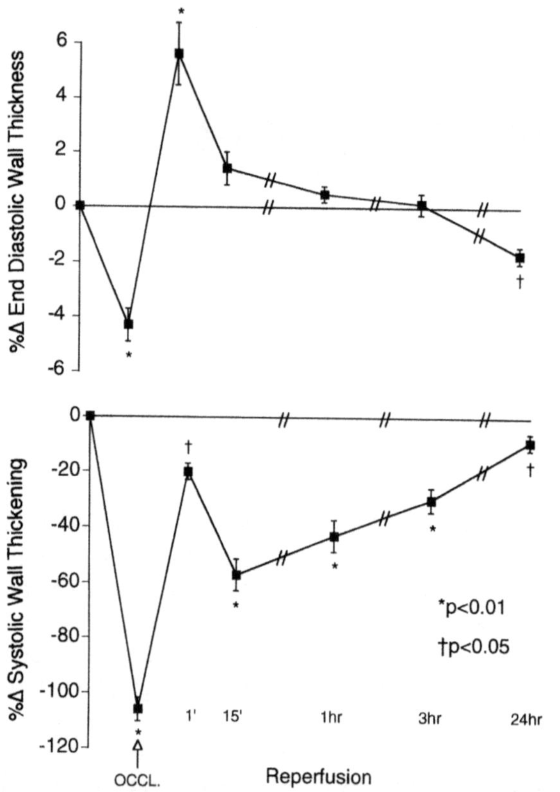

Fig. 1 Effects of a 15-min coronary occlusion and subsequent reperfusion at 1, 15, 60, and 180 min on average (± SEM) changes for end-diastolic wall thickness and systolic wall thickening. Significant changes are denoted by symbols. With coronary occlusion end-diastolic wall thickness and systolic wall thickening fell significantly. With coronary artery reperfusion there was a transient rebound, and then prolonged stunning, i.e., end-diastolic wall thickness was not significantly above control, but systolic wall thickening remained significantly depressed for at least 3 h. (Reprinted with permission from the American Physiological Society).

After relief of the stress, e.g., after cessation of exercise, regional myocardial function remains depressed and gradually recovers, which is indicative of myocardial stunning (6). A similar situation occurs following relief of a prolonged coronary artery stenosis (8).

In the presence of normal coronary arteries

The blood supply to the myocardium can be compromised even in situations of completely patent coronary arteries. One example occurs in the presence of severe cardiac hypertrophy. The hypertrophied heart is characterized by reduced subendocardial coronary reserve (5), although the luminal area of the coronary arteries is essentially normal, and there is no transmural difference in arteriolar or capillary density (1), suggesting that the limited subendocardial coronary reserve has as its mechanism an important hemodynamic component (4). With the stress of exercise, regional subendocardial wall motion was impaired in the hypertrophied heart, which is associated with a decline in the endo/epi blood flow ratio (5) (Fig. 3). With cessation of exercise, blood flow is rapidly restored to pre-exercise baseline levels transmurally, resulting in normalization of the endo/epi ratio, yet subendocardial wall motion remains depressed and requires hours to recover fully, which is reminiscent of myocardial stunning (5). Thus, even in the presence of normal coronary arteries, an imbalance between myocardial O_2 supply and demand can occur resulting in ischemia, which upon resolution can result in delayed recovery of regional myocardial function, i.e., myocardial stunning.

Myocardial stunning as the mechanism underlying myocardial hibernation

Studies in patients have pointed out that many instances of chronically depressed myocardial function cannot be explained by irreversible damage and infarcted myocar-

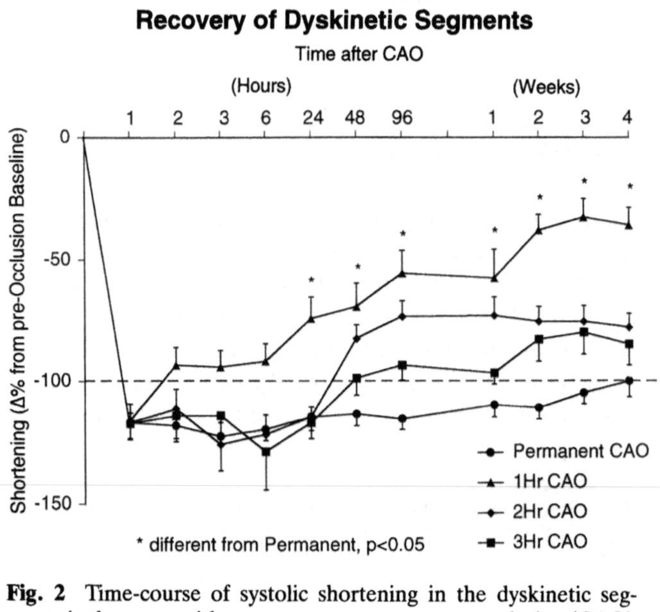

Fig. 2 Time-course of systolic shortening in the dyskinetic segments in the group with permanent coronary artery occlusion (CAO) (circles) or the group with 1 hr CAO (triangles), the group with 2 hr CAO (diamonds), and the group with 3 hr CAO(squares). Systolic shortening is expressed as percent change from pre-coronary artery occlusion (COA) baseline. Values depressed by over 100 % represent paradoxical systolic motion. The asterisks represent responses different from those in the permanent CAO group. (Reprinted with permission from the American Heart Association).

dium. With the advent of coronary artery bypass therapy, dyskinetic areas of myocardium rapidly regain normal myocardial function. This is one piece of evidence that prompted Rahimtoola to develop the concept of hibernating myocardium (9). Hibernating myocardium is recognized as chronically depressed regional myocardial function in the absence of irreversible injury (9). The sine qua non for hibernating myocardium is depressed regional myocardial blood flow. The underlying hypothesis is that regional hypofunction results from an adaptive response to reduced myocardial flow at rest whereby the heart downgrades its metabolic and contractile function in order to restore perfusion-contraction matching, thereby averting the evolution towards necrosis. Recent studies in patients (12) and experimental animals (11) have challenged this concept. Vanoverschelde et al., using PET technology to quantify regional myocardial perfusion, have demonstrated that resting flour in hibernating segments is in most instances normal. It is not always so clear that blood flow is actually reduced in clinical studies, in part because of the difficulty in making such precise measurements *in vivo* in patients. Recently, Shen and Vatner utilized a model of gradually increasing severity of coronary artery stenosis in the conscious pig with ameroid-induced coronary constriction (11). In that study, regional myocardial function in the ameroid-dependent zone was reduced by approximately 60 %, but blood flow was not depressed (Fig. 4). Since blood flow was not depressed, the depression in function could not be attributed to myocardial hibernation. With close inspection of continuous records of regional wall motion in the pigs with chronic coronary artery constriction, it was observed that brief episodes of stress resulted in prolonged periods of depressed myocardial function. The depressed function clearly followed episodes of myocardial O_2 supply/ demand imbalance and were characteristic of myocardial stunning (Fig. 5). These studies challenge the concept of myocardial hibernation and potentially lead to a redefinition of this phenomenon. It is conceivable that the clinical

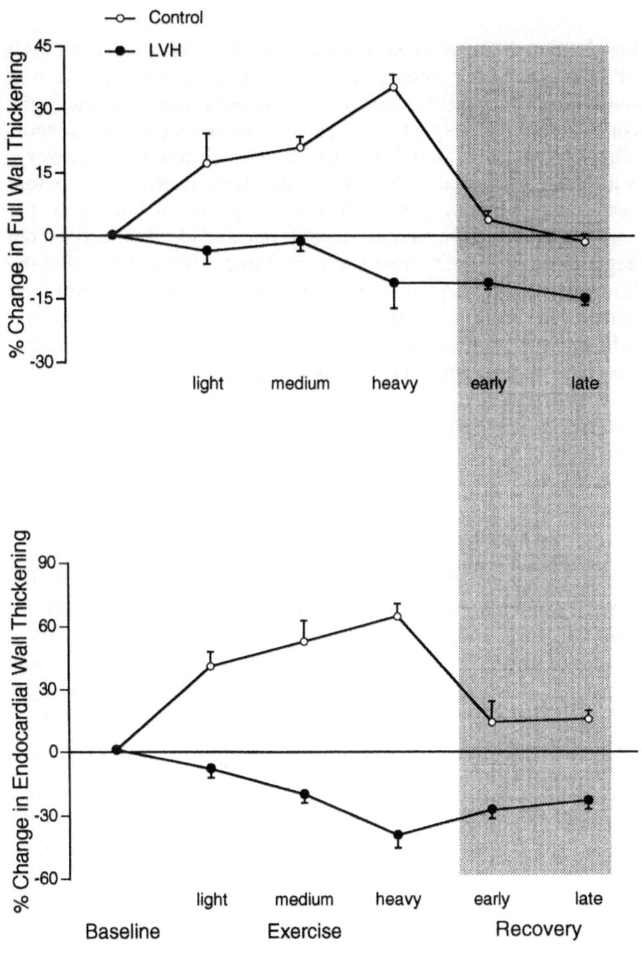

Fig. 3 Graphs showing responses to exercise for left ventricular (LV) full wall thickening (upper panel) and subendocardial wall thickening (lower panel). These responses are shown as percent changes from baseline values for control dogs and dogs with LV hypertrophy (LVH). Baseline values are in parentheses. Full and subendocardial wall thicknesses increased significantly in the control dogs with progressive levels of exercise. Subendocardial wall thickening actually fell during exercise in LVH dogs. Late in recovery, full and subendocardial thickening remained significantly depressed compared with baseline values in LVH dogs. (Reprinted with permission from the American Heart Association).

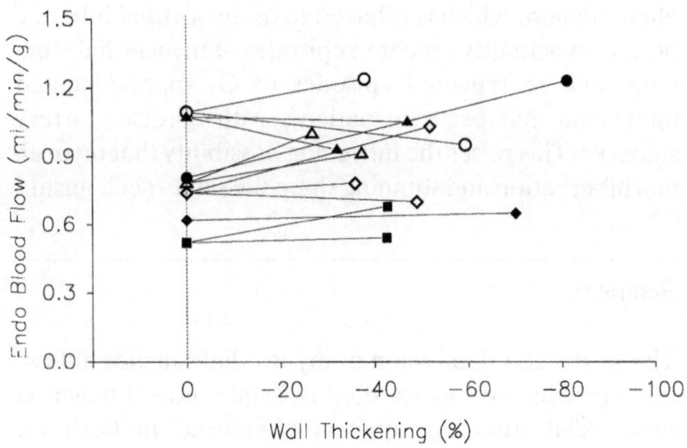

Fig. 4 Graph shows the relation between the decrease in wall thickening (abscissa) and simultaneous endocardial (ENDO) blood flow measurements (ordinate). In this figure, there are 13 measurements of blood flow made in the seven pigs bracketing the time of peak reduction in wall thickening. Note that there were major decrease in wall thickening ranging from 27 % to 81 % but little decreases in any of the 13 measurements of blood flow. (Reprinted with permission from the American Heart Association).

phenomenon, which is referred to as myocardial hibernation, is in actuality repeated episodes of myocardial stunning, due to repeated episodes of O_2 supply/demand imbalance that occur in patients with coronary artery stenoses. This raises the intriguing possibility that myocardial hibernation and stunning share the same mechanism.

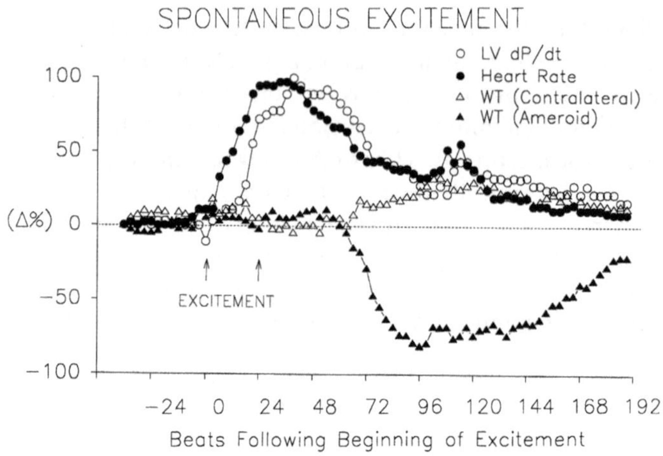

Fig. 5 Graph shows a beat-by-beat analysis of left ventricular (LV) dP/dt (open circles), heart rate (closed circles), and systolic wall thickening (WT) distal to the ameroid (closed triangles) and in the contralateral regions (open triangles) in a conscious pig during spontaneous excitement, the duration of which is denoted by the arrows. Values are expressed as percent change from control, i.e., before excitement. However, the reduction in systolic WT distal to the ameroid followed the increase in heart rate and LV dP/dt and did not begin until after excitement had terminated. This suggests that the functional deficit was caused by an imbalance in oxygen supply and demand in response to the hemodynamic changes rather than by a primary reduction in coronary blood flow. (Reprinted with permission from the American Heart Association).

Summary

The prolonged depression of myocardial function following episodes of myocardial ischemia now known as myocardial stunning, appears ubiquitous in both the experimental and clinical settings. With recent therapies designed to ameliorate ischemic myocardium, e.g., coronary artery bypass, coronary thrombolysis, coronary angioplasty, the inexorable progression from ischemia to necrosis has been averted more successfully and frequently, which permits appearance of myocardial stunning to become clearer. Myocardial stunning occurs in the presence of a multitude of inciting stimuli to myocardial ischemia, including a fixed stenosis, relief from stenosis or even in the presence of reduced coronary reserve, without a coronary stenosis. It will be potentially most interesting to determine if myocardial stunning also belies the hibernating myocardium and is, in fact, its actual mechanism.

References

1. Bishop SP, Powell PC, Hasebe N, Shen Y-T, Patrick TA, Hittinger L, Vatner SF Coronary vascular morphology in pressure-overload left ventricular hypertrophy (submitted for publication)
2. Braunwald E, Kloner RA (1982) The stunned myocardium: prolonged, postischemic ventricular dysfunction. Circulation 66: 1146–1149
3. Heyndrickx GR, Millard RW, McRitchie RJ, Maroko PR, Vatner SF (1975) Regional myocardial functional and electrophysical alterations after brief coronary artery occlusion in conscious dogs. J Clin Invest 56: 978–985
4. Hittinger L, Mirsky I, Shen Y-T, Patrick TA, Bishop SP, Vatner SF (1995) Hemodynamic mechanisms responsible for reduced subendocardial coronary reserve in dogs with severe left ventricular hypertrophy. (Circulation, in press)
5. Hittinger L, Shannon RP, Kohin S, Manders WT, Kelly P, Vatner SF (1990) Exercise induced subendocardial dysfunction in dogs with left ventricular hypertrophy. Circ Res 66: 329–343
6. Homans DC, Sublett E, Lindstrom P, Nesbitt T, Bach RJ (1988) Subendocardial and subepicardial wall thickening during ischemia in exercising dogs. Circulation 78: 1267–1276
7. Lavallee M, Cox D, Patrick TA, Vatner SF (1983) Salvage of myocardial function by coronary artery reperfusion 1, 2 and 3 hours after occlusion in conscious dogs. Circ Res 53: 235–247
8. Matsuzaki M, Gallagher KP, Kemper WS, White F, Ross J Jr (1983) Sustained regional dysfunction produced by prolonged coronary stenosis: gradual recovery after reperfusion. Circulation 68 (1): 170–182
9. Rahimtoola SH (1989) The hibernating myocardium. Am J Heart 117: 211–221
10. Serruys PW, Jaski B, Piscione F, ten Kate F, de Feyter P, van den Brand M, Hugenholtz P (1986) Early changes in wall thickness and epicardial wall motion during percutaneous angioplasty in man. Similarities with in vitro and in vivo model. In coronary angioplasty: A controlled model for ischemia. p. 19–31. Eds. Serruys PW, Meester GT, Martinus Nijhoff, Publishers
11. Shen Y-T, Vatner SF (1995) Mechanism of impaired myocardial function during progressive coronary stenosis in conscious pigs: Hibernation vs. stunning. Circ Res 76: 479–488
12. Vanoverschelde JL, Wijns W, Depré C, Essamri B, Heyndrickx GR, Borgers M, Bol A, Melin JA (1993) Mechanisms of chronic regional postischemic dysfunction in humans: New insights from the study of non-infarcted collateral dependent myocardium. Circulation 87: 1513–1523

69 – 74

R. Bolli

Common methodological problems and artifacts associated with studies of myocardial stunning in vivo

Key words Myocardial stunning – "hypersensitive" myocardium – methodological problems

Introduction

Since the original description of myocardial stunning by Heyndrickx et al. in 1975 (6), the number of studies dealing with this phenomenon has continued to increase, to the point that myocardial stunning is now one of the most common problems addressed in experimental cardiology. Each year new drugs or manipulations are added to the lengthening list of interventions that are claimed to attenuate myocardial stunning. This is somewhat reminiscent of the situation that occurred with infarct size limitation in the 1970s and 1980s, when a bewildering array of interventions were claimed to reduce infarct size, and their list kept increasing at a relentless pace. In view of the disastrous outcome of the infarct size limitation saga (the vast majority of the claims were not subsequently substantiated), this similarity is worrisome. We have now come to realize that the main reason for the fiasco of infarct size limitation was the presence of methodological problems in many published studies. To prevent a similar outcome for studies of myocardial stunning it is important that the most common methodological problems and artifacts associated with these studies be recognized and dealt with appropriately. The purpose of this brief review is to identify them and suggest possible approaches for avoiding their interference. The discussion is limited to studies of regional stunning in vivo.

As a general concept, the stunned myocardium is a "hypersensitive" myocardium; that is, every factor that affects contractile performance in the normal, healthy myocardium can be expected to have a greater impact on the stunned, convalescent myocardium.

This concept has two implications. First, numerous variables that are known to influence normal cardiac function have considerable influence on the stunned myocardium. These variables need to be carefully measured and taken into account. Second, the fact that in a given study a variable has no influence on the nonischemic zone does not mean that it has no significant influence on the reperfused zone, since the sensitivity to this variable may be greater in the reperfused region than in the nonischemic region.

Listed below are the most important variables that affect myocardial stunning.

Collateral blood flow during ischemia

The degree of myocardial perfusion during ischemia is a major determinant of the severity of myocardial stunning after reperfusion (1, 2). In conscious dogs there is a close direct relationship between collateral flow during coronary occlusion and wall thickening after reperfusion, which is best described by exponential regression models (2). Such a relationship predicts that in the low-flow range even small differences in collateral flow result in large differences in postischemic wall thickening (1, 2, 8, 10). In

Supported in part by NIH R01 grants HL-43151 and HL-55757.

Dr. R. Bolli (✉)
Division of Cardiology
University of Louisville
Louisville, Kentucky 40292, USA

open-chest animals this relationship is looser, probably because of the many confounding influences associated with these preparations (such as variations in temperature); nevertheless, a linear direct relationship between collateral flow and postischemic contractile performance is usually appreciable in these models (5, 8, 12, 13).

Recommendation

When myocardial stunning is studied in dogs, collateral flow must be measured in every animal (obviously, this is unnecessary in species that lack preformed coronary collateral vessels). As a minimum, it must be verified that the average collateral flow is similar in the different groups of dogs compared; the optimal approach would probably be an analysis of covariance in which collateral flow is the covariate.

Myocardial temperature

Myocardial temperature is an enormously important determinant of the severity of myocardial stunning, and unfortunately one that is often overlooked or ignored. The powerful influence of temperature on postischemic regional function was demonstrated by Triana et al. (11) in open-chest dogs. These authors found that when no effort was made to keep the animals normothermic, esophageal temperature fell to an average of 33.7° C at 4 h of reperfusion after a 15-min occlusion; at this time raising the temperature from 33.8° to 36.6° C resulted in a dramatic deterioration in systolic wall thickening in the stunned myocardium from 65 % to – 52 % of baseline values (11) (Fig. 1). For each 1° C increase in temperature between 33.8° and 36.6° C, thickening fraction in the reperfused region decreased by an average of 43 % of baseline values (Fig. 2). In the nonischemic region the increse in temperature from 33.8° to 36.6° C did not produce any change in thickening fraction (Fig. 2), indicating that temperature has a selective depressant effect on the stunned myocardium (11). Thus, even small and unnoticed fluctuations in body temperature after reperfusion have a profound influence on the outcome of studies of myocardial stunning. It is important to stress that if no efforts are made to maintain body temperature in open-chest animals, the animals become hypothermic within a few hours, which artifactually enhances the recovery of regional wall motion (11). It should also be noted that although the temperature present during ischemia undoubtedly affects postischemic dysfunction, major changes in the severity of myocardial stunning can be produced by the temperature present *after* reperfusion, regardless of the temperature present *during* ischemia.

Recommendation

It is imperative that myocardial or body temperature be measured and controlled strictly during experiments

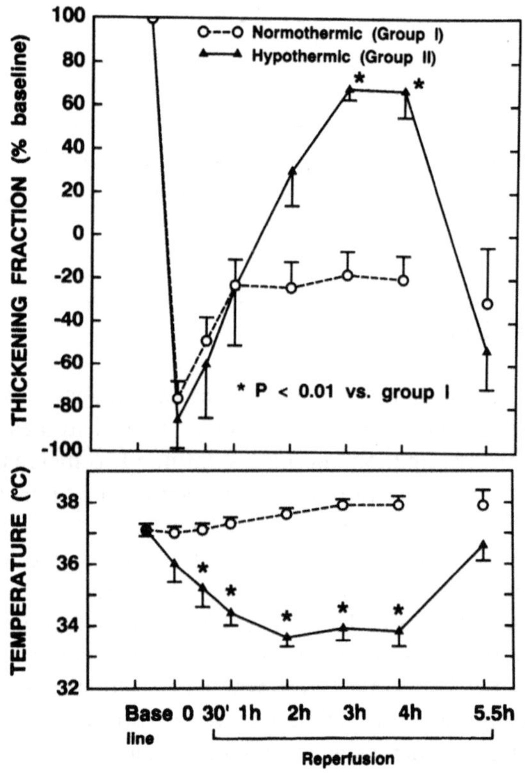

Fig. 1 The systolic thickening fraction in the ischemic/reperfused region (*top panel*) and esophageal temperature (*bottom panel*) 5 min after coronary occlusion (O) and at selected times after reperfusion in normothermic open-chest dogs (group I; n = 30) and hypothermic open-chest dogs (group II; n = 5). Thickening fraction is expressed as percentage of baseline values. In group I the esophageal temperature was kept between 37° and 38° C by using a heating blanket and by covering the animal; in group II, no effort was made to control esophageal temperature. After 4 h of reperfusion, in group II the temperature was raised by 2.8° C by covering the animal and by using heating blankets (this required ~1.5 h). Note that the increase in temperature was associated with a striking decrease in thickening fraction in the stunned myocardium. This decrease was not due to a spontaneous deterioration of the open-chest preparation after 4 h of reperfusion because in eight dogs in group I thickening fraction remained stable between 4 h (–32 ± 24 % of baseline) and 5.5 h (–31 ± 26 %). The thickening fraction and the temperature in these eight dogs are represented by the isolated open circles at 5.5 h of reperfusion. (From [11]).

focusing on myocardial stunning. One can obtain literally any result that one wishes simply by manipulating body temperature!

Position of the ultrasonic crystals with respect to the border zone

Another major determinant of the results of studies of stunning that is usually overlooked is the distance between the ultrasonic crystals and the border of the ischemic-reperfused bed. Buda et al. (4) found that the "tethering" effect exerted by the ischemic myocardium on the adjacent nonischemic myocardium during coronary artery occlusion resulted in a zone of hypofunction but normal perfusion extending approximately 8 – 9 mm on either lateral border. We have observed that this tethering effect is even more pronounced after reperfusion, such that regional contractile performance in the stunned region is artifactually enhanced when the crystals are placed within approximately 1 cm from the perfusion boundary. Thus, one can markedly "improve" the recovery of regional wall thickening simply by positioning the ultrasonic crystals close to the perfusion border between ischemic and nonischemic regions. This becomes a real problem when the ischemic zone is very small because it is difficult to position the crystals farther than 1 cm from the perfusion boundaries.

It is important to stress that the influence of the tethering effect is larger after reperfusion (when active contraction is decreased but still present) than during ischemia (when active contraction is totally absent). Consequently, the presence of dyskinesis during ischemia should not be used as evidence that there is no tethering effect after reperfusion.

Recommendation

Care must be taken to place the crystals farther than 1 cm from the perfusion boundaries. Furthermore, the distance of the crystals from the perfusion boundaries should be measured at postmortem examination. Crystals found to be less than 1 cm from the boundary should not be used.

Fig. 2 *Left panel,* relationship between the change in thickening fraction in the ischemic/reperfused region (*vertical axis*) and the change in esophageal temperature (*horizontal axis*) after 4 h of reperfusion in five hypothermic open-chest dogs (group II). In these animals temperature was raised by 2.8° C by covering the animals and by using heating blankets; this increase in temperature was associated with a striking decrease in thickening fraction in the stunned myocardium. The decrement in thickening fraction averaged 43 % of baseline values for each 1° C increase in temperature between 33.8° and 36.6° C. Temperature had little effect on the nonischemic region. Therefore, the changes in temperature exerted a selective depressant effect on the mechanical function of the stunned myocardium. *Right panel,* relationship between thickening fraction in the ischemic/reperfused region and in the nonischemic region and esophageal temperature in a dog in group II after 4 h of reperfusion. In this dog temperature was raised from 35.6° C at 4 h of reflow to 38.3° C 82 min later, and measurements were repeated for every 0.6° C increase in temperature. Note that stepwise increases in temperature were associated with stepwise decreases in thickening fraction in the stunned myocardium but not in the nonischemic myocardium. Even small increases in temperature resulted in substantial decreases in wall thickening, indicating a sensitive coupling between body temperature and function in stunned myocardium. (From [11).

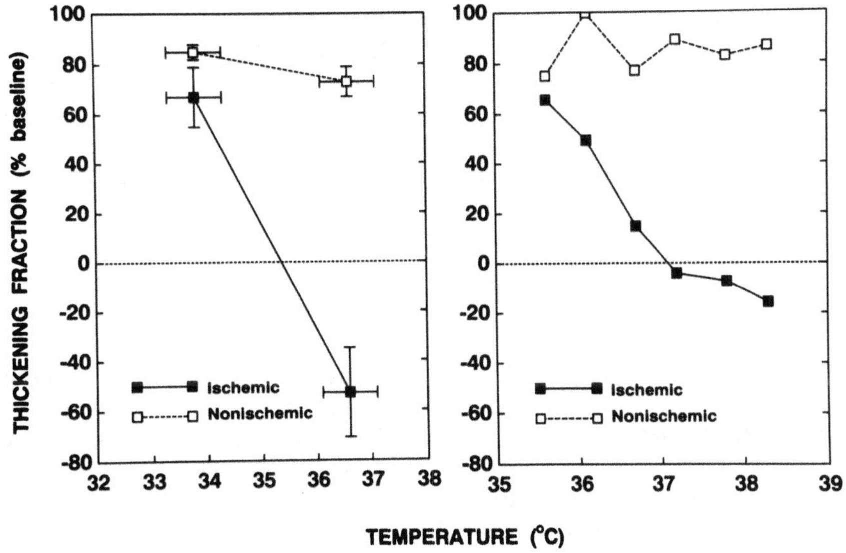

Baseline level of regional myocardial function

In our experience, in some open-chest dogs (but not in conscious dogs) regional myocardial function under baseline conditions is abnormally low (i.e., systolic thickening fraction is <15 %). This probably indicates some abnormality in the myocardium, which makes it unsuitable to be studied. We found that when baseline thickening fraction is less than 15 %, the myocardium invariably fails to recover after reperfusion.

Recommendation

Myocardial segments with baseline thickening fraction less than 15 % should not be used in studies of myocardial stunning. One can be certain that they will not recover!

Depth of anesthesia

When pentobarbital or other barbiturates are used, one must be concerned about the myocardial depressant effects of these drugs. This is particularly a problem when supplemental doses of barbiturates are given during the course of the experiment to maintain the depth of anesthesia. For example, immediately after the administration of a supplemental bolus of pentobarbital the performance of a stunned myocardial region may deteriorate markedly. The depth of anesthesia also affects myocardial stunning in the opposite way. If the animal is not sufficiently anesthetized, this results in increased levels of circulating catecholamines, which increases the mechanical performance of the stunned myocardium. Under these conditions there is usually an increase in heart rate and blood pressure, which can serve as markers of inadequate anesthesia.

Recommendation

One should attempt to maintain adequate and consistent levels of anesthesia in different animals. In addition, whenever possible, supplemental doses of anesthetics should be given immediately *after* taking the measurement of regional myocardial function rather than immediately before.

Size of the ischemic-reperfused region

The size of the ischemic-reperfused region affects myocardial stunning in two ways. First, a small region makes it difficult to avoid placing the crystals in the functional border zone, as mentioned above. Second, a large ischemic region is more likely to bulge out during systole and therefore to be associated with dyskinesis. When an effort is made to keep the ischemic zone sizes within a narrow range, the size of the ischemic area is not an independent determinant of the severity of stunning (2). However, if the range of the ischemic zone sizes is large, it is our experience that this becomes an independent determinant.

Recommendation

An effort should be made to obtain similar ischemic zone sizes in different animals. The size of the ischemic zone should be measured to verify that it is comparable in different groups. Animals with ischemic zones less than 15 % of left ventricular weight should not be used: in our experience these animals almost invariably exhibit a good recovery.

Heart rate

Because the diastolic filling time per minute is inversely related to heart rate, and because a decrease in filling time results in a decrease in end-diastolic length, increases in heart rate are usually associated with a deterioration in function of the stunned myocardium. This can be easily tested by comparing myocardial performance in stunned myocardium at spontaneous heart rates and during pacing at faster rates; one often notices a deterioration in segment shortening or wall thickening.

Recommendation

Heart rate should obviously be measured, and one should ensure that it is comparable between different groups of animals.

Arterial pressure

Changes in afterload have a marked effect on the contractile performance of the stunned myocardium. It is possible to "improve" the contractile performance simply by decreasing systolic arterial pressure and, conversely, to "worsen" the recovery by increasing arterial pressure.

Recommendation

It is essential that systolic arterial pressure be measured, and that it be similar in the different groups of animals being compared. If an intervention is studied which is likely to change arterial pressure, measures should be taken to prevent or minimize these changes (e.g., aortic constriction). An even better but more cumbersome approach would be to use load-independent parameters of contractile performance.

Myocardial blood flow

Stahl et al. (9) reported that increases in blood flow in the stunned myocardium were associated with increases in contractile performance, suggesting a "Gregg phenomenon". In our experience this effect is somewhat erratic and perhaps dependent on the severity of myocardial stunning. In hypokinetic stunned myocardium after a 10-min coronary occlusion, the intravenous infusion of adenosine increased wall thickening dramatically (from 5.1 % to 17.7 %) with no change in systolic arterial pressure (10). (Interestingly, the same infusion of adenosine before ischemia had little or no effect [10] again indicating the "hypersensitivity" of stunned myocardium to exogenous influences.) In akinetic stunned myocardium after 15-min occlusion, the intravenous infusion of adenosine 4 h after reperfusion increased wall thickening from 1.4 % to 7.3 %, but this was due at least in part to a marked decrease in systolic arterial pressure (3). In severely dyskinetic myocardium (thickening fraction –30 % of baseline) after a 15-min occlusion, intracoronary adenosine had no appreciable affect on wall thickening despite a greater than fourfold increase in coronary flow (8). Thus, it appears that the effect of coronary flow is relatively greater when the severity of myocardial stunning is relatively mild.

Recommendation

If there are major differences in coronary flow among dogs, these could play a role in modulating myocardial stunning, particularly if the severity of stunning is relatively mild. However, coronary flow is not likely to be important when the differences in flow are not very large. It is a good idea to measure postreperfusion flow in order to exclude such large differences.

Preload

As is the case for normal myocardium, preload has an important effect on the contractile performance of stunned myocardium.

Recommendation

The rate of fluid replacement should be standardized in all animals. When possible, measurements of end-diastolic length should be reported. If these are not possible, measurements of left atrial pressure or left ventricular end-diastolic pressure should be reported.

These are the most important variables to consider in studies of myocardial stunning. In addition, it is a good idea to exclude dogs with anemia (hematocrit less than 30%), hypoxemia (PO_2 less than 60 mmHg), acidosis (arterial pH less than 7.30), heart worm infestation, or other pathological conditions. Although no specific data are available to support this recommendation, it appears that these pathological conditions have the potential to influence myocardial stunning. Obviously the decision to exclude expensive animals (such as dogs) for one of these reasons is difficult, due to financial considerations.

As is apparent from this discussion, studies of myocardial stunning in vivo are quite difficult and expensive if one seeks to avoid all of the potential sources of artifact. (In our laboratory we end up excluding 30 – 50 % of the dogs used for acute open-chest studies and a similar proportion of the dogs used for chronic studies, due to technical problems or one of the reasons specified above). Although following these recommendations can be costly and time consuming, I believe it is necessary in order to prevent erroneous conclusions.

References

1. Bolli R (1990) Mechanism of myocardial "stunning". Circulation 82: 723–738
2. Bolli R, Zhu WX, Thornby JI, O'Neill PG, Roberts R (1988) Time-course and determinants of recovery of function after reversible ischemia in conscious dogs. Am J Physiol 254: H102–H114
3. Bolli R, Triana JF, Jeroudi MO (1990) Prolonged impairment of coronary vasodilation after reversible ischemia: evidence for microvascular "stunning". Circ Res 67: 332–343
4. Buda AJ, Zotz RJ, Gallagher KP (1986) Characterization of the functional border zone around regionally ischemic myocardium using circumferential flow-function maps. J Am Coll Cardiol 8: 150–158
5. Gross GJ, Farber NE, Hardman HF, Warltier DC (1986) Beneficial actions of superoxide dismutase and catalase in "stunned" myocardium of dogs. Am J Physiol 250: H372–H377
6. Heyndrickx GR, Millard RW, McRitchie RJ, Maroko PR, Vatner SF (1975) Regional myocardial function and electrophysiological alterations after brief coronary artery occlusion in conscious dogs. J Clin Invest 56: 978–985
7. Sekili S, McCay PB, Li XY, Zughaib M, Sun JZ, Tang XL, Thornby JI, Bolli R (1993) Direct evidence that the hydroxyl radical plays a pathogenetic role in myocardial "stunning" in the conscious dog and that stunning can be markedly attenuated without subsequent adverse effects. Circ Res 73: 705–723
8. Sekili S, Jeroudi MO, Tang XL, Zughaib M, Sun JZ, Bolli R (1995) Effect of adenosine on myocardial "stunning" in the dog. Circ Res 76: 82–94
9. Stahl LD, Aversano TR, Becker LC (1986) Selective enhancement of function of stunned myocardium by increased flow. Circulation 74: 845–851
10. Triana JF, Bolli R (1991) Decreased flow reserve in "stunned" myocardium after a 10-minute coronary occlusion. Am J Physiol 261: H793–H804
11. Triana JF, Li XY, Jamaluddin U, Thornby JI, Bolli R (1991) Postischemic myocardial "stunning": identification of major differences between the open-chest and the conscious dog and evaluation of the oxygen radical hypothesis in the conscious dog. Circ Res 69: 731–747
12. Zughaib ME, Abd-Elfattah AS, Jeroudi MO, Sun JZ, Sekili S, Tang XL, Bolli R (1993) Augmentation of endogenous adenosine attenuates myocardial "stunning" independently of coronary flow or hemodynamic effects. Circulation 88: 2359–2369
13. Zughaib ME, Tang XL, Schleman M, Jeroudi MO, Bolli R (1994) Beneficial effects of MDL 74,405, a cardioselective water soluble alpha-tocopherol analogue, on the recovery of function of stunned myocardium in intact dogs. Cardiovasc Res 28: 235–241

75 – 77

D. J. Hearse

Stunning: Three questions and concerns

Key words Stunning – ischaemia – reperfusion injury

Introduction

Of all the manifestations of left ventricular dysfunction, myocardial stunning must be the most exhaustively investigated. More drugs have been evaluated in the canine model of stunning than in any other model but, despite this, several fundamental questions about this phenomenon remain unanswered. In the following, I pose three questions and anticipate some of the answers.

Is stunning really the defenitive example of "reperfusion injury"?

I, as others, have written on the penomenon termed "reperfusion injury", discussing its nature and even its existence (3). Reperfusion injury can be simply defined as deleterious events, occurring *during* reperfusion (and arising as a *consequence* of reperfusion) that subtract from the benefits of the restoration of flow and thereby increase tissue injury over and above that substained during the preceding period of ischaemia. Stunning is frequently cited as a classic example of such injury, and evidence for the existence of a deleterious component of reperfusion usually derives from the observation that interventions given *only* during reperfusion are able to attenuate stunning. Thus Bolli et al. (1) have shown that a free radical scavenger given only (and transiently) at the time of reperfusion can dramatically attenuate stunning in the canine heart. However, can this *really* be taken as definitive evidence of the existence of reperfusion injury? Whilst the administration of a drug after a period of ischaemia cannot lessen the amount or nature of the injury sustained during that period, I remain sceptical that such experiments provide *definitive* proof for the existence of reperfusion injury. If my following arguments are correct, it becomes important so question whether stunning is necessarily an example of reperfusion injury (a situation that would in no way diminish the significance of stunning).

It seems to me that a finite amount of time is always required for tissue to recover from a transient pathological insult. Why then should a piece of myocardium that has sustained reversible (but nonetheless metabolically and functionally devastating) ischaemic injury be expected to recover fully and immediately on the restoration of flow? Why should the myocyte be denied a reasonable period to re-instate its metabolic and ionic homeostasis before returning to full contractile activity? Can we not view the stunned myocardium as a well-regulated tissue undergoing a controlled period of convalescence? Why can we not assume that the salutory effects of interventions given at the time of reperfusion are merely accelerating the recovery of some (as yet unknown) metabolic process sustained during ischemia in a manner akin to an aspirin hastening the departure of an alcoholic hangover? Would anyone argue that part of the hangover is a consequence of stopping drinking? Why should we not consider stunning as an "ischaemic hangover"?

It follows from the above argument that it is impossible to prove the existence of a deleterious component of

Prof. Dr. J. Hearse (✉)
Cardiovascular Research
The Rayne Institute
St. Thomas' Hospital
London SE1 7EH, United Kingdom

reperfusion simply by *adding* an intervention at the time of reperfusion and looking for benefit. We may, however, stand a better chance if we endeavour to attenuate stunning (or any other putative manifestation of reperfusion injury) by *removing* a component of the reperfusion process and demonstrating clear benefit. Such experiments are more difficult to devise, but some do exist, such as transient leucocyte depletion at the time of reperfusion – and what a controversial field this has become!

Even if reperfusion injury does exist, and assuming that it makes a contribution to stunning, we should ask: what fraction of the contractile deficit should be attributed to reperfusion injury and what fraction reflects convalescence from the injury sustained during the period of ischaemia? With rare exceptions (2) this question is hardly ever discussed – despite the likelihood that the answer could be of major importance to understanding the mechanisms of stunning. The fact that interventions given (sometimes in combination) at the time of reperfusion, have never been shown to totally abolish the phenomenon, must add to the common-sense view that a *substantial proportion* of the contractile deficit must be attributable to convalescence from ischaemic injury. The recent studies showing that the pre-ischaemic administration alone of interventions such as ATP-sensitive potassium channel openers can result in a substantial attenuation of post-ischaemic stunning, can only add weight to this argument. In the absence of any data, should we perhaps agree that as much as half of the contractile deficit of stunning may be unrelated to reperfusion injury?

Has something been omitted from the description of stunning?

Figure 1A is representative of many hundreds of figures in the literature, and is fully consistent with the accepted definition of stunning as a post-ischaemic contractile deficit that takes hours or days to normalise. Almost without exception investigators portray the recovery profile as one the *progressively improves* from a very low value at the onset of reperfusion. However, this does not adequately portray the dynamic nature of the contractile recovery during the early moments of reperfusion, when a potentially important, but generally ignored, event occurs. Most investigators, know that the profile for functional recovery is in fact *biphasic* (Figure 1B) with an early, and *often complete,* recovery of contractile function. This recovery is, however, transient, and after a few minutes contractile function declines again (sometimes to zero) to be followed by a very slow recovery. Possibly, most investigators do not record function until 15 min or so into the reperfusion period. Nonetheless, failure to record or discuss this early recovery must be to the detriment of our understanding of myocardial stunning.

It could be argued that the early and rapid recovery might be a consequence of some transient inotropic stimulus such as reperfusion-induced release of catecholamines or intracellular calcium overload; certainly the stunned heart possesses considerable inotropic reserve. However, an alternative interpretation is that the heart has the potential to recover rapidly and fully from the ischaemia-induced injury, but this is halted and reversed by the onset of reperfusion injury, which accounts for the secondary decline in function. Is it a coincidence that the curtailment of the early recovery of function appears to coincide temporally with the burst of free radical production that has often been suggested as responsible for the induction of

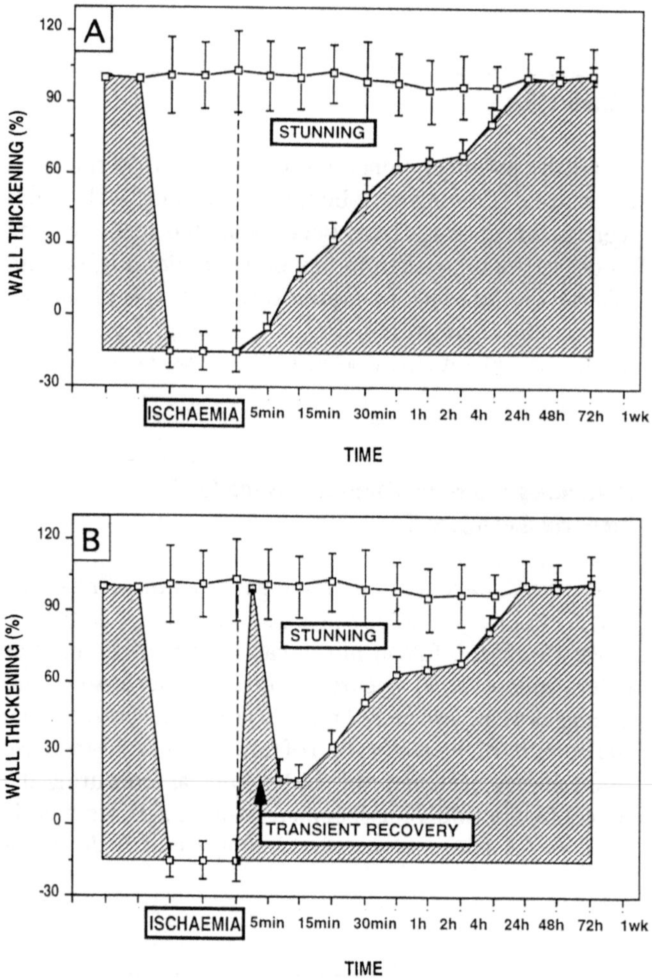

Fig. 1 **A** Traditional representation of the recovery profile for myocardial stunning. **B** The more complete representation of the profile showing the early, transient, hyperdynamic phase that is rarely reported or discussed in the literature.

reperfusion injury? I have discussed this possibility in detail elsewhere (5).

Could the cause of the delay lie in the nucleus?

Perhaps the most surprising feature of stunning (be it convalescence from ischaemia or recovery from reperfusion injury) is the protracted length of the recovery period, which may exceed by 100-fold the duration of the initiating insult. Recovery times of 24 h or more are far greater than would be expected for the re-establishment of ionic homeostasis or the restoration of normal levels of metabolites. Certainly there is convincing evidence that the disturbances of energy metabolism that accompany stunning do not underlie the impairment of function. Similarly the intracellular content and distribution of key ions such as calcium appear to revert to normal soon after the onset of reperfusion. It has, however, been suggested (4) that the nature of calcium transients and the sensitivity of the myofibrils to calcium may remain perturbed for some time. Disturbances in the *control* of ion movements or reactivity of contractile proteins are indicative of some malfunction in the structure and function of the proteins involved. This raises the intriguing possibility that some event during ischaemia or reperfusion (possibly free radical-induced oxidant stress) may injure some contractile or ion translocating proteins.

Since I have discussed this possibility in detail elsewhere (2), suffice it to say here that I advance the hypothesis that contractile or ion translocating proteins (such as the sodium-calcium exchanger, the sodium pump and the calcium-regulating proteins of the sarcoplasmic reticulum), that have thiol groups involved in the regulation of their function, may be particularly vulnerable to modification by reperfusion-induced oxidant stress. Oxidation of such thiol groups might lead to reversible or irreversible damage to the protein, and this in turn, might lead to a reduction, an increase or a total loss of its ion regulating or contractile properties. However, as the oxidant stress subsides and the cell seeks to re-establish its normal redox status, some of these oxidative changes may be reversed so allowing a rapid recovery of normal protein function. Other oxidative changes may be irreversible, and under such conditions, the restoration of normal function may require the synthesis of new proteins. Nuclear gene expression, protein synthesis and incorporation of the new proteins into membranes or myofibrils. This may take many hours and could well account for the prolonged time required for full recovery from stunning. During this period, an incomplete complement of ion-regulating proteins and/or a mixture of normally and abnormally regulated contractile proteins might well result in ever-changing ion transients and aberrant electromechanical behaviour. With the powerful tools at their disposal, it should be possible for molecular biologists to address this hypothesis with comparative ease.

References

1. Bolli R, Jeroudi MD, Patel BS, Aruoma OI, Halliwell B, Lai EK, McCay PB (1989) Marked reduction of free radical generation and contractile dysfunction by antioxidant therapy begun at the time of reperfusion. Evidence that myocardial "stunning" is a manifestation of reperfusion injury. Circulation Research 65: 607–622
2. Hearse DJ, Bolli R (1992) Reperfusion induced injury: manifestations, mechanisms and clinical relevance. Cardiovascular Research 26: 101–109
3. Hearse DJ (1991) Stunning: a radical review. Drugs and Cardiovascular Therapy 5: 853–876
4. Krause SM, Jacobus WE, Becker LC (1989) Alterations in cardiac sarcoplasmic reticulum calcium transport in the postischaemic "stunned" myocardium. Circulation Research 65: 526–530
5. Manche A, Edmondson SJ, Hearse DJ (1995) Dynamics of early post-ischaemic myocardial functional recovery: evidence for reperfusion injury. Circulation 92: (in press)

78–80
© Steinkopff Verlag 1996

G. J. Gross

Do ATP-sensitive potassium channels play a role in myocardial stunning?

Key words K_{ATP} channels – myocardial stunning – action potential shortening – endogenous cardioprotection – glibenclamide

Introduction

Single or multiple brief periods (5–20 min) of myocardial ischemia followed by reperfusion have been shown to result in prolonged abnormalities in systolic or diastolic contractile function, tissue blood flow, cell ultrastructure, and adenine nucleotide content (4). This phenomenon has been shown to occur in many animal species including man (3, 4). The most common mechanisms proposed to be responsible for the prolonged postischemic dysfunction are thought to be the result of oxygen free radical induced damage to cardiac membranes which may result in a transient intracellular calcium overload during the late phase of coronary occlusion and during the initial phase of reperfusion (3). In support of this hypothesis several investigators have shown that oxygen radical scavengers such as superoxide dismutase and catalase (3) and calcium channel blockers (8) both attenuate stunning and enhance the recovery of wall motion during reperfusion. Based upon these findings and the proposed theory concerning the pathogenesis of stunning any pharmacological agent which is able to reduce intracellular calcium overload by a variety of direct or indirect mechanisms should be capable of enhancing the recovery of wall function in stunned myocardium.

G. J. Gross, Ph. D. (✉)
Professor of Pharmacology and Toxicology
Medical College of Wisconsin
8701 Watertown Plank Road
Milwaukee, Wisconsin 53226, USA

Myocardial K_{ATP} channels

In 1983 Noma (9) discovered a unique potassium channel in cardiac myocytes that is sensitive to changes in intracellular ATP concentrations, and he named this selective ion channel the ATP-sensitive potassium channel (K_{ATP}). Subsequently Noma (9) suggested that this K_{ATP} channel serves an endogenous cardioprotective role in the heart by a numbert of mechanisms schematically diagrammed in Fig. 1. The primary electrophysiological effect of opening the K_{ATP} channel during ischemia or hypoxia is the shortening of the cardiac action potential due to accelerated phase 3 repolarization. In addition, the membrane potential may also be maintained at a more negative level by K_{ATP} channel opening, and both of these effects would result in less calcium influx via voltage-gated L-type calcium channels and sodium-calcium exchange. Based on these theoretical considerations the present review discusses the evidence for a potential endogenous cardioprotective role of the K_{ATP} channel in myocardial stunning. Even though the mechanisms may not be identical in both models, results from in vitro models in which global ischemia is used to produce stunning, and those from in vivo models of regional ischemia are discussed in the context of the K_{ATP} channel and its role in the pathogenesis of myocardial stunning.

K_{ATP} channels and stunned myocardium

The results of a number of in vitro studies performed primarily by Grover and his colleagues (7) in isolated buffer-perfused rat hearts have shown that several K_{ATP} channel openers enhance the recovery of left ventricular developed pressure, reduce lactic dehydrogenase release, and preserve adenine nucleotide concentrations following

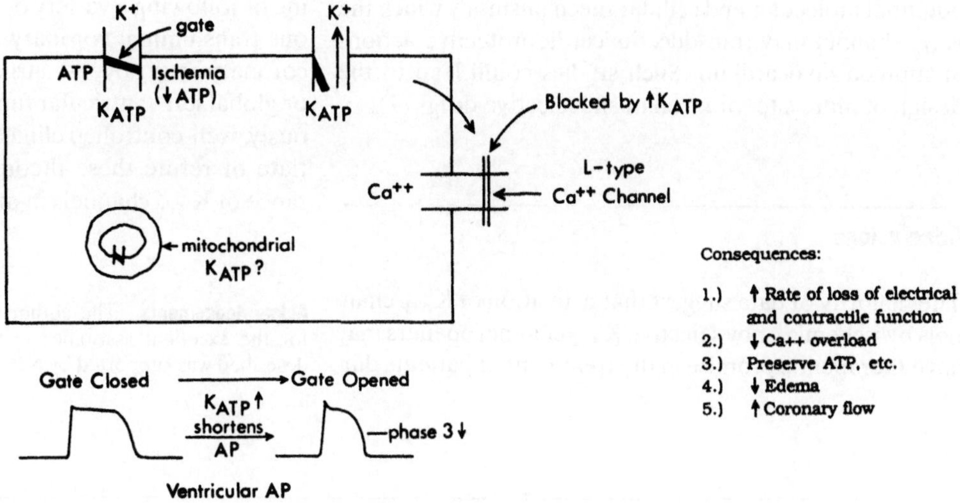

Fig. 1 A schematic diagram depicting potential mechanisms by which activation of K_{ATP} channels produce a cardioprotective effect in stunned myocardium.

global ischemia and reperfusion (7). These beneficial effects were blocked by the selective K_{ATP} channel antagonists glibenclamide and sodium 5-hydroxydecanoate (5-HD). However, in control hearts, glibenclamide and 5-HD had no effect on indices of injury which questioned the importance of endogenous K_{ATP} channel activation as a protective mechanism in this model. In contrast, Cole et al. (5), using a buffer-perfused right ventricular wall preparation, demonstrated that glibenclamide produced a deterioration in the recovery of contractile function following a short period of no-flow ischemia and reperfusion, whereas the K_{ATP} opener pinacidil resulted in an enhanced recovery of contractile function. These effects appeared to be related to the ability of glibenclamide to prevent action potential shortening during the ischemic period and to that of pinacidil to accelerate the rate of shortening. The results obtained with glibenclamide suggest that K_{ATP} channel opening during ischemia produces an endogenous protective effect in this model. The reasons for these differences between the rat and guinea pig models in vitro are not clear but may be related to experimental conditions, protocols, species, or other unknown factors. Since the rat has a higher heart rate as compared to the guinea pig, it is possible that changes in action potential duration are less important in mediating the actions of K_{ATP} openers and antagonists in this species and other mechanisms may be more important.

Data obtained in models of myocardial stunning produced by regional ischemia in vivo have also yielded equivocal results concerning the importance of endogenous myocardial K_{ATP} channel activation as a cardioprotective mechanism. Results obtained from our laboratory in a canine model of stunning in which a single 15-min period of occlusion followed by 3 – 4 h of reperfusion was used to produce postischemic dysfunction, showed that two K_{ATP} openers, nicorandil and aprikalim, markedly enhance the recovery of regional segment shortening (1, 2). In the case of nicorandil the drug was given only prior to and during the occlusion period whereas with aprikalim the drug was infused prior to, during occlusion, and throughout reperfusion. When aprikalim was administered only at reperfusion, it had no significant effect on the recovery of segment function, which suggests that the K_{ATP} channel needs to be activated either prior to and/or during ischemia to be effective. In both cases the beneficial effects of both K_{ATP} openers were blocked by glibenclamide which suggests a K_{ATP} channel mechanism. The dose of glibenclamide which was used to block the beneficial effects of aprikalim and nicorandil had no effect on stunning in control animals, again questioning the importance of endogenous K_{ATP} channel activation in the pathogenesis of stunning in this model. On the other hand, a higher dose of glibenclamide and tolbutamide produced a worsening of functional recovery in the stunned canine heart (2), which suggests that the K_{ATP} channel may have a cardioprotective role in this model after all. In support of these findings, Yao et al. (10) recently showed that a low dose of glibenclamide worsened the recovery of postischemic dysfunction in a model of repetitive stunning in dogs and blocked the shortening of the monophasic action potential during ischemia. Conversely, administration of a K_{ATP} opener, aprikalim, accelerated the shortening of action potential duration during the brief periods of ischemia used to produce stunning and enhanced functional recovery. These results support the previous findings of Cole et al. (5) obtained in isolated guinea pig right ventricular wall and clearly suggest an important role for K_{ATP} channels as an endogenous protective mechanism during repetitive periods of stunning in the canine heart. However, more studies are needed to further probe for potential molecular and cellular mechanisms by which the K_{ATP} channel may transduce its cardioprotective actions in stunned myocardium. Such studies could lead to the design of more site- or mechanism-selective drugs (7).

Conclusions

The majority of data suggest that activation of K_{ATP} channels by ischemia or by selective K_{ATP} channel openers may have therapeutic promise in the treatment of patients during or following a variety of procedures such as percutaneous transluminal coronary angioplasty, thrombolysis, or coronary artery bypass surgery in which impaired regional or global left ventricular function may be the result. Obviously, well-controlled clinical trials are needed to substantiate or refute these theoretical claims as to the importance of K_{ATP} channels in myocardial stunning (3).

Acknowledgements The author wishes to thank Ms. Carol Knapp for the excellent assistance in typing this manuscript. The work described was supported by NIH Grant HL 08311.

References

1. Auchampach JA, Cavero I, Gross GJ (1992) Nicorandil attenuates myocardial dysfunction associated with transient ischemia by opening ATP-dependent potassium channels. J Cardiovasc Pharmacol 20: 765–771
2. Auchampach JA, Maruyama M, Cavero I, Gross GJ (1992) Pharmacological evidence for a role of ATP-dependent potassium channels in myocardial stunning. Circulation 86: 311–319
3. Bolli R (1991) Oxygen-derived free radicals and myocardial reperfusion injury: an overview. Cardiovasc Drug Ther 5: 249–268
4. Braunwald E, Kloner RA (1982) The stunned myocardium: prolonged postischemic ventricular dysfunction. Circulation 66: 1146–1149
5. Cole WC, McPherson CD, Sontas D (1991) ATP-regulated K^+ channels protect the myocardium against ischemia/reperfusion damage. Cir Res 69: 571–581
6. Gross GJ, Auchampach JA (1992) Role of ATP-dependent potassium channels in myocardial ischemia. Cardiovasc Res 26: 1011–1016
7. Grover GJ (1994) Protective effects of ATP-sensitive potassium channel openers in models of myocardial ischaemia. Cardiovasc Res 28: 778–782
8. Heusch G (1992) Myocardial stunning: a role for calcium antagonists during ischaemia? Cardiovasc Res 26: 14–19
9. Noma A (1983) ATP-regulated K channels in cardiac muscle. Nature 305: 147–148
10. Yao Z, Cavero I, Gross GJ (1993) Activation of cardiac K_{ATP} channels: an endogenous protective mechanism during repetitive ischemia. Am J Physiol 264: H495–H504

81–84
© Steinkopff Verlag 1996

E. Marban
W. D. Gao

Stunned myocardium: a disease of the myofilaments?

Key words Intracellular calcium – myofilament Ca^{2+} sensitivity – myocardial ischemia – reperfusion

Introduction

Stunned myocardium is the first clinically relevant disorder of excitation-contraction coupling whose pathophysiology has been successfully elucidated by the application of contemporary cellular methods. Direct measurements of intracellular calcium in the stunned myocardium have revealed normal calcium levels during activation, but these normal levels of calcium are dramatically uncoupled from the accompanying contractions. The demonstration that normal intracellular calcium levels result in weak contractions implicates a lesion of the myofilaments in stunned myocardium. Here we review briefly the experimental basis for this conclusion; for a more complete treatment, please refer to Gao et al. (11). We then attempt to resolve the following paradox: if the myofilaments are desensitized to calcium, how is it that the stunned myocardium can still increase its force in response to positively inotropic stimuli?

Supported by the National Institutes of Health (R01 HL44065 to E.M.), and the American Heart Association (International Research Followship to W.D.G.).

E. Marban, M.D. Ph. D. (✉) · W. D. Gao
Division of Cardiology
Department of Medicine
The Johns Hopkins University School of Medicine
Room 844, Ross Building
720 Rutland Avenue
Baltimore, Maryland 21205, USA

Excitation-contraction coupling in stunned myocardium

For days to weeks following a severe but brief ischemic insult myocardial contractility is decreased. This reversible form of dysfunction, known as stunning (5), has been subjected to extensive investigation at various levels of integration. Although there is a general consensus that free radicals are involved in the pathogenesis of stunning (4), the site of the lesion in excitation-contraction coupling is still a matter of some debate. Electrical activation is normal (12), so that the basis for stunned myocardium must lie in either of two broad mechanistic categories. First, the availability of activator Ca^{2+} might be restricted. Such an effect could be mediated by abnormal Ca^{2+} entry into (or removal from) the cytosol due to lesions in one or more cellular Ca^{2+}-handling pathways. Alternatively, the responsiveness of the contractile machinery to Ca^{2+} might be blunted such that the myocardium generates less force for any given Ca^{2+} transient; in this case the availability of Ca^{2+} need not be the limiting factor.

Direct measurements of $[Ca^{2+}]_i$ in stunned perfused hearts have revealed that $[Ca^{2+}]_i$ is not reduced during twitch contractions (6, 16). In addition, estimates of maximal Ca^{2+}-activated force in perfused hearts have shown a reduction which accounts for at least half of the decrease in developed pressure observed after stunning (15). We have recently confirmed and extended these results in intact experimental preparations devoid of complications from the superimposed effects of vascular turgor and loading. Our measurements of $[Ca^{2+}]_i$ and force in thin ventricular trabeculae from nonischemic and stunned rat hearts reveal that Ca^{2+} transients are not reduced in stunned myocardium; during steady-state Ca^{2+} activation the alterations consist of both a decrease in maximal force and desensitization (i.e., a rightward shift of the $[Ca^{2+}]_i$-force relationship). Simple changes of cross-bridge attachment and detachment rates in a quantitative model of myofilament interaction reproduced the salient features of the contractile dysfunction of stunned myocardium (11).

Whether the decreased Ca^{2+} responsiveness of the myofilaments is due to decreased maximal Ca^{2+}-activated force or decreased Ca^{2+} sensitivity, or both, is controversial. Kusuoka et al. (15) argued that both of these fundamental aspects of myofilament function are depressed in postischemic hearts. Hofmann et al. (13) observed decreased Ca^{2+} sensitivity but no resolvable change in maximal Ca^{2+}-activated force in skinned single cell-sized fragments of porcine stunned myocardium, but there was a large variation in the absolute values of the maximal force (ranging from about 55 % to approx. 150 % of the mean value). Carrozza et al. (6) concluded that only the maximal Ca^{2+}-activated force was depressed.

The mechanism underlying the decreased Ca^{2+} responsiveness is not known at present. Some results from skinned myocardium suggest that stunning reflects alterations within the myofilaments themselves (13). However, another study showed no changes in the force-$[Ca^{2+}]_i$ relationship in skinned trabeculae from rat hearts reperfused after 40 min of ischemia (7). In addition to structural modification of the myofilaments, other mechanisms may influence the Ca^{2+} sensitivity of stunned myocardium in vivo. For example, it has been reported that $[Mg^{2+}]_i$ is elevated in stunned myocardium (14, 18). Mg^{2+} is known to be an important factor affecting the force-Ca^{2+} relationship (10). There is also abundant evidence implicating oxygen free radicals in the pathogenesis of myocardial stunning (4). Besides their effects on Ca^{2+} homeostasis, oxygen free radicals also promote the production of hydrogen peroxide, which is then decomposed by the catalase/peroxidase system resulting in decreases in the content of reduced glutathione and increases in oxidized glutathione (9). Oxidized glutathione has been shown to decrease Ca^{2+} sensitivity in skinned cardiac muscles, while reduced glutathione has the opposite effect (2); thus, changes in the redox state of cytosolic glutathione may contribute to the desensitization of the stunned myofilaments. Clearly, additional studies are needed to determine the relative importance of "soluble" vs. structural factors in the diminished Ca^{2+} responsiveness of stunned myocardium.

Pathophysiological and therapeutic implications

The last decade has witnessed a major transition, from a supporting role to center stage, in our recognition of the pathophysiological importance of the myofilaments: the contractile proteins have now been implicated in fundamental disease processes ranging from hypertrophy-associated sudden death (17) to the stunned myocardium. Various lines of evidence now point to the cardiac myofilaments as the primary culprits in heritable forms of hypertrophic cardiomyopathy (8). While the first molecular

Fig. 1 Steady-state force-$[Ca^{2+}]_i$ relationship (open circles) and peak force-peak $[Ca^{2+}]_i$ relationship (filled circles) of a control trabecula (**A**) and a stunned trabecula (**B**). The trabeculae were superfused with Krebs-Henseleit solution at room temperature, pH 7.4 (see ref 11 for details of experimental procedures). $[Ca^{2+}]_i$ was measured using fura-2 salt which was microinjected ionotophoretically into the muscles. Steady-state force-$[Ca^{2+}]_i$ relations were obtained by stimulating the muscles at 10 Hz in the presence of ryanodine (5 μM). The varied tetani were achieved at different external $[Ca^{2+}]$s (0.5 – 20 mM). Peak force and peak $[Ca^{2+}]_i$ transient relations were obtained at external $[Ca^{2+}]$s of 0.5, 1.0, 1.5, and 2.0 mM.

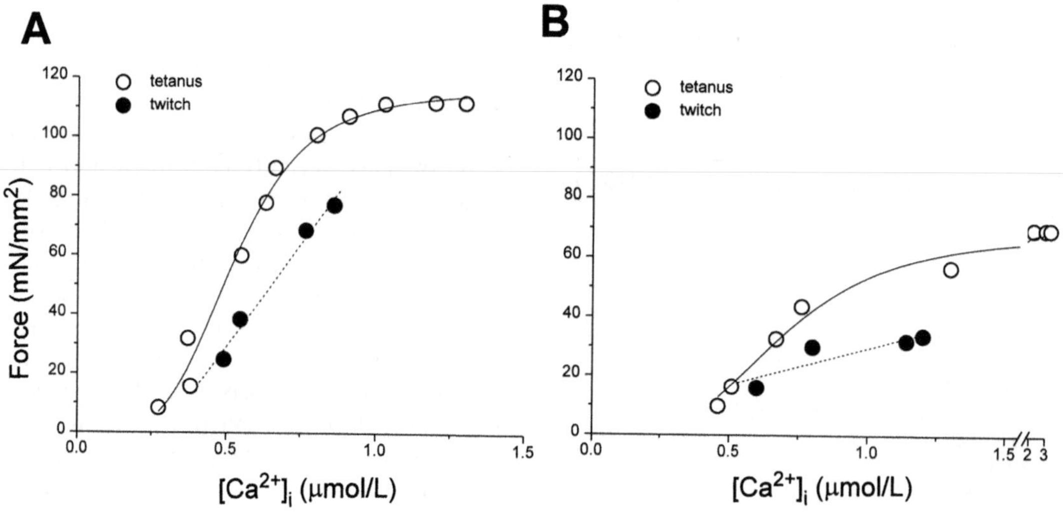

abnormalities to be described were point mutations of the thick filament protein myosin (19), similar phenotypes can result from lesions of at least two thin filament proteins (21). Altered patterns of expression of various contractile protein isoforms accompany ordinary congestive heart failure, but the functional significance of these changes relative to abnormalities of Ca^{2+} handling remains to be clarified (1).

Our work supports the view that stunned myocardium represents an acquired, reversible disease of the myofilaments. As such, treatment with Ca^{2+} sensitizers is not only effective (20) but also rational.

Moderate positive inotropic therapy is known to be capable of improving the ability of stunned myocardium to generate force (3). This retained responsiveness to catecholamines and to elevations of extracellular calcium seems paradoxical given the conclusion that the myofilaments are less sensitive to intracellular calcium. Two considerations help to resolve this apparent paradox. First, the upstream mechanisms that control $[Ca^{2+}]_i$ appear to be largely intact. Figure 1 shows peak $[Ca^{2+}]_i$ versus twitch force (filled symbols) and steady-state $[Ca^{2+}]_i$ versus tetanic force (open symbols), at various levels of extracellular Ca^{2+}. In both control (A) and stunned myocardium (B), $[Ca^{2+}]_i$ increases appropriately when external calcium is elevated. Second, the stunned myocardium (and normal myocardium) recruits only a fraction of its maximal force during physiological contractions. Refer once again to Fig. 1 and compare the levels of force during physiological twitch contractions (filled symbols) to the corresponding levels of maximal force achieved under steady-state conditions. In both control and stunned myocardium, physiological contractions recruit only 20 – 60 % of maximal force. The levels of $[Ca^{2+}]_i$ achieved during twitches do not come close to saturating the force-generating capacity of the myofilaments. Thus, inotropic interventions that increase $[Ca^{2+}]_i$ can increase force even in stunned heart.

Acknowledgements We thank Dr. Hideo Kusuoka for many helpful discussions.

References

1. Atar D, Gao WD, Marban E (1994) Alterations of excitation-contraction coupling in stunned myocardium and in failing myocardium. J Mol Cell Cariol (in press)
2. Bauer SF, Schwarz K, Ruegg JC (1989) Glutathione alters calcium responsiveness of cardiac skinned fibers. Basic Res Cardiol 84: 591–596
3. Becker LC (1993) Inotropic agents and stimulation of stunned myocardium. In: Koner RA, Przyklenk K (eds) Stunned myocardium: properties, mechanisms and clinical manifestations. Dekker, New York, pp 267–280
4. Bolli R (1990) Mechanism of myocardial "stunning". Circulation 80: 723–738
5. Braunwald E, Kloner RA (1982) The stunned myocardium: Prolonged, post-ischemic ventricular dysfunction. Circulation 66: 1146–1149
6. Carrozza Jr JP, Bentivegna LA, Williams CP, Kuntz RE, Grossman W, Morgan JP (1992) Decreased myofilament responsiveness in myocardial stunning follows transient calcium overload during ischemia and reperfusion. Circ Res 71: 1334–1340
7. Dietrich DLL, van Leeuwen GR, Stienen GJM, Elzinga G (1993) Stunning does not change the relation between calcium and force in skinned rat trabeculae. J Mol Cell Cardiol 25: 541–549
8. Dietz HC 3rd, Pyeritz RE (1994) Molecular genetic approaches to the study of human cardiovascular disease. Am Rev Physiol 56: 763–796
9. Ferrari R, Ceconi C, Curello S, Cargnoni A, Alfieri O, Pardini A, Marzollo P, Visioli O (1991) Oxygen free radicals and myocardial damage: Protective role of thiol-containing agents. Am J Med 91 (suppl 3C): 95S–105S
10. Gao WD, Backx PH, Azan-Backx MD, Marban E (1994) Myofilament Ca^{2+} sensitivity in intact versus skinned rat ventricular muscle. Circ Res 74: 408–415
11. Gao WD, Atar D, Backx PH, Marban E (1995) Relationship between intracellular calcium and contractile force in stunned myocardium: direct evidence for decreased myofilament Ca^{2+} responsiveness and altered diastolic function in intact ventricular muscle. Circ Res 76: 1036–1048
12. Hanich RF, Levine JH, Prood C, Weiss JL, Gallans DJ, Spear JF, Moore EN (1993) Electrophysiologic recovery in postischemic, stunned myocardium despite persistent systolic dysfunction. Am Heart J 25: 23–32
13. Hofmann PA, Miller WP, Moss RL (1993) Altered calcium sensitivity of isometric tension in myocyte-sized preparations of porcine postischemic stunned myocardium. Circ Res 72: 50–56

14. Kirkels JH, van Echteld CJA, Ruigrok TJC (1989) Intracellular magnesium during myocardial ischemia and reperfusion: possible consequences for postischemic recovery. J Mol Cell Cardiol 21: 1209–1218
15. Kusuoka H, Porterfield JK, Weisman HF, Weisfeldt ML, Marban E (1987) Pathophysiology and pathogenesis of stunned myocardium: depressed Ca^{2+} activation of contraction as a consequence of reperfusion-induced cellular calcium overload in ferret hearts. J Clin Invest 79: 950–961
16. Kusuoka H, Koretsune Y, Chacko VP, Weisfeldt ML, Marban E (1990) Excitation-contraction coupling in postischemic myocardium: does failure of activator Ca^{2+} transients underlie "stunning"? Circ Res 66: 1268–1276
17. Maron BJ, Fananapazir L (1992) Sudden cardiac death in hypertrophic cardiomyopathy. Circulation 85: 157–163
18. Murphy E, Steenbergen C, Levy LA, Raju B, London RE (1989) Cytosolic free magnesium levels in ischemic rat heart. J Biol Chem 264: 5622–5627
19. Seidman CE, Seidman JG (1991) Mutations in cardiac myosin heavy chain genes cause familial hypertrophic cardiomyopathy. Mol Biol Med 8: 159–166
20. Soei LK, Sassen LMA, Fan DS, van Veen T, Krams R, Verdouw PD (1994) Myofibrillar Ca^{2+} sensitization predominantly enhances function and mechanical efficiency of stunned myocardium. Circ 90: 959–969
21. Thierfelder L, Watkins H, MacRae C, Lamas R, McKenna W, Vosberg HP, Seidman JG, Seidman CE (1994) Alpha-tropomyosin and cardiac troponin T mutations cause familial hypertrophic cardiomyopathy: a disease of the sarcomere. Cell 77: 701–712

85–87
© Steinkopff Verlag 1996

W. Schaper

Stunned myocardium, an opinionated review

Key words Stunned myocardium – distance measurement – sonomicrometer crystals

The discovery of stunned myocardium (5) was made possible by a new technical device: the measurement of distance by sonomicrometer crystals (3). Stunned myocardium cannot be readily detected by the naked eye and even the micrometer trace must be analyzed for correct phase.

A subtle change of contractility

I say this to emphasise that stunning is a subtle change from the normal pattern of contraction: if the amplitude of the shortening phase of contraction in an *in situ* beating dog or pig heart is reduced by 50 %, we call it marked, i.e., at that time the development of force is completely unaltered (7). When so-called stunning is produced in a buffer perfused isolated heart preparation, the investigators usually reduce the development of force, which is a much more severe type of damage and may be the underlying cause for contrasting views on its molecular mechanisms.

The reduction in the amplitude of shortening does not become apparent immediately after the onset of reperfusion: return to function is usually normal, sometimes even overshooting and supernormal. It takes a few minutes of reperfusion before the stable period of stunning begins. This is suggestive for reperfusion damage, but one has to take into consideration the complexity of the many systems that are perturbed at the beginning of reperfusion: tissue catecholamine concentration is high and might contribute to the supernormal phase, the high extracellular potassium is quickly flushed out, sodium and calcium enter the cell in addition to the oxygen derived radicals that are probably generated in the mitochondria upon the sudden flush of oxygen.

Prof. Dr. W. Schaper (✉)
(W. G. Kerckhoff-Institut)
Max-Planck-Institut für physiologische und klinische Forschung
Abt. Experimentelle Kardiologie
Benekestraße 2
61231 Bad Nauheim

Calcium homeostasis is changed

There exists general consensus that stunned myocardium is the expression of a disturbance of calcium homeostasis, but there is controversy about the actual mechanism. Two dissenting schools exist: those favoring a disturbance of the system that regulates calcium availability (sarcoplasmic reticulum, calcium binding proteins, pumps) versus those who favor a change in calcium sensitivity of the myofibrils. Ito et al. (7) have shown that the sensitivity to added calcium in the *in situ* beating stunned dog heart is unchanged. Dietrich et al. (2) have shown that skinned fibers of the stunned rat heart exhibit a normal dose response to calcium. Kusuoka et al. (9) infer from unchanged calcium transients that the calcium sensitivity must have changed in buffer perfused force-depressed preparations. Fraß et al. (4) studied gene expression in stunned myocardium of the pig and found overexpression of the calcium binding proteins SERCA-2, phosholamban, calsequestrin and calmodulin and they concluded from this that these molecules had been damaged during ischemia and that the observed overexpression was a repair reaction.

Regulation or paralysis?

An alternative explanation could be that the relative overexpression of phospholamban with regard to SERCA-2 may play a key role in maintaining stunning for hours and sometimes days: overexpression of phospholamban, by controlling the calcium pump, would effectively reduce the calcium availability at the sarcomere and it is imaginable that this is a regulated phenomenon using phospholamban as a molecular switch.

It is easy to imagine that repeated stunning, leading to chronic overexpression of Plb, might constitute the molecular switch that also causes hibernating myocardium.

Radicals on the go?

The prevailing view with regard to the pathomechanism of stunning is damage by oxygen derived radicals. This might not be the whole answer because Bolli (1) had shown that treatment with a combination of the most potent radical scavengers cures most but not all of the contractile defect. This would mitigate for an additional causative agent for which there are no clues available at present.

A unifying theory?

Brief coronary occlusions also cause ischemic preconditioning and repeated brief occlusions may be the cause of hibernating myocardium. Years ago the debate seemed to have been closed with regard to the question whether stunning and ischemic preconditioning are different symptoms for the same molecular process. Stunning could be easily cured or prevented by drugs, notably calcium antagonists, but preconditioning persisted and it was inferred that these are two unrelated phenomena. Today, I would question the discriminating power of that argument, because the disturbance is so slight (*vide supra,* only shortening is involved) and small changes in pre- and afterload may diminish it in a cosmetic way.

Recent research into the causes of ischemic preconditioning has discovered molecular mechanisms that may explain both systolic dysfunction as well as myocardial protection. One of the underlying themes regarding the sequelae of brief occlusions is the observation that enzyme systems rearrange during reperfusion in a way that their activity becomes translocated from the cytosol to the sarcolemma or that sarcolemmal activity increases. This had been shown for proteinkinase C (PKC) (12), for the inducible NO-synthase of myocytes (10) for 5'-nucleotidase and for the inhibitory G-protein (11). The sarcolemmal Na^+/H^+ exchanger as well as other ion channels also change their activity during ischemia and reperfusion (13) and most of these system (exception: Na^+/H^+ exchanger which goes in the wrong direction) would also tend to depress contractility, reduce oxygen requirements and favor survival under conditions of long coronary occlusions.

Is oxygen wasted in stunning?

Oxygen requirements of the stunned myocardium have long been a matter of debate. Ito et al. (14) showed that in the phase of stable stunning subendocardial blood flow was 30 % below that of the control region at identical venous oxygen saturations from which they concluded that MVO_2 must have decreased by a similar degree. Other groups showed either no change or even an increase. A subsequent paper from Schaper's laboratory (8) showed that in the pig MVO_2 was increased in the early phase of reflow but no measurements were carried out hours into the reperfusion. A recent paper by Ito (6) showed that stunning produced in the pig heart by ramp-decrease of flow showed a significant decrease of MVO_2 during the stable phase of stunning. From a theoretical point of view the oxygen sparing effect of stunning should not be very marked since it is the development of force that uses most of the oxygen, whereas changes in the shortening phase have little impact.

New genes?

Reverse genetics offers a wonderful possibility and perspective to screen for new and known gene activity without a working hypothesis: mRNA is reverse transcribed and differentially displayed (ischemic/reperfused versus control) and differentially expressed cDNAs are sequenced. Our own attempts in this field (Ralph Knöll, 15) were surprisingly successful in a quantitative way: about 600 clones can be expected to be differentially expressed in reperfused tissue. Of the 60 clones that we have sequenced so far, about 50 % are unknown. To ascribe a function for the unknown – and still to be discovered – proteins will not be an easy task. Working hypotheses do have their merits, we realize.

Summary

Brief coronary occlusions cause stunning and ischemic preconditioning, the molecular mechanisms of which are insufficiently known. A marked reprogramming of sarcolemmal functions (including those of the sarcoplasmic reticulum) seems to occur and may be the basis for many of the observed phenomena. A bewilderingly complex pattern of gene expression emerges from mRNA-studies with reperfused tissue which at present does not permit a focussed or coherent view of mechanisms.

References

1. Bolli R (1990) Mechanism of myocardial "stunning". Circulation 82: 723–738
2. Dietrich DLL, Elzinga G (1992) Energetic determinants of stunning and cell damage following reoxygenation of rabbit myocardium. J Mol Cell Cardiol 24: 1277–1290
3. Franklin DL, Kemper WS, Patrick T, McKown D (1973) Technique for continuous measurement of regional myocardial segment dimensions in chronic animal preparations. Fed Proc 32: 343
4. Fraß O, Sharma HS, Knöll R, Duncker DJ, McFalls EO, Verdouw PD, Schaper W (1993) Enhanced gene expression of calcium regulatory proteins in stunned porcine myocardium. Cardiovasc Res 27: 2037–2043
5. Heyndrickx GR, Millard RW, McRitchie RJ, Maroko PR, Vatner SF (1975) Regional myocardial, functional, and electrophysiological alterations after brief coronary occlusion in conscious dogs. J Clin Invest 56: 978–985
6. Ito B (1995) Gradual onset of myocardial ischemia results in reduced myocardial infarction. Circulation 91: 2058–2070
7. Ito B, Tate H, Kobayashi M, Schaper W (1987) Reversibly injured, postischemic canine myocardium retains normal contractile reserve. Circ Res 61: 834–846
8. Kobayashi M, Schmidt T, Schaper W (1987) Regional myocardial oxygen consumption and segmental function in "stunned" myocardium of the pig. Circulation 76 (Suppl IV): 1510 (abstr)
9. Kusuoka H, Kitakaze M, Koretsune Y, Inoue M, Marban E (1991) Pathophysiology and pathogenesis of contractile failure in stunned myocardium. Japan Circ J 55: 878–884
10. Michel T, Li GK, Busconi L (1993) Phosphorylation and subcellular translocation of endothelial nitric oxide synthase. Proc Natl Acad Sci 90: 6252–6256
11. Niroomand F, Strasser R (1995) Impaired functions of inhibitory G-proteins. Circ Res 76: 861–870
12. Nishizuka J (1984) The role of protein kinase C in cell surface signal transduction and tumour promotion. Nature 308: 693–697
13. Sack S, Mohri M, Schwarz ER, Arras M, Schaper J, Ballagi-Pordány G, Scholz W, Lang HJ, Schölkens BA, Schaper W (1994) Effects of a new NA^+/H^+ antiporter inhibitor on postischemic reperfusion in pig heart. J Cardiovas Pharmacol 23: 72–78
14. Schaper W, Ito BR (1988) The energetics of "stunned" myocardium. In: JW de Jong (eds) Myocardial Energy Metabolism, Martinus Nijhoff Publishers, Boston Lancaster Dordrecht, pp 203–213
15. Knöll R, Zimmermann R, Berwing K, Arras M, Schaper W (1995) Characterization of differential expressed genes following short coronary occlusions. JMCC 6: A 145

88–90

R. Lerch

Myocardial stunning: the role of oxidative substrate metabolism

Key words Stunning – myocardial oxygen consumption – glucose – free fatty acids

Introduction

"In contrast to several previous studies about reperfusion after short periods of ischemia myocardial function did not return completely to control within 30 minutes." The editor's invitation to provide a personal view on myocardial stunning gives this author the unexpected satisfaction to read the main conclusion of his doctoral thesis in the journal which rejected the manuscript 20 years ago with the argument that this observation, in a dog model of transient ischemia (7), was probably an artifact.

In the meantime the existence of persistent depression of contractile function following a short period of ischemia, after the unequivocal documentation by Heyndrickx et al., is generally acknowledged and referred to as "stunning". The initial hypothesis of a primary defect in energy metabolism is presently rejected by most authors because (a) myocardial content of creatine phosphate is often increased in stunned myocardium (7), (b) stunned myocardium promptly responds to inotropic stimulation (3), and (c) accelerated restoration of myocardial ATP content by administration of precursor molecules does not influence recovery of contractile function. At present the two most favored hypotheses to explain stunning at the subcellular level are (a) impairment of sarcoplasmic reticulum function and (b) reduction in calcium responsiveness of the myofilaments. Both of these lesions may be caused either by oxygen-derived free radicals or transient cytosolic calcium overload or a combination of both. Although insufficient energy production by intermediary metabolism seems not to limit contractile function after short periods of ischemia, at least two observations related to oxidative metabolism merit consideration. The following short comment focuses on these two metabolic aspects.

Dr. R. Lerch (✉)
Cardiology Center
University Hospital
1211 Geneva 14, Switzerland

Coupling between oxidative metabolism and contractile function

In a number of studies recovery of myocardial oxygen consumption in reversibly dysfunctioning postischemic myocardium exceeded in extent the recovery of indices of contractile performance. In in vivo models of myocardial stunning the percentage reduction in regional systolic segment length shortening early during reperfusion is consistently greater than that of myocardial oxygen consumption, suggesting less efficient oxygen use in terms of contractile function. However, because systolic segment length shortening does not direcly reflect regional work, it has been argued that inefficiency of oxidative metabolism may be only apparent (2, 8). In fact, McFalls et al. (8) have observed in a porcine model of stunning that the reduction in regional work, estimated from pressure segment length loops, closely matches the reduction of myocardial oxygen consumption. This suggests that systolic segment length shortening may underestimate regional contractile performance, possibly because of asynchrony of contraction (2).

Nevertheless, we (4) and others have observed that myocardial oxygen consumption is also higher relative to tension-based indices in isovolumically beating isolated hearts reperfused after global ischemia. Furthermore, studies assessing different levels of work load have found a shift in the relationship between myocardial oxygen consumption and the rate-pressure product towards higher oxygen consumption (10). These observations strongly suggest that a disturbance in coupling between mechanical function and oxidative metabolism does exist in stunned myocardium.

The mechanism responsible for the dissociation between contractile function and oxidative metabolism in stunned myocardium is presently not known. The fact that contractile function can be recruited by inotropic interventions in globally ischemic-reperfused heart preparations argues against mitochondrial uncoupling (3). It is tempting to speculate that respiratory energy is dissipated at the site of the primary defect responsible for contractile dysfunction. Accordingly, damaged myofibrils may hydrolyze ATP without tension development. Alternatively, ATP may be used to support increased activity of the sarcoplasmic reticulum Ca^{2+}-ATPase caused by primary upregulation of the Ca^{2+} pump (6), by increased calcium transient to compensate for reduced myofibrillar responsiveness (5), or by cycling of calcium due to opening of the release channels.

Rapid recovery of substrate metabolism despite persistent depression of contractile function is clinically employed as index for the documentation of myocardial viability in reperfused hypocontractile regions by positron emission tomography with labeled metabolic substrates or substrate analogs. Although it is obvious that metabolic activity is low or absent in necrotic myocardium, we believe that normalization of oxidative metabolic rate is not an unequivocal sign of reversibility of myocardial damage during the early reperfusion period. In fact we have observed in isolated red blood cell perfused rat hearts that myocardial oxygen consumption initially recovers to a comparable extent in stunned hearts and in hearts reperfused after 40 – 60 min of now-flow ischemia leading to predominately irreversible injury (4). In advanced myocardial injury stimulation of myocardial oxygen consumption seems to be related to intracellular calcium movement because reduced metabolic efficiency returned to normal in the presence of ruthenium red, which lowers both mitochondrial calcium uptake and sarcoplasmic reticulum calcium release (1).

Influence of metabolic substrate on recovery of contractile function

Stunned myocardium is capable of oxidizing both free fatty acids and glucose. Although in some studies a transient increase in glucose oxidation has been observed early during reperfusion (4), free fatty acids remain the predominate substrate for oxidative metabolism because oxidation of glucose is still largely inhibited in the presence of exogenous fatty acids. There is evidence from experiments in isolated heart preparations that the substrate pattern of oxidative metabolism may influence contractile recovery of moderately injured hearts, in which contractile dysfunction in mainly attributable to stunning. Lopaschuk's group has observe in isolated working rat hearts perfused with medium containing 1.2 mM palmitate and 11 mM glucose, and subjected to 25 min of no-flow ischemia, that contractile function (expressed as product of heart rate and developed left ventricular pressure) was reduced to less than 60 % of the preischemic value during reperfusion without intervention, but recovered almost completely when glucose oxidation was stimulated pharmacologically or by removal of palmitate from the perfusate (9). The mechanism responsible for the favorable effect of glucose oxidation is not yet clarified. Proposed mechanisms include rapid restoration of the cytosolic phosphorylation potential by glycolytic production of ATP, removal of protons from the cytoplasm by oxidation of lactate mediated by activation of the pyruvate dehydrogenase reaction, and acceleration of reenergization of the mitochondria. All these metabolic effects may favorably influence recovery of ion homeostasis and reduce cytosolic calcium overload early during reperfusion.

In summary, although insufficient recovery of energy metabolism can be virtually excluded as primary defect underlying myocardial stunning, interrelations exist between the myocyte lesion and oxidative substrate metabolism. Metabolic interventions may influence contractile recovery of stunned myocardium, possibly by modification of the severity of reperfusion-induced myocyte injury.

References

1. Benzi R, Lerch R (1992) Dissociation between contractile function and oxidative metabolism in postischemic myocardium: attenuation by ruthenium red administered during reperfusion. Circ Res 71: 567–576
2. Chiu WC, Kedem J, Scholz PM, Weiss HR (1994) Regional asynchrony of segmental contraction may explain the "oxygen consumption paradox" in stunned myocardium. Bas Res Cardiol 89: 149–162
3. Görge G, Papageorgiou I, Lerch R (1990) Epinephrine-stimulated contractile and metabolic reserve in postischemic rat myocardium. Bas Res Cardiol 85: 595–605
4. Görge G, Chatelain P, Schaper J, Lerch R (1991) Effect of increasing degrees of ischemic injury on myocardial oxidative metabolism early after reperfusion in isolated rat hearts. Circ Res 68: 1681–1692
5. Kusuoka H, Koretsune Y, Chacko VP, Weisfeldt ML, Marban E (1990) Excitation-contraction coupling in post-ischemic myocardium. Does failure of activator Ca^{2+} transients underlie stunning? Circ Res 66: 1268–1276
6. Lamers JMJ, Duncker DJ, Bezstarosti K, McFalls EO, Sassen LMA, Verdouw PD (1993) Increased activity of sarcoplasmic reticular calcium pump in porcine stunned myocardium. Cardiovasc Res 27: 520–524
7. Lerch R, Villiger B, Riedhammer H, Meier WE, Rutishauser W (1975) Left ventricular function and creatine phosphate content during reperfusion (abstract). Circulation 51 and 52 (supplement II): II-208
8. McFalls EO, Duncker DJ, Krams R, Sassen LMA, Hoogendoorn A, Verdouw PD (1992) Recruitment of myocardial work and metabolism in regionally stunned porcine myocardium. Am J Physiol 263: H1724–H1731
9. McVeigh JJ, Lopaschuk GD (1990) Dichloroacetate stimulation of glucose oxidation improves recovery of ischemic rat hearts. Am J Physiol 259: H1079–H1085
10. Zimmer SD, Ugurbil K, Michurski SP, Mohanakrishnan P, Ulstad VK, Foker JE, From AHL (1989) Alterations in oxidative function and respiratory regulation in the post-ischemic myocardium. J Biol Chem 264: 12402–12411

91–93

B. Renstrom
A. J. Liedtke

Adjustments in competitive substrate utilization in stunned myocardium during early reperfusion

Key words Fatty acid – glucose – pyruvate, lactate metabolism

The purpose of this precis is to state and support a personal viewpoint concerning intermediary metabolism and substrate utilization in stunned and reperfused myocardium following an interval of nonnecrotizing myocardial ischemia. The data in support of this viewpoint were derived from an intact, working pig heart preparation which includes extracorporeal control of regional coronary perfusion, and which has been used in our laboratory for almost two decades. Metabolism was characterized using steady-state labeling of myocardium with tracer isotopes including [U-^{14}C]palmitate, [9,10-^{3}H]palmitate, [6-^{14}C] glucose, [5-^{3}H]glucose, [2-^{14}C]pyruvate, [^{14}C]lactate, and [1-^{14}C]acetate either singly or in combination. Myocardium was rendered mild to moderately ischemic for 30 – 40 min in separate protocols and then aerobically reperfused for 40 – 60 min. Rates of substrate utilization and/or oxidation were routinely measured during the preischemic period, the ischemic interval, and as emphasized in this overview the subsequent period of metabolic adjustments during aerobic reperfusion. The composite data compiled from these experiments indicate that in stunned myocardium metabolism is in rapid transition with greater restoration of aerobic oxidation than mechanical function, a hierarchical shift in preferred substrate relationships back toward aerobic utilization with beneficial washout of noxious amphiphiles, and an overshoot in fatty acid oxidation, presumably due to persistent alterations in regulatory mechanisms affected by the preceding ischemic stress.

In select reperfusion studies and depending somewhat on the levels of exogenous fatty acid substrate in perfusate, fatty acid oxidation approximately doubled over preischemic values (6). This augmentation occurred in part from fatty acids made available from release of intracellular stores, principally triacyclglycerols, as we showed (8) and in part from increased uptake of exogenous substrate as demonstrated by Saddik and Lopaschuk (12). This rapid ascendancy in fatty acid preference, however, does not imply a substrate immunity from the normal regulatory inhibitions imposed by competing substrates. In separate studies we provided to recovering myocardium excess propionate to influence the kinetics of anaplerotic entrance to the citric acid cycle (4). This competing substrate effected a 38 % decrease in the oxidation of fatty acids which was not explained by the scavenging of coenzyme A units otherwise destined for fatty acid activation. It has been argued from data collected in isolated preparations that the resurgency in fatty acid oxidation is of no benefit but rather a negative inotropic influence on mechanical recovery (1, 7). However, in our intact model using whole blood perfusate this was not the case (6).

A second objective in our experiments was to place in perspective the role of carbohydrate substrate utilizations using glucose, pyruvate, and lactate as representative analogues and to define their relationships to those of fatty acids as regulated substrates. Glucose flux and glu-

This work was supported in part by PHS Grants HL-32350 and HL-41914, the Rennebohm Foundation of Wisconsin, the Oscar Mayer Cardiovascular Research Fund, and American Heart Association Grants 92-729 of the National Center and 91-GA-11/92-GS-26 of the Wisconsin Affiliate (the Dave McClain Research Grant).

B. Renstrom · Dr. A. J. Liedtke (✉)
Cardiology Section
University of Wisconsin Hospital and Clinics
600 Highland Avenue, H6/372
Madison, Wisconsin 53792-3248, USA

cose oxidation were highly suppressed during preischemia, presumably due to allosteric and product inhibitions imposed by the preferred use of fatty acids (2, 3, 9). In moderately ischemic pig hearts with a 60 % reduction in regional coronary flow, glycolysis rose nearly tenfold, and even glucose oxidation was increased slightly (2, 9). When multiple exposures of brief ischemic pretreatments were applied in protocols designed to simulate preconditioning (2), flux rates for glycolysis were significantly reduced. During reperfusion, glucose utilization and oxidation fell toward normal preischemic values and lactate release into perfusate, which had been observed during ischemia, reverted to lactate extraction, consistent with aerobic myocardium. Increased levels of glucose in perfusate tended to maintain somewhat higher rates of glycolysis in reperfusion (3). The shift in glucose utilization toward normal preischemic levels were compatible with the allosteric and product inhibitions imposed by the rebound in fatty acid metabolism. To further test this hypothesis, oxfenicine (S-4-hydroxyphenylglycine), an inhibitor of fatty acid utilization and specifically of carnitine palmitoyltransferase I, was administered in separate studies (9). With relief of the regulatory influence of fatty acids, glucose oxidation appropriately increased twofold in stunned myocardium.

It was suggested also that pyruvate and lactate oxidation responded predictably to the regulatory influences of fatty acids (10, 11). Utilization rates of both substrates were decreased from preischemic levels during withdrawal of oxygen supply in moderate ischemia but remained depressed during aerobic reperfusion. Treatment with oxfenicine in separate studies caused an appropriate restoration of pyruvate oxidation during reflow to near preischemic values (10).

It is noteworthy that if one compares the metabolic adjustments in stunned, acutely reperfused myocardium with those of an acutely reperfused, chronic pig model simulating hibemating myocardium (5), important distinctions are evident. In the latter group heart rate was increased, but oxidative capacity was maintained and myocardial oxygen consumption was higher than in acutely developed sham hearts paced at similar rates. Fatty acid oxidation was in the aerobic range compatible with values obtained in acute experiments during early reperfusion following moderate ischemia (6). In chronic hearts, however, in contrast to stunned hearts, glycolytic flux during reflow remained elevated and was sixfold greater than rates in acute sham hearts. This latter finding suggests a disruption in the normal regulatory controls of fatty acid utilization upon constituent steps within the glycolytic pathway.

In summary, in stunned and reperfused myocardium after a reversible period of moderate ischemia rapid adjustments in substrate utilization occur dominated by the return of the preferred use of long-chain fatty acids for energy metabolism. This recovery of fatty acid oxidation may include an overshoot above preischemic aerobic values. Mechanisms of regulation are maintained among substrates such that glucose, pyruvate, and lactate utilization are normally suppressed during reperfusion but may be up-regulated by the inhibition of fatty acid oxidation. Patterns of glucose utilization appear different between stunned and hibernating myocardium.

References

1. Johnston DL, Lewandowski ED (1991) Fatty acid metabolism and contractile function in the reperfused myocardium: multinuclear NMR studies of isolated rabbit hearts. Circ Res 68: 714–725
2. Liedtke AJ, Renstrom B, Hacker TA, Nellis SH (1995) The effects of moderate ischemic pretreatment of myocardial substrate utilization. Am J Physiol, in press
3. Liedtke AJ, Renstrom B, Nellis SH (1992) Correlation between [5-^{3}H]glucose and [U-^{14}C]deoxyglucose as markers of glycolysis in reperfused myocardium. Circ Res 71: 689–700
4. Liedtke AJ, Renstrom B, Nellis SH (1993) Kinetics of acetate in the setting of competitive substrate inhibition. Circulation (suppl I) 88: I-427 (manuscript in preparation)
5. Liedtke AJ, Renstrom B, Nellis SH, Subramanian R (1994) Myocardial function and metabolism in pig hearts after relief from chronic partial coronary stenosis. Am J Physiol 267 (Heart Circ Physiol 36): H1312–H1319
6. Liedtke AJ, DeMaison L, Eggleston AM, Cohen LM, Nellis SH (1988) Changes in substrate metabolism and effects of excess fatty acids in reperfused myocardium. Circ Res 62: 535–542
7. Lopaschuk GD, Wall SR, Olley PM, Davies NJ (1988) Etomoxir, a carnitine palmitoyltransferase I inhibitor, protects heart from fatty acid-induced ischemic injury independent of changes in long chain acylcarnitine. Circ Res 63: 1036–1043
8. Nellis SH, Liedtke AJ, Renstrom B (1991) Distribution of carbon flux within fatty acid utilization during myocardial ischemia and reperfusion. Circ Res 69: 779–790

9. Renstrom B, Nellis SH, Liedtke AJ (1989) Metabolic oxidation of glucose during early myocardial reperfusion. Circ Res 65: 1094–1101

10. Renstrom B, Liedtke AJ, Nellis SH (1990) Mechanisms of substrate preference for oxidative metabolism during early myocardial reperfusion. Am J Physiol 259 (Heart Circ Physiol 28): H317–H323

11. Renstrom B, Nellis SH, Liedtke AJ (1990) Metabolic oxidation of pyruvate and lactate during early myocardial reperfusion. Circ Res 66: 282–288

12. Saddik M, Lopaschuk GD (1992) Myocardial triglyceride turnover during reperfusion of isolated rat hearts subjected to a transient period of global ischemia. J Biol Chem 267: 3825–3831

94–96

L. C. Becker

Is stunned myocardium ischemic on a microvascular level?

Key words Myocardial stunning – resting flow – contractile reserve – beta-adrenergic agonists – free radical hypothesis

Introduction

An early hypothesis for myocardial stunning held that contractile dysfunction was caused by neutrophil-mediated microvascular occlusions which produced focal areas of myocardial ischemia. Although this hypothesis appeared to go against the basic tene that blood flow was normal, or nearly normal in stunned myocardium, an interesting model resembling stunning was described by Hori et al. (1) in which coronary microsphere embolization was used to produce progressive microvascular occlusion and resting contractile dysfunction. Like stunned myocardium, resting flow remained normal and, although resting function was depressed, contractile reserve could be recruited by beta-adrenergic agonists. However, maximal flow reserve progressively declined as the microvasculature became obliterated. Resting flow was maintained at normal levels by local release of adenosine from ischemic areas, resulting in hyperemia of surrounding normal regions.

In the past few years, the free radical hypothesis for myocardial stunning has taken precedence (2), and less attention has been paid to the vasculature. However, free radical scavengers reduce but generally do not eliminate myocardial dysfunction resulting from brief periods of ischemia. It is therefore possible that other factors, such as abnormalities of the microvasculature, are playing a role in myocardial stunning.

Dr. L. C. Becker (✉)
Department of Medicine
The Johns Hopkins Medical Institutions
600 N. Wolfe Street
Baltimore, MD 21287, USA

Is the vasculature abnormal in stunned myocardium?

Whether the blood vessels are normal or abnormal in stunned myocardium has been controversial. Resting flow is often said to be mildly depressed, but this is usually attributed to autoregulation of flow secondary to resting contractile dysfunction. Nicklas and Gips (3) introduced the concept of "vascular stunning". Following 15 min of coronary artery occlusion in the dog, flow reserve, elicited by post-occlusion hyperemia or intracoronary adenosine, was reduced by about 30 %. Bolli et al. (4) confirmed these observations, reporting that 15 min of ischemia in the dog led to prolonged increases in resting vascular resistance and decreases in maximal flow reserve lasting at least 4 hr.

However, other laboratories have not found "vascular stunning" in mechanically stunned myocardium. Jeremy et al. (5) reported that after 10 min of ischemia in the dog, resting function was depressed, but coronary flow reserve was almost identical to baseline values when tested with intracoronary adenosine or after a 100 second coronary occlusion. Duncker et al. (6) found that myocardial stunning produced by 15 min of low flow ischemia in swine increased the slope of the pressure-maximal coronary flow relationship, indicating a *reduction* rather than an increase in minimal coronary resistance. This finding was attributed to decreased extravascular compressive forces secondary to myocardial stunning. McFalls et al. (7) also showed that the coronary vasodilator response to ATP, an endothelium dependent dilator, and adenosine were unchanged following myocardial stunning in swine.

The discrepancy between the Nicklas and Bolli studies and the others is probably related to the duration of ischemia used to produce mechanical stunning. The longer duration in the first two studies may have caused more vascular injury or more tissue edema, leading to more vascular compression. In any event, if "vascular stunning" exists, it can clearly be dissociated from mechanical stunning and is unnecessary to explain the contractile dysfunction that is so much a characteristic of stunned myocardium. In Bolli's study (4), the severity of the vascular derangement was unrelated to the severity of the contractile depression.

The microvasculature in stunned myocardium

The weight of physiological evidence is against microvascular obstruction in most models of stunned myocardium. Maintenance of normal coronary flow reserve implies that the microvasculature is patent and is capable of normal vasodilation. Stahl et al. (8) reported that after stunning produced by ten 5 minute coronary occlusions in the dog, microvascular injection studies with microfil or drawing ink demonstrated normal patency of arterioles and capillaries. Several laboratories have now reported that neutrophils, the putative mediator of the hypothesized microvascular occlusions, are not involved in myocardial stunning (9, 10). Removal or neutralization of neutrophils through filtration, cytotoxic drugs or antibodies has no effect on the severity of contractile dysfunction following brief ischemia.

Flow and stunned myocardium

Although the microvasculature is patent, resting flow is normal, and flow reserve is maintained in stunned myocardium, an increase in flow following administration of a vasodilator can recruit contractile function (7, 11). This phenomenon does not occur, or at least does not occur to nearly the same extent, in normal unstunned myocardium. This observation suggests that the stunned myocardium is somehow ischemic, despite normal resting flow and normal flow distribution by microspheres. Microspectrophotometry of stunned dog myocardium has demonstrated an excess of veins $< 100\ \mu m$ diameter with very low ($< 20\ \%$) oxygen saturations indicating foci of either impaired microvascular perfusion or increased oxygen consumption (8). Vasodilators could increase the function of stunned myocardium by improving oxygen delivery to presumed ischemic foci. Alternatively, there could be enhancement of lactate washout. McFalls et al. (7) reported continuous production of lactate from the stunned swine heart 30 minutes after restoration of flow. Lactate may contribute to contractile dysfunction, and removal of lactate from microvascular foci of ischemia could thereby improve mechanical function. Functional improvement of stunned myocardium during increased flow does not appear to be related to reduced afterload (11) or to the Gregg phenomenon, with increased stretch of the contractile fibers (11). Since the microvasculature is not obstructed, the beneficial effects of vasodilators on mechanical function could be related to a relief of abnormal microvascular constriction or spasm, which in turn could be caused by the local release of vasoconstrictor substances, such as endothelin. A "microvascular spasm" hypothesis that could partially explain the dysfunction of stunned myocardium is attractive because it accounts for several otherwise unexplained observations, including lactate production, foci with very low oxygen saturation, and improved function following vasodilator administration. Further studies are required to evaluate the validity and importance of the "microvascular spasm" hypothesis.

Conclusions

Stunned myocardium generally has normal resting flow and most studies have documented normal flow reserve. "Vascular stunning" (reduced vasodilator capacity) can be produced by ischemia, but the duration required is longer than that required to produce mechanical stunning. The two phenomenon can therefore be dissociated and are essentially unrelated. Nevertheless, despite evidence of normal microvascular patency in stunned myocardium, there are observations consistent with the existence of microvascular foci of ischemia, possibly related to vascular spasm or constriction, and this may explain the finding that increased flow in stunned myocardium may partially, or even largely, reverse the mechanical dysfunction. The "microvascular spasm" hypothesis may explain a significant portion of the dysfunction of stunned myocardium and deserves further study.

References

1. Hori M, Inoue M, Kitakaze M, Koretsune Y, Iwai K, Tamai J, Ito H, Kitabakate A, Sato T, Kamada T (1986) Role of adenosine in hyperemic response of coronary blood flow in microembolization. Amer J Physiol 250: H509–H518
2. Bolli R (1990) Mechanism of myocardial "stunning". Circulation 82: 723–738
3. Nicklas JM, Gips S (1989) Decreased coronary flow reserve after transient myocardial ischemia in dogs. J Am Coll Cardiol 13: 195–199
4. Bolli R, Triana JF, Jeroudi MO (1990) Prolonged impairment of coronary vasodilation after reversible ischemia. Evidence for microvascular "stunning". Circ Res 67: 332–343
5. Jeremy RW, Stahl L, Gillinov M, Litt M, Aversano TR, Becker LC (1989) Preservation of coronary flow reserve in stunned myocardium. Am J Physiol 256: H1301–H1310
6. Duncker DJ, McFalls EO, Krams R, Verdouw PD (1992) Pressure-maximal coronary flow relationship in regionally stunned porcine myocardium. Am J Physiol 262: H1744–H1751
7. McFalls EO, Duncker DJ, Krams R, Ward H, Gornick C, Verdouw PD (1991) Endothelium dependent vasodilatation following brief ischemia and reperfusion in anaesthetized swine. Cardiovasc Res 25: 659–665
8. Stahl LD, Weiss HR, Becker LC (1988) Myocardial oxygen consumption, oxygen supply/demand heterogeneity and microvascular patency in regionally stunned myocardium. Circulation 77: 865–872
9. Jeremy RW, Becker LC (1989) Neutrophil depletion does not prevent myocardial dysfunction after brief coronary occlusion. J Am Coll Cardiol 13: 1155–1163
10. Juneau CF, Ito BR, del Balzo U, Engler RL (1993) Severe neutrophil depletion by leucocyte filters or cytotoxic drug does not improve recovery of contractile function in stunned porcine myocardium. Cardiovasc Res 27: 720–727
11. Stahl LD, Aversano TR, Becker LC (1986) Selective enhancement of function of stunned myocardium by increased flow. Circulation 74: 843–851

97–99

P. G. Camici

Absolute myocardial blood flow in chronic left ventricular dysfunction

Key words Coronary artery disease – myocardial ischemia – ventricular dysfunction – positron emission tomography

Introduction

Myocardial regions with chronic wall motion abnormalities, subtended by stenotic arteries, may improve function after coronary revascularization. This was thought to represent a condition in which myocardial contractility and metabolism are reduced to match the reduced blood supply (7).

The hypothesis that myocardial hypoperfusion is the basis of chronic left ventricular dysfunction has recently been challenged by Vanoverschelde et al. (10), who demonstrated that baseline myocardial blood flow (MBF) measured with positron emission tomography (PET) was normal in segments subtended by occluded coronary arteries in patients with angina but without previous infarction. These authors suggested that repeated episodes of ischemia rather than chronic hypoperfusion is the basis of myocardial hibernation in these patients.

However, in most cases chronic ventricular dysfunction is detected in patients with previous infarction. In these patients wall motion abnormalities may be the result of permanent anatomical damage and/or a state of hibernation. The aim of the present study was to measure absolute regional myocardial blood flow in patients with chronic left ventricular dysfunction and previous infarction undergoing bypass surgery.

Prof. P. G. Camici (✉)
Cyclotron Unit
MRC Clinical Sciences Centre
Hammersmith Hospital
Du Cane Road
London W12 ONN, United Kingdom

Methods

The patient population consisted of 30 patients (2 women and 28 men; age 56 ± 11 years) with at least one chronically dysfunctional left ventricular region subtended by a diseased coronary artery amenable to revascularization. All patients had suffered a previous myocardial infarction at least 6 months before the study. Global and regional left ventricular function was assessed before and 4–6 months after bypass using radionuclide ventriculography.

All PET scans were performed using an ECAT 931-08/12 scanner (CTI, Knoxville, TN, USA). After the transmission scan the blood pool was imaged using ^{15}O-labelled carbon monoxide, which labels erythrocytes through the formation of carboxyhemoglobin. After 15 min to allow for decay of ^{15}O radioactivity to background levels MBF was measured using inhaled [^{15}O] CO_2, which is rapidly converted to [^{15}O] H_2O by carbonic anhydrase in the lungs (1). Unlike other implementations, this model provides MBF values per milliliter of perfusable tissue (not per milliliter of region of interest), based on the assumption that the uptake of [^{15}O] H_2O in scar tissue is negligible compared to that in normal myocardium (1). Therefore in a myocardial region consisting of an admixture of normal and necrotic tissue this model predominantly measures flow to the residual normal myocardium (5). At variance, the flow measured with other methods, for example, [^{13}N] NH_3, represents an average flow per unit of mass of tissue as with the microsphere technique (2).

Results and discussion

A total of 247 segments were analyzed. Of these, 114 were dysfunctional and 133 had a normal function. After surgery 10 segments worsened, and they were excluded from the PET data analysis, leaving a total of 107 dysfunctional and 130 normal segments. Of the 107 dysfunctional segments 59 had a functional improvement after surgery while 48 were unchanged. MBF in the 130 segments with normal function was 0.92 ± 0.25 ml min^{-1} g^{-1}. MBF was 0.87 ± 0.31 ml min^{-1} g^{-1} in the 59 segments that improved after bypass (NS vs. normal segments) and 0.82 ± 0.40 ml/ min^{-1} g^{-1} in the 48 segments that were unchanged after surgery ($p < 0.05$ vs. normal segments).

This study demonstrates that most of the chronically dysfunctional myocardial segments have MBF values, measured with [^{15}O] H_2O and PET, within the normal range (Fig. 1). If a cut-off value of 0.67 ml min^{-1} g^{-1} (mean MBF – 1 SD in normally contracting myocardium) is used to identify the low flow segments, only a small proportion (10 – 20 %) of the dysfunctional regions appear to by hypoperfused. The latter cut-off value of 0.67 ml min^{-1} g^{-1} is identical to that proposed by Bergmann et al. (3) and very similar to that (0.70 ml min^{-1} g^{-1}) proposed by Perrone-Filardi et al. (6), both obtained in normal subjects using [^{15}O] H_2O and PET. The present finding indicates that in this series of patients with previous myocardial infarction chronic left ventricular dysfunction was not characterized by a reduced baseline MBF. In patients with coronary artery disease coronary flow reserve decreases as the degree of stenosis is increased and is abolished for stenoses equal to 80 % or more of the luminal diameter (9). Under these circumstances any increase in cardiac workload above baseline conditions cannot be met by an adequate increase in MBF, leading to myocardial ischemia. Therefore it is possible that in patients with severe coronary artery disease the limited flow reserve leads to the development of myocardial ischemia even for small increases of oxygen demand such as those associated with ordinary daily activities (4). In this case frequently repeated bouts of ischemia rather than chronically reduced MBF could be the basis of chronic left ventricular dysfunction.

In several other studies MBF has been assessed with PET using [^{13}N] NH_3. In 22 Patients 86 ± 38 h after acute myocardial infarction (8) flow in viable (PET with fluorodeoxyglucose) infarcted segments was higher (0.6 ± 0.2 ml min^{-1} g^{-1}) than in non-viable segments (0.3 ± 0.1 ml min^{-1} g^{-1}; $p < 0.05$). In another series (8) of 15 patients with reperfused anterior infarction who were studied 42 ± 25 days after the acute event MBF averaged 0.8 ± 0.1 ml min^{-1} g^{-1} in remote segments, 0.7 ±0.2 ml min^{-1} g^{-1} in adjacent segments and 0.5 ± 0.1 ml min^{-1} g^{-1} in segments at the center of the infarcted area. Similar findings have been reported recently in 26 patients with

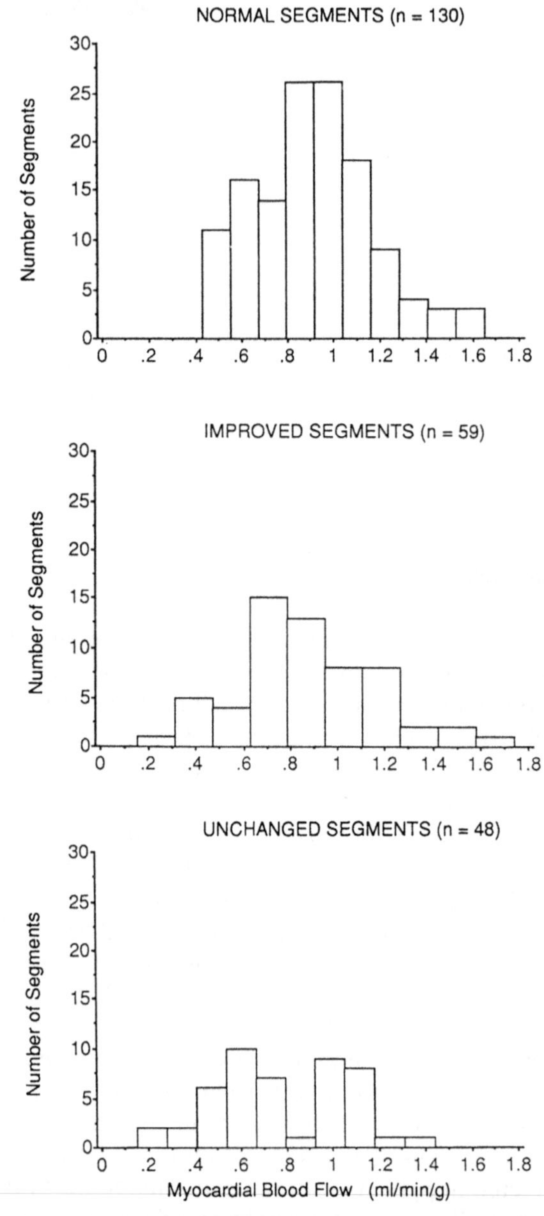

Fig. 1 Frequency of distribution of MBF in normal segments (*top panel*), in dysfunctional segments which improved after revascularization (*middle panel*) and in dysfunctional segments which did not improve after revascularization (*bottom panel*). MBF in normal segments ranges between 0.4 and 1.6 ml min^{-1} g^{-1} perfusable tissue, although in more than 90 % of the segments MBF are more than 0.6 ml min^{-1} g^{-1} perfusable tissue. The distribution of MBF values in the dysfunctional segments (both improved and unchanged) is similar to that found in the normal segments although in a minority of dysfunctional segments MBF is very low (i.e. <0.4 ml min^{-1} g^{-1} perfusable tissue).

chronic healed infarction studied 44 ± 65 months after the event (8). To be able to compare our data with those obtained with [^{13}N] NH_3 our MBF values (expressed as flow per milliliter of perfusable tissue) (5) were multiplied by tissue fraction (1) to yield values of milliliter per unit mass of tissue (8). The flow values obtained after this conversion were similar to those measured with [^{13}N] NH_3 i.e. 0.71 ± 0.23 ml min^{-1} g^{-1} in normal segments, 0.64 ± 0.27 ml min^{-1} g^{-1} in segments which improved after surgery and 0.61 ± 0.33 ml min^{-1} g^{-1} ($p < 0.05$ vs. normal segments) in segments which did not improve after surgery.

References

1. Araujo LI, Lammertsma AA, Rhodes CG, McFalls EO, Iida H, Rechavia E, Gallassi AR, De Silva R, Jones T, Maseri A (1991) Non-invasive quantification of regional myocardial blood flow in normal volunteers using oxygen-15 labeled carbon dioxide and positron emission tomography. Circulation 83: 875–885
2. Bellina RC, Parodi O, Camici P, Salvadori PA, Taddei L, Fusani L, Guzzardi R, Klassen GA, L'Abbate A, Donato L (1990) Simultaneous in vitro and in vivo validation of nitrogen-13 ammonia for the assessment of regional myocardial blood flow: J Nucl Med 31: 1335–1343
3. Bergmann SR, Herrero P, Markham J, Weinheimer CJ, Walsh MN (1989) Noninvasive quantitation of myocardial blood flow in human subjects with oxygen-15-labelled water and positron emission tomography. J Am Coll Cardiol 14: 639–652
4. Deanfield JE, Selwyn AP, Chierchia S, Maseri A, Ribeiro P, Krikler S (1983) Myocardial ischaemia during daily life in patients with stable angina: its relation to symptoms and heart rate changes. Lancet 753–758
5. Lammertsma AA, De Silva R, Araujo LI, Jones T (1992) Measurement of regional myocardial blood flow using $C^{15}O_2$ and positron emission tomography: comparison of tracer models. Clin Phys Physiol Meas 13: 1–20
6. Perrone-Filardi P, Bacharach SL, Dilsizian V, Marin-Neto JA, Maurea S, Arrighi JA, Bonow RO (1994) Clinical significance of reduced regional myocardial glucose uptake in regions with normal blood flow in patients with chronic coronary artery disease. J Am Coll Cardiol 23: 608–616
7. Rahimtoola SH (1985) A perspective on the three large multicenter randomized clinical trials of coronary bypass surgery for chronic stable angina. Circulation 72 (suppl V): V123–V135
8. De Silva R, Camici PG (1994) The role of positron emission temography in the investigation of coronary circulatory function in man. Cardiovasc. Research 28 (11): 1595–1612
9. Uren NG, Melin JA, De Bruyne B, Wijns W, Baudhuin T, Camici PG (1994) Relation between myocardial blood flow and the severity of coronary artery stenosis. N Engl J Med 330: 1782–1788
10. Vanoverschelde J-L J, Wijns W, Depre C, Essamri B, Heyndrickx GR, Borgers M, Bol A, Melin J (1993) Mechanisms of chronic regional postischemic dysfunction in humans. New insights from the study of noninfarcted collateral-dependent myocardium. Circulation 87: 1513–1523

100 – 102

L. Mandinov
P. Kaufmann
O. M. Hess

Coronary vasomotion of the stunned myocardium

Key words Coronary vasomotion – myocardial stunning – quantitative coronary angiography – endothelial stunning – PTCA

The term "stunned" moycardium describes a dysfunction of the myocardium which may persist for hours, days or even weeks after restoration of coronary blood flow following thrombolysis, percutaneous transluminal coronary angioplasty (PTCA) or aorto-coronary bypass grafting (7, 9). The "stunned" myocardium is characterized – despite marked dyskinesis – by near normal levels of myocardial perfusion and normal or even enhanced oxygen consumption (2), probably due to higher oxygen requirements of the contractile elements. Thus, a mismatch between function and flow exists which has been recognized to be a characteristic finding of the "stunned" myocardium. However, coronary reperfusion may result in an attenuation of the endothelial response to coronary vasodilators such as acetylcholine, bradykinin, etc. (3). It is well established that prolonged myocardial ischemia is associated with irreversible myocardial damage and profound structural and functional derangements of the coronary microvasculature which may persist even if perfusion is restored (1). Local vasoactive substances such as the endothelium-dependent relaxing factor (EDRF) also play an important role in the regulation of myocardial perfusion. EDRF is a potent vasodilator which is released from the coronary endothelium but is reduced in patients with atherosclerotic plaques or hypercholesterolemia (= endothelial dysfunction). Since there are shear-stress dependent flow receptors, EDRF is released proportionally to coronary flow, i.e., the higher the flow the larger the artery and vice versa. However, flow regulation is dependent on several factors such as perfusion pressure, peripheral resistance, sympathetic activation, oxygen saturation, metabolic factors etc. EDRF is synthetized in the endothelial cells and is rapidly broken down during ischemia by superoxide radicals which inactivate EDRF and, thus, decrease flow-induced vasodilation (6). Neutrophil aggregation may further contribute to this process by the release of proteolytic enzymes which can convert oxygen to superoxide anions, i.e., oxygen free radicals. These radicals may injure the endothelium when generated in large amounts such as during ischemia (4) and may sensitize the smooth vasculature to contraction by alpha-adrenergic mechanisms (8).

Prof. O. M. Hess (✉) · L. Mandinov · P. Kaufmann
Department of Internal Medicine
University Hospital
8091 Zurich, Switzerland

Coronary artery dimensions in the "stunned" myocardium

In the ischemic myocardium coronary vasoconstriction has been reported in the experimental animal with a reduction in coronary artery size of approximately 30 % (11). The reduction in coronary artery dimensions has been attributed to the decrease in flow and the activation of the alpha-adrenergic system during ischemia (5). In contrast to the acutely ischemic myocardium, coronary flow has been reported to be normal in the "stunned" myocardium but impaired coronary vasodilation due to microvascular "stunning" was described in the experimental animal (1).

Determination of coronary artery dimensions in patients with unstable angina pectoris, respectively acute myocardial infarction (group 1) showed reduced vessel dimensions distally to the stenosed or occluded coronary artery (Table 1). This narrowing of the distal vessel segment could be attributed to the aforementioned reduction

Table 1 Clinical data in acute and chronic ischemia

	group 1*	group 2
n	12	21
age (years)	56 ± 11	51 ± 7
gender M/F	11/1	20/1
NYHA-class:		
– II	–	13 (62 %)
– III	–	8 (38 %)
– IV	12 (100 %)	
acute ischemic events:		
– unstable angina	3 (25 %)	–
– myocardial infarction	9 (75 %)	–
chronic ischemic events:		
– myocardial infarction	–	18 (86 %)
– stable angina	–	3 (14 %)
presence of collateral flow	4 (33 %)	9 (43 %)

* = "stunned" myocardium

in coronary blood flow and/or the enhanced alpha-adrenergic stimulation during ischemia in the "stunned" myocardium. After successful PTCA and recanalization of the coronary artery (in the presence of a "stunned" myocardium) distal coronary artery dimensions remained smaller than the proximal reference vessels.

In contrast, coronary vessel segments in patients with severe stenotic lesions but without acute myocardial ischemia (group 2) distal vessel segments were similar in size to the proximal reference vessels (Fig. 1). Thus, abnormal coronary vasomotion can be observed in the "stunned" myocardium which is not seen in the normally perfused myocardium before and after PTCA.

Mechanisms of enhanced vasomotor tone in the "stunned" myocardium

These findings can be explained by several mechanisms: 1) "Stunning" of the endothelium with reduced release of EDRF (= ischemic endothelial dysfunction); 2) Enhanced sympathetic stimulation with increased circulating levels of catecholamines; 3) Reduced coronary flow reserve with an increased peripheral vascular resistance (= microvascular "stunning").

Thus, altered coronary vasomotion of the distal vessel segment in the "stunned" myocardium can be attributed to several factors but may represent a reversible ischemic dysfunction of the endothelium, since follow-up examinations after PTCA (10) have shown normalization of coronary vasomotion 4 months after revascularization. Release of oxygen free radicals which may interfere with the normal endothelial function and inactivate EDRF seem to play a major role in this process (8). Changes in resting flow cannot be completely ruled out as a mechanism for this alteration in vasomotion, but resting flow has been found to be increased after PTCA (= postischemic hyperemia) and, thus, a larger rather than a smaller coronary artery size would have been expected after acute revascularization. Enhanced sympathetic stimulation has been reported during acute ischemia (5, 11) which may render the ischemic endothelium especially sensitive for vasoconstrictory influences. However, in the nonischemic myocardium (Fig. 1) the distal coronary artery dimensions remained largely unchanged by PTCA, indicating that this factor is probably of minor importance for the disturbance of coronary vascular tone in the "stunned" myocardium although coronary vasoconstriction has been reported after PTCA.

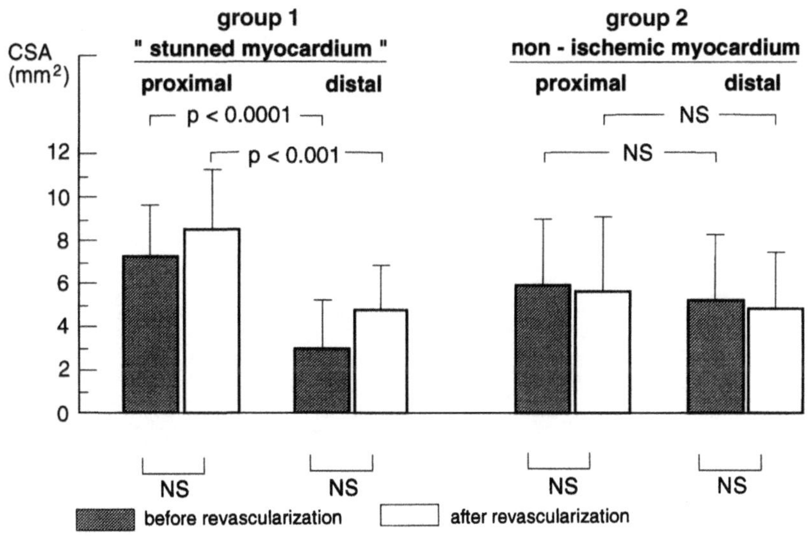

Fig. 1 Coronary cross-sectional area (CSA) of the proximal and distal segment of a stenotic coronary artery in patients with acute ischemia ("myocardial stunning" = group 1) and in patients without acute ischemia but severe coronary stenosis (group 2) before (closed bar) and after (open bar) PTCA. Please note that the distal vessel segment is smaller before as well as after PTCA in patients with "myocardial stunning" but remains unchanged in control patients without acute ischemia.

Conclusion

Abnormal coronary vasomotion can be observed in the "stunned" myocardium which can be explained by a reversible ischemic dysfunction of the coronary endothelium. However, other mechanisms such as a reduced coronary flow reserve due to microvascular "stunning" or an enhanced sympathetic stimulation could also be responsible for the occurrence of abnormal vasomotion in the "stunned" myocardium.

References

1. Bolli R, Triana JF, Jeroudi MO (1990) Prolonged impairment of coronary vasodilation after reversible ischemia. Evidence for microvascular "stunning". Circ Res 67: 332–343
2. Dean EN, Shlafer M, Nicklas JM (1990) The oxygen consumption paradox of "stunned myocardium" in dogs. Basic Res Cardiol 85 (2): 120–131
3. Gross GR, O'Rourke ST, Pelc LR, Warltier DC (1992) Myocardial and endothelial dysfunction after multiple, brief coronary occlusion: role of oxygen radicals. Am J Physiol 263: H1703–H1709
4. Gryglewsky RJ, Ashton DS, Moncada S (1986) Superoxide anion is involved in the breakdown of the endothelium-derived vascular relaxing factor. Nature 320: 454–456
5. Heusch G (1989) Koronare Vasomotion bei Myokardischämie. Z Kardiol 78: 485–499
6. Kaneko M, Hayashi H, Kobayashi A et al. (1991) Stunned myocardium and oxygen free radicals – sarcolemmal membrane damage due to oxygen free radicals. Jpn Circ J 55 (9): 885–892
7. Kloner RA, Przyklenk K, Kay GL (1994) Clinical evidence for stunned myocardium after coronary artery bypass surgery. J Card Surg 9 (3 Suppl): 397–402
8. Lawson DL, Mehta JL, Nichols WW, Mehta P, Donnelly WH (1990) Superoxide radical-mediated endothelial injury and vasoconstriction of rat thoracic aortic rings. J Lab Clin Med 115: 541–548
9. Sone T, Tsubot H, Sassa H (1991) Clinical study of the stunned myocardium. Jpn Circ J 55 (9): 904–912
10. Suter TM, Buechi M, Hess OM, Haemmerli-Saner C, Gaglione A, Krayenbuehl HP (1992) Normalization of coronary vasomotion after percutaneous transluminal coronary angioplasty? Circulation 85: 86–92
11. Vassalli G, Bracht Ch, Bischoff R, Schulz R, Heusch G, Hess OM (1995) Epicardial coronary artery vasoconstriction during acute myocardial ischemia: Reversibility by calcium-antagonists. JACC 73A (abstract)

103 – 105

Y. Birnbaum
R. A. Kloner

Therapy for myocardial stunning

Key words Diastolic dysfunction – myocardial ischemia – stunning – systolic dysfunction – therapy

Introduction

Myocardial stunning, or postischemic dysfunction, is defined as delayed recovery of systolic and/or diastolic function of viable myocardium despite restoration of coronary flow after an ischemic insult (4). The severity and duration of myocardial stunning is highly dependent on the duration and severity of the previous ischemic insult (2). Thus, clinically significant myocardial stunning can be seen only after severe ischemic insult, especially after reperfusion therapy for acute myocardial infarction and during the recovery period after coronary artery bypass surgery (2). However, in the former condition some of the cases of delayed recovery of function may be attributed to delayed improvement of perfusion by either delayed recanalization or recuitment of collaterals, and in the latter condition a delayed recovery from hibernation or new ischemic insult due to acute occlusion of the bypass grafts may be the reason for the continuous myocardial dysfunction (2). Thus, in the clinical setting pure myocardial stunning should be diagnosed only after simultaneous demonstration of persistent mechanical dysfunction despite restoration of normal coronary perfusion. Myocardial stunning has also been described following less severe ischemia induced by partial coronary stenosis following exercise in both animals and humans (2). This form of myocardial stunning following exercise treadmill testing may serve as a marker of severe multivessel coronary artery disease (2). It might be that in daily life uncontrolled effort induced ischemia may result in prolonged and clinically relevant myocardial stunning in patients with severe coronary artery disease.

Several mechanisms may be involved in the generation of myocardial stunning. There might be a difference in the mechanism of stunning that results after brief ischemic episodes and stunning that appears after prolonged ischemia with partial myocardial necrosis (3). The two major hypotheses that have been proposed to explain the etiology of postischemic myocardial dysfunction are: oxygen free radical generation, abnormal calcium homeostasis, or some combination of these (3).

Prevention of myocardial stunning

Antioxidants

According to experimental models, myocardial stunning can be prevented by administration of antioxidative agents just prior to reperfusion, especially after brief ischemic episodes. However, in the clinical setting the goal is to prevent severe and prolonged periods of myocardial stunning which follow lengthy ischemic episodes as seen in acute myocardial infarction or postcardiac surgery. The role of free radicals in myocardial stunning induced by prolonged ischemic periods is less clear. Some authors have reported that allopurinol, a blocker of free radical production, improved cardiac performance and reduced cardiac complications in patients undergoing coronary artery bypass surgery (6). However, these studies included a small number of patients. Until now no other

Dr. Y. Birnbaum (✉) · R. A. Kloner
The Heart Institute
Good Samaritan Hospital
616 South Witmer Street
Los Angeles, California 90017, USA

controlled clinical trial has documented the efficacy of antioxidants in the clinical setting of prolonged myocardial ischemia. A clinical trial of recombinant human superoxide dismutase coupled with primary angioplasty at the time of acute myocardial infarction did not show significant benefit on left ventricular function (7).

Calcium channel blockers

Calcium antagonists have a potential role in prevention of stunning by blocking the transient hypercalcemic phase immediately after reperfusion that might be the mechanism for myocardial stunning. Another potential mechanism is their free radical scavenging effect (9). Various experimental models of global or brief regional myocardial ischemia and reperfusion have demonstrated that calcium antagonists, given especially prior to occlusion but also during reperfusion, enhance the recovery of contractile function. However, the results following long ischemic episodes are conflicting (9). The effect of calcium antagonists on myocardial stunning has been evaluated in only small clinical trials. Adding nifedipine or diltiazem to cardioplegic solutions resulted in improved myocardial metabolism and hemodynamic status (9). Calcium antagonists improved recovery of myocardial dysfunction induced by prolonged balloon inflation during angioplasty (11).

Other agents

The evidence for efficacy of beta blockers to augment recovery of myocardial stunning is equivocal. Several studies have shown that stable analogs of prostacyclin enhances the recovery of myocardial function upon reperfusion. Angiotensin-converting enzyme (ACE) inhibitors have been demonstrated to enhance recovery of function following ischemia-reperfusion insult (10). However, the mechanism is not clear. The SH-containing agents captopril and zofenopril have been shown consistently to ameliorate stunning, possibly by their antioxidant properties. However, even other ACE inhibitors that do not contain the SH group, such as enalapril, are effective in some experimental models of stunning. However, the protective effect of enalapril was blocked by infusion of indomethacin. Thus, a prostaglandin-mediated mechanism may be important (10). Although there is direct clinical evidence that ACE inhibitors reduce mortality and improve left ventricular function, there is no direct clinical evidence of a beneficial effect on myocardial stunning. There is some experimental evidence that ubiquinone (coenzyme Q_{10}) augments recovery of function after an ischemic insult. A small randomized clinical study demonstrated better preservation of the myocardium and enhanced recovery of function post cardiac surgery, using hypothermic cardioplegic arrest in patients pretreated with ubiquinone (5). Although the mechanism is not clear, the effect may be due to the antioxidant properties of ubiquinone.

Augmentation of myocardial function

Stunned myocardium retains its contractile reserves. Following infusion of various positive inotropic agents, transient augmentation of global and regional function is observed. Various beta-mimetic agents are effective in enhancement of contractility and improvement of diastolic relaxation in the ischemic-reperfused zone, without further depletion of ATP stores (1). However, due to downregulation of the beta-receptors the effect may be lost after 24 h of infusion. Thus these agents are less effective when the recovery of postischemic dysfunction is delayed over several days or weeks. Recently the use of extracorporeal life support devices has been reported as a mean to overcome prolonged and severe cardiogenic shock after acute myocardial dysfunction (8).

In conclusion, myocardial stunning is an important cause of severe and prolonged reversible myocardial dysfunction. Evidence of clinical efficacy of various modalities for prevention of myocardial stunning is lacking. Transient augmentation of myocardial function by beta-mimetic agents, or use of various mechanical assisting devices may help to overcome the critical period of myocardial depression.

References

1. Becker LC (1993) Inotropic agents and stimulation of stunned myocardium. In: Kloner RA, Przyklenk K (eds) Stunned myocardium: properties, mechanisms and clinical manifestations. Dekker, New York, pp 267–279
2. Birnbaum Y, Kloner R (1995) Clinical aspects of myocardial stunning. Coronary Artery Dis (in press)
3. Bolli R (1990) Mechanism of myocardial "stunning". Circulation 82: 723–738
4. Braunwald E, Kloner RA (1982) The stunned myocardium: prolonged postischemic ventricular dysfunction. Circulation 66: 1146–1149
5. Chen YF, Lin YT, Wu SC (1994) Effectiveness of coenzyme Q10 on myocardial preservation during hypothermic cardioplegic arrest. J Thorac Cardiovasc Surg 107: 242–247
6. Coghlan JG, Flitter WD, Clutton SM, Panda R, Daly R, Wright G, Ilsley CD, Slater TF (1994) Allopurinol pretreatment improves postoperative recovery and reduced lipid peroxidation in patients undergoing coronary artery bypass grafting. J Thorac Cardiovasc Surg 107: 248–256
7. Flaherty JT, Pitt B, Gruber JW, Heuser RR, Rothbaum DA, Burwell LR, George BS, Kereiakes DJ, Deitchman D, Gustafson N, Brinker JA, Becher LC, Mancini J, Topol E, Werns SW (1994) Recombinant human superoxide dismutase (h-SOD) fails to improve recovery of ventricular function in patients undergoing coronary angioplasty for acute myocardial infarction. Circulation 89: 1982–1991
8. Kurose M, Okamoto K, Sato T, Kukita I, Taki K, Goto H (1994) Emergency and long-term extracorporeal life support following acute myocardial infarction: rescue from severe cardiogenic shock related to stunned myocardium. Clin Cardiol 17: 552–557
9. Przyklenk K, Kloner RA (1993) Calcium antagonists as treatment for the stunned myocardium. In: Kloner RA, Przyklenk K (eds) Stunned myocardium: properties, mechanisms and clinical manifestations. Dekker, New York, pp 281–301
10. Przyklenk K, Kloner RA (1993) "Cardioprotection" by ACE-inhibitors in acute myocardial ischemia and infarction? Basic Res Cardiol 88 (suppl 1): 139–154
11. Sheiban I, Tonni S, Marini A, Trevi GP (1993) Left ventricular dysfunction following transient ischaemia induced by transluminal coronary angioplasty. Beneficial effects of calcium antagonists against post-ischaemic myocardial stunning. Eur Heart J (suppl A) 14: 14–21

106–108

R. Schulz
T. Ehring
G. Heusch

Stunned myocardium: inotropic reserve and pharmacological attenuation

Key words Myocardial ischemia – reperfusion – inotropic reserve calcium antagonists – ACE inhibitors

Definition of stunned myocardium

Brief episodes of myocardial ischemia, too short in duration to cause irreversible damage, may nevertheless result in a prolonged impairment of contractile function upon reperfusion (9). This phenomenon has been termed stunned myocardium by Braunwald and Kloner (2). In stunned myocardium contractile function remains depressed despite fully or almost fully restored blood flow. The rate of recovery of function during reperfusion depends on the severity of blood flow reduction during the preceding ischemia (1).

Energetics of stunned myocardium and recruitment of an inotropic reserve

Decreases in myocardial energy-rich phosphates during ischemia with only slow repletion of ATP during reperfusion have been demonstrated and related to the prolonged myocardial dysfunction. However, enhanced repletion of myocardial ATP by infusion of nucleotide precursors does not enhance myocardial function during reperfusion. Also, even while baseline contractile function of the reperfused myocardium is depressed, it retains the capacity to respond to various inotropic interventions such as postextrasystolic potentiation (3), infusion of inotropic drugs (8), and cardiac sympathetic nerve stimulation (8). The increment in contractile function of reperfused myocardium in response to cardiac sympathetic nerve stimulation or intravenous norepinephrine infusion is identical throughout the entire reperfusion period and does not differ from the control response, thus excluding an impairment of sympathetic neurotransmission as the underlying mechanism of postischemic contractile dysfunction (8).

R. Schulz · T. Ehring · Prof. Dr. G. Heusch (✉)
Abteilung für Pathophysiologie
Zentrum für Innere Medizin
Universitätsklinikum Essen
Hufelandstraße 55
45122 Essen

Calcium antagonists in stunned myocardium

An apparent paradox characterizing the stunned myocardium is the role of calcium ions. On the one hand, an increase in cytosolic calcium is thought to be causally involved in the development of postischemic contractile failure. On the other hand, inotropic interventions which act ultimately through an increase in cytosolic calcium increase the contractile function of stunned myocardium.

There is unequivocal evidence from both in vitro and in vivo studies that pretreatment with calcium antagonists before ischemia improves the recovery of contractile function during reperfusion, i.e., attenuates myocardial stunning (7). The potential benefit from calcium antagonists when given during reperfusion remains somewhat controversial (7). The consistent attenuation of stunning by pretreatment with calcium antagonists cannot be explained by an improvement in myocardial blood flow during ischemia or reperfusion or by more favorable hemodynamic conditions but appears to be related to an attenuated calcium overload during early ischemia (Fig. 1a) (4). While cellular calcium overload might therefore play a major role in the pathogenesis of myocardial stunning, the precise mechanism by which ischemic cellular calcium overload depresses contractile function during reperfusion remains unclear at present.

So far, the potential clinical use of treatment with calcium antagonists in attenuating myocardial stunning is therefore limited to controlled interventions involving ischemia-reperfusion such as PTCA. On the other hand, patients under treatment with calcium antagonists experience not only a reduction in the severity of ischemia but also a better recovery of contractile function after termination of ischemia.

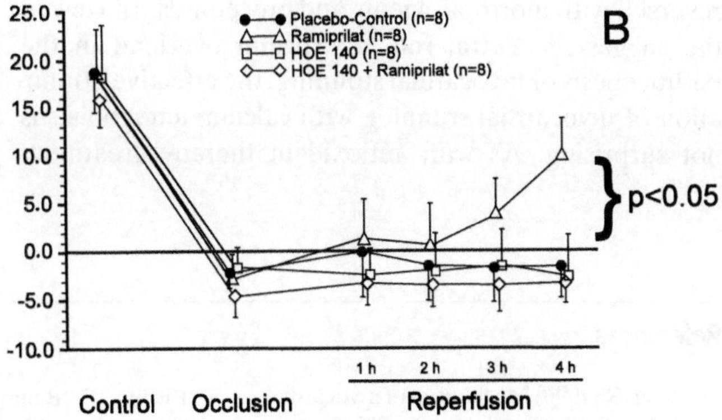

Fig. 1B Only in the dogs that received ramiprilat did posterior systolic wall thickening recover significantly during 4 h reperfusion. The bradykinin B_2 receptor antagonist HOE 140 abolished the beneficial effect of ramiprilat alone. (From [5])

ACE inhibitors in stunned myocardium

The attenuation of myocardial stunning by several angiotensin-converting enzyme (ACE) inhibitors has been demonstrated in a number of experimental studies in vitro and in vivo (Fig. 1b) (5). While in isolated hearts the cardioprotective effect of the ACE inhibitor ramiprilat appears to be mediated by prostaglandins and NO, a signal cascade of bradykinin and prostaglandins, but not NO is mediating such cardioprotection in the in situ heart (5). This cardioprotection by ramiprilat is prevented by the cyclo-oxygenase inhibitor indomethacin (5). Therefore, in the clinical setting of ischemia/reperfusion an interference with the cyclo-oxygenase inhibitor aspirin, which is widely used to prevent platelet aggregation, could be expected. However, in a recent study from our laboratory the attenuation of myocardial stunning by ramiprilat was not prevented by aspirin in dosages which were nevertheless sufficient to inhibit platelet aggregation (10).

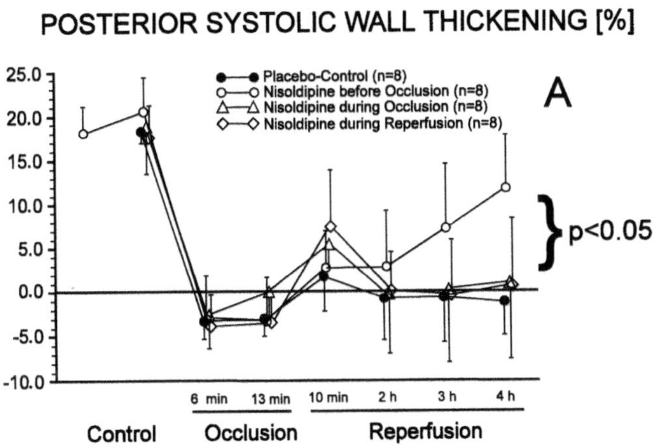

Fig. 1A Only after pretreatment with the calcium antagonist nisoldipine did posterior systolic wall thickening recover significantly during 4 h of reperfusion. (From [4])

Identification of stunned myocardium

In contrast to dysfunctional, irreversibly damaged myocardium, stunned myocardium retains an inotropic reserve. To further distinguish stunned from viable, hibernating myocardium, i.e., myocardium characterized by contractile dysfunction during persistent ischemia, either regional myocardial blood flow must be measured or the metabolic changes associated which an inotropic challenge be analyzed. The recruitment of an inotropic reserve in hibernating myocardium is at the expense of metabolic recovery (11) while in stunned myocardium no metabolic deterioration occurs during inotropic stimulation (6). Therefore, metabolic imaging using positron-emission tomography may help not only to identify viable, dysfunctional myocardium, but also to distinguish hibernating from stunned myocardium and predict the success of reperfusion procedures.

Therapy of stunned myocardium

Myocardial stunning per se requires no therapy at all, since by definition blood flow is normal and contractile function recovers spontaneously. If, however, myocardial stunning is severe, involves large parts of the left ventricle and thus impairs global left ventricular function, it can be reversed with inotropic agents and procedures. In view of the suggested central role of calcium overload in the pathogenesis of myocardial stunning, the effective attenuation of myocardial stunning with calcium antagonists is not surprising. As with antioxidant therapy, treatment with calcium antagonists is most effective when started before ischemia (4). ACE inhibition also attenuates myocardial stunning (5). There are as yet, however, no controlled clinical data on the efficacy of these therapies, but both approaches are in principle clinically applicable.

References

1. Bolli R (1990) Mechanism of myocardial "stunning". Circulation 82: 723–738
2. Braunwald E, Kloner RA (1982) The stunned myocardium: prolonged, postischemic ventricular dysfunction. Circulation 66: 1146–1149
3. Ehring T, Heusch G (1991) Postextrasystolic potentiation does not distinguish ischaemic from stunned myocardium. Pfluegers Arch 418: 453–461
4. Ehring T, Böhm M, Heusch G (1992) The calcium antagonist nisoldipine improves the functional recovery of reperfused myocardium only when given before ischemia. J Cardiovasc Pharmacol 20: 63–74
5. Ehring T, Baumgart D, Krajcar M, Hümmelgen M, Kompa S, Heusch G (1994) Attenuation of myocardial stunning by the ACE-inhibitor ramiprilat through a signal cascade of bradykinin and prostaglandins, but not nitric oxide. Circulation 90: 1368–1385
6. Görge G, Papageorgiou I, Lerch R (1990) Epinephrine-stimulated contractile and metabolic reserve in postischemic rat myocardium. Basic Res Cardiol 85: 595–605
7. Heusch G (1992) Myocardial stunning: a role for calcium antagonists during ischaemia? Cardiovasc Res 26: 14–19
8. Heusch G, Frehen D, Kröger K, Schulz R, Thämer V (1988) Integrity of sympathetic neurotransmission in stunned myocardium. J Appl Cardiol 3: 259–272
9. Heyndrickx GR, Millard RW, McRitchie RJ, Maroko PR, Vatner SF (1975) Regional myocardial functional and electrophysiological alterations after brief coronary artery occlusion in conscious dogs. J Clin Invest 56: 978–985
10. Sakka S, Ehring T, Rose J, Skyschally A, Heusch G (1995) Aspirin does not prevent the attenuation of myocardial stunning by the ACE-inhibitor ramiprilat. Pflügers Archiv 429: R103 (Abstract)
11. Schulz R, Guth BD, Pieper K, Martin C, Heusch G (1992) Recruitment of an inotropic reserve in moderately ischemic myocardium at the expense of metabolic recovery: a model of short-term hibernation. Circ Res 70: 1282–1295

109–111
© Steinkopff Verlag 1996

G. Ambrosio

The elusive difference between hibernation and stunning in patients

Key words Hibernation – stunning

Hibernation and stunning both refer to reversible contractile impairment of otherwise viable myocardium. Since they entail different therapeutic approaches, it is important to distinguish these conditions. Hibernation is the *concomitant* reduction of myocardial flow *and* contractility, whereas stunning is contractile impairment persisting for some time *after* perfusion has been restored (8). However, this description may represent a simplification of reality. In many patients the clinical picture is more complex, as these conditions often blend into each other.

Unlike experimental models, in which ischemia is induced in normal hearts, ischemic episodes in patients typically occur in myocardium perfused through a stenosed artery. This fact may obscure differences between stunning and hibernation. If one accepts the concept that hibernation is caused by stenosis severe enough to reduce blood flow at rest, it follows that in some patients transient episodes of ischemia (and hence stunning) are superimposed on hibernation (Fig. 1). In this case it is difficult to establish how much contractile impairment is caused by either mechanism (14). A similar argument has been raised to question the very existence of hibernation. It has been argued that myocardium distal to a severely stenotic artery may undergo repeated episodes of ischemia because flow cannot increase to match increases in myocardial oxygen demand that occur during daily activity (4). According to this theory, what appears as hibernating myocardium is the result of multiple episodes of ischemia, and therefore dysfunctional regions are instead "chronically" stunned. In either case it is difficult to judge whether impaired contractility in areas of viable myocardium distal to a coronary artery stenosis truly represents hibernation (which can benefit only from revascularization), as opposed to residual stunning from ischemic episodes, which recovers spontaneously.

These issues have become clinically relevant since the concept of stunning has extended from the initial observations after acute coronary artery occlusion to encompass other conditions of transient ischemia. Effort angina is a frequent cause of transient myocardial ischemia in patients with coronary artery disease, and there is now evidence that stunning can follow exercise-induced ischemia (1, 9). Furthermore, repeated episodes of exercise-induced ischemia can have a cumulative effect (7), in which case the dysfunction lasts much longer. This phenomenon may affect our ability to interpret the significance of regional dysfunction in patients. One option is that of reevaluating regional function of a patient after some time. However, ischemia is often clinically "silent", and therefore we may have no clues to relate the moment of evaluation with the timing of the last ischemic episode. Thus regional contractile impairment which apparently persists might still represent stunning rather than hibernation.

The issue is complicated by the fact that, unless regional contractility and perfusion status are *simultaneously* assessed, it is hard to differentiate in the clinical setting stunning from contractile abnormalities deriving from hibernation, or even from dysfunction accompanying silent ischemia (2, 14). For example, Renkin et al. (13) have described patients with unstable angina in whom contractile impairment was significantly less after resolu-

Dr. G. Ambrosio, M.D., Ph. D. (✉)
Sezione di Cardiologia "R"
Dipartimento di Medicina Clinica
Universita' di Perugia
Via Eugubina 42
06122 Perugia, Italy

tion of the acute episode than in other patients also admitted for unstable angina and with apparently similar angiographic data. PTCA was subsequently performed in all patients, but function improved only in the former group. Those findings suggest that unstable angina induced stunning in both groups, and that PTCA improved flow (and function) of hibernating myocardium, which was the underlying condition only in a subgroup of patients. In another study regional wall motion was assessed early after acute myocardial infarction treated with thrombolytic therapy, and at late follow-up in patients who were either revascularized or treated with medical therapy (3). Revascularization was associated with marked recovery of function. However, smaller but significant recovery was also observed in patients receiving medical therapy alone, consistent with resolution of stunning. Further recovery after revascularization suggests resolution of additional contractile impairment due to hibernation.

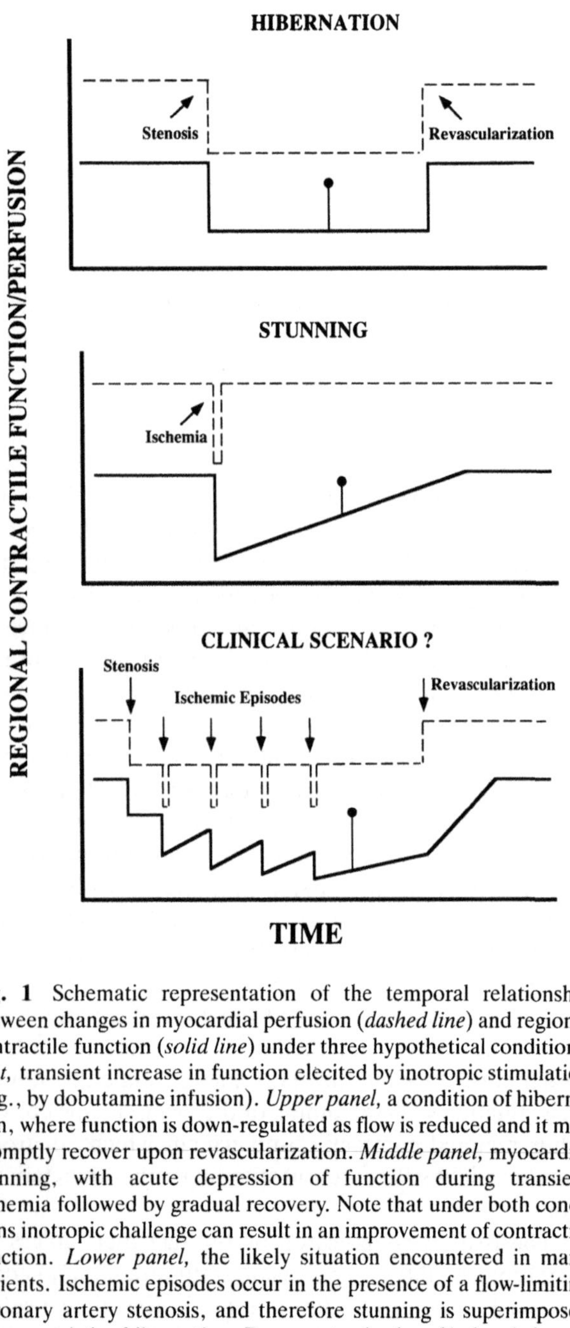

Fig. 1 Schematic representation of the temporal relationship between changes in myocardial perfusion (*dashed line*) and regional contractile function (*solid line*) under three hypothetical conditions. *Dot,* transient increase in function elecited by inotropic stimulation (e.g., by dobutamine infusion). *Upper panel,* a condition of hibernation, where function is down-regulated as flow is reduced and it may promptly recover upon revascularization. *Middle panel,* myocardial stunning, with acute depression of function during transient ischemia followed by gradual recovery. Note that under both conditions inotropic challenge can result in an improvement of contractile function. *Lower panel,* the likely situation encountered in many patients. Ischemic episodes occur in the presence of a flow-limiting coronary artery stenosis, and therefore stunning is superimposed over preexisting hibernation. Recurrent episodes of ischemia have a cumulative effect, thus prolonging the time required for stunning to disappear. Here the relative importance of hibernation is overestimated. Furthermore, while complete recovery of function do not occur unless normal flow is restored, this does not promptly ensue after revascularization. Adapted from (2).

Recently attempts have been made to identify hibernating myocardium based upon its ability to recruit inotropic reserve. Indeed, infusion of dobutamine may improve function in hypocontracting but viable regions, whereas myocardial scars show no improvement. However, while clinically useful to differentiate reversibly from irreversibly dysfunctional areas, this approach does not provide information about perfusion, and therefore it does not discriminate between hibernation and stunning, since stunned myocardium may also respond to inotropic interventions (5). This problem is illustrated in a study by Pierard and coworkers (12). They analyzed regional function at rest and during dobutamine infusion early after thrombolysis in patients with acute myocardial infarction who were also reevaluated after several months. Lack of improvement during dobutamine infusion could clearly identify irreversibly injured myocardium. However, of all patients in whom dobutamine improved function, those with normal perfusion in the dysfunctional region went on to spontaneously recover function over time, while patients showing reduced perfusion had no subsequent recovery at follow-up. These findings suggest that in the former group recruitment of inotropic reserve occurred in stunned regions, whereas in other patients depressed function which responded to dobutamine might have been due to hibernation, which persisted at follow-up because revascularization was not performed.

Another factor which may contribute to blur the boundaries between hibernation and stunning is that, although normalization of function upon revascularization is the tenet of hibernation, the time course of recovery is largely unknown. Experimental evidence suggests that recovery of function after prolonged underperfusion is a relatively slow process (10). Myocytes in biopsies from underperfused, hypocontracting myocardium appear in a "de-differentiated" state, with reduced density of contractile elements (6). This finding implies that recovery of function upon revascularization may not be immediate, since it should wait for reestablishment of normal contractile machinery. These speculations find support in clinical observations. Nienaber et al. (11) analyzed recovery of contractility, flow, and metabolism after PTCA in myocardium perfused through a severely stenotic artery. While flow normalized immediately after PTCA, function and metabolism did not, and recovered over 2 – 3 months. We do not know whether recovery was delayed because hibernating myocardium takes time to readjust itself to the new condition, or whether it was hampered by occurrence of stunning, perhaps induced by PTCA itself. In either case, these data confirm that the clinical scenario may be more complex than anticipated, and that hibernation may often coexist with (or be followed by) a condition of delayed functional recovery, akin to stunning.

References

1. Ambrosio G, Losi MA, Perrone-Filardi P, Betocchi S, Pace L, Soricelli A, Piscione F, Salvatore M, Chiariello M, Weiss JL (1993) Persistence of contractile impairment in the absence of flow abnormalities after exercise: evidence for myocardial stunning in patients with stable angina. Circulation 88: 1–646
2. Ambrosio G et al., Perrone Filardi P (1994) Myocardial hibernation and stunning: what is their practical significance? Myocard Ischemia 6: 19–32
3. Barilla F, Gheorghiade M, Alam M, Khaja F, Goldstein S (1991) Low-dose dobutamine in patients with acute myocardial infarction identifies viable but not contractile myocardium and predicts the magnitude of improvement in wall motion abnormalities in response to coronary revascularization. Am Heart J 122: 1522–1531
4. Bolli R (1993) Myocardial "stunning" in man. Circulation 86: 1671–1691
5. Bolli R, Zhu WX, Myers ML, Hartley CJ, Roberts R (1985) Beta-adrenergic stimulation reverses postischemic myocardial dysfunction without producing subsequent functional deterioration. Am J Cardiol 56: 964–968
6. Borgers M, Ausma J (1995) Structural aspects of the chronic hibernating myocardium in man. Basic Res Cardiol 90: 44–46
7. Homans DC, Laxson DD, Sublett E, Lindstrom P, Bache RJ (1989) Cumulative deterioration of myocardial function after repeated episodes of exercise-induced ischemia. Am J Physiol 256: H1462–H1471
8. Kloner RA, Przyklenk K (1991) Hibernation and stunning of the myocardium. New Engl J Med 325: 1877–1879
9. Kloner RA, Allen J, Cox TA, Zheng Y, Ruiz CE (1991) Stunned left ventricular myocardium after exercise treadmill testing in coronary artery disease. Am J Cardiol 68: 329–334
10. Matsuzaki M, Gallagher KP, Kemper WS, White F, Ross J Jr (1983) Sustained regional dysfunction produced by prolonged coronary stenosis: gradual recovery after reperfusion. Circulation 68: 170–182
11. Nienaber CA, Brunken RC, Sherman CT, Yeatman LA, Gambhir SS, Child JS, Phelps ME, Schelbert HR (1991) Metabolic and functional recovery of ischemic human myocardium after coronary angioplasty. J Am Coll Cardiol 18: 966–978
12. Pierard LA, De Landsheere CM, Berthe C, Rigo P, Kulbertus HE (1990) Identification of viable myocardium by echocardiography during dobutamine infusion in patients with myocardial infarction after thrombolytic therapy: comparison with positron emission tomography. J Am Coll Cardiol 15: 1021–1031
13. Renkin J, Wijns W, Ladha Z, Col J (1990) Reversal of segmental hypokinesis by coronary angioplasty in patients with unstable angina, persistent T wave inversion, and left anterior descending coronary artery stenosis. Additional evidence for myocardial stunning in humans. Circulation 82: 913–921
14. Ross J Jr (1995) Myocardial hibernation, stunning, or both? Basic Res Cardiol 90: 41–43

112–114

R. Ferrari

Commentary on myocardial stunning and its clinical relevance

Key words Myocardial stunning – myocardial ischaemia – myocardial reperfusion

Introduction

Left ventricular dysfunction is in most cases the consequence of myocardial ischaemia. It may occur transiently after a short episode of ischaemia and is usually reversible. It may persist over hours or even days in patients after an episode of ischaemia followed by reperfusion, leading to the so-called condition of stunning (1).

Stunning is defined as a transient left ventricular dysfunction that persists after reperfusion despite the absence of irreversible damage and despite restoration of normal or near normal coronary flow (2). This definition implies that: (a) stunning is a transient, fully reversible abnormality provided that sufficient time is allowed for recovery; (b) stunning is a mild, sublethal injury which must be kept distinct from the irreversible damage occurring in myocardial infarction; and (c) stunned myocardium has a normal or near normal coronary flow. Thus, the hallmark of this condition is the presence of a flow – function "mismatch", with normal flow but abnormal function. This is quite in contrast to the other forms of reversible myocardial dysfunction, such as ischaemia and hibernation, in which depressed flow and function are matched.

A clear definition is desirable and important, but its application to the clinical condition is often problematic. Diagnosis of stunning in patients requires demonstration of two major points: (a) the dysfunctional myocardium has normal or near normal coronary flow; and (b) the contractile abnormality is reversible with time. This implies that it is possible to measure accurately regional myocardial function and blood flow in humans, which obviously is not the case.

To fulfil the second point, before making diagnosis of stunning the physician should allow sufficient time for the myocardium to recover. This suggests myocardial stunning is a well – tolerated condition, and that its diagnosis is important retrospectively but does not imply a decision – making process for clinical management of the patient. It could be argued that in some high-risk situations stunning can become dangerous. In clinical practice stunning is dangerous when the degree and the extent of the left ventricular dysfunction is associated with a low output syndrome. Under these circumstances, however, therapy with inotropic and afterload – reducing agents is a common approach, independently of the diagnosis of stunning (3).

It has been suggested that recognition of stunning may be important in high-risk conditions (such as thrombolysis after acute myocardial infarction and reperfusion after cardiac surgery or transplantation) because the physician could try to prevent it from occurring (3). Experimentally stunning can be prevented by calcium antagonists administered before ischaemia or by anti-oxidants given just before reflow (2). At present no controlled clinical

This work was supported by National Research Council (C.N.R.) – targeted project "Prevention and Control Disease Factors" n. 93.00656. PF 41/115. 19070 and by a CNR target project on "Biotechnology and Bioinstrumentation"

Prof. R. Ferrari (✉)
Cattedra di Cardiologia
Universita' degli Studi di Brescia
c/o Spedali Civili
P. le Spedali Civili, 1
25123 Brescia, Italy

data on the efficacy of these therapies are available. It is also essential to identify the high-risk conditions which need to be treated to avoid unnecessary therapy in a vast population for the benefit of a few patients.

Left ventricular dysfunction due to repetitive stunning

Patients with coronary artery disease experience recurrent episodes of ischaemia, often silent, in the same territory (4). If the myocardium is not able to recover completely between the frequent episodes, its function remains consistently depressed (5). Often recurrent ischaemia is a consequence of recurrent coronary artery spasm (5). Thus some of the chronic alterations in regional function that have been ascribed to hibernation could in fact be caused by stunning, resulting from repetitive episodes of ischaemia (3). For clinical decision making in these patients it is useful to obtain a series of information in addition to the distinction whether the dysfunctioning myocardium is stunned or hibernating. First, it is important to establish whether the dysfunctioning myocardium is viable, and whether it is normally perfused or hypoperfused. Second, it is useful to test the contractile reserve of the akinetic myocardium. Third, and perhaps more importantly, it is essential to establish by coronary angiography whether the perfusion defect is susceptible to interventional or pharmacological correction. All this information allows correct management of the left ventricular dysfunction, independently of whether it is the result of stunning or hibernation.

Stunning after angioplasty and resolution of coronary artery spasm

In our experience this is a rare phenomenon, probably in relation to the short period of regional ischaemia occurring under these conditions. The available evidence agrees that reperfusion in the setting of PTCA or of Prinzmetal's angina is well tolerated and usually does not cause postischaemic systolic dysfunction. Angioplasty may induce diastolic abnormalities resulting in a transient decrease in left ventricular compliance. This abnormality, however, is usually well tolerated.

Stunning after acute myocardial infarction and unstable angina

The studies assessing recovery of left ventricular function in acute myocardial infarction after thrombolysis and/or PTCA uniformly suggest a delayed improvement (7 – 10 days) after reperfusion (6). The severity of the residual stenosis appears to be an important determinant of the rate of recovery after thrombolytic therapy (7).

Postischaemic left ventricular dysfunction is also likely to occur in patients with acute myocardial infarction who have not been treated with thrombolysis or PTCA, as coronary reperfusion may occur spontaneously. Similarly, stunning is likely in patients with unstable angina, as this syndrome is caused by transient episodes of severe ischaemia and reperfusion, not associated with irreversible damage (8). Both these conditions have been associated with reversible wall motion abnormalities which could reflect stunning. However, the same abnormalities could also be caused by hibernation, ongoing silent ischaemia or both. Unfortunately, appropriate controlled studies monitoring the time course of the ventricular dysfunction and coronary flow are still lacking.

During acute myocardial infarction it is not uncommon to observe ventricular dysfunction which in turn causes a mitral incompetence. A test with echocardiography and increasing doses of dobutamine may be important. If dobutamine improves function without causing further ischaemia, the dysfunctioning myocardium is probably well perfused and therefore likely to be stunned. Transient administration of a positive inotropic agent causes a clear and substained improvement of ventricular function with resolution of the valvular dysfunction and improvement in global ejection fraction.

Stunning after open heart surgery

There is a consensus that a transient depression of myocardial function is common after cardiopulmonary bypass (3, 6). Probably the surgeons were aware of this possibility long before the description of stunning, as they successfully used calcium or positive inotropic agents to stimulate those hearts having difficulty in recovering after reperfusion despite the absence of evidence of myocardial necrosis. Most likely the stunning is consequent on a period of global and total ischaemia. This type of ventricular dysfunction is reversible within 24 – 48 h in most cases.

We have demonstrated that, as in the case of thrombolysis, the dysfunction is related to the duration of the previous ischaemic period and to the degree of oxidative stress occurring on reperfusion (9).

It has been suggested that postsurgical stunning in subgroups of high-risk patients with poor preoperative ventricular function, prolonged aortic cross-clamping time, or with unstable angina before surgery, could have adverse effects on morbidity and mortality. Clinical trials are in progress regarding the possibilities of preventing stunning (with calcium antagonist and antioxidants) under these conditions. It must be considered, however, that the high operative risk of such patients may be also related to the higher incidence of reversible damage during the operation.

Finally, stunning could also develop in the course of cardiac transplantation as the heart is subjected to prolonged ischaemia followed by reperfusion. There is considerable and largely anecdotal evidence that cardiac function is reversibly depressed in the first hours or days after transplantation, but controlled studies have not been performed.

Studies with two-dimensional echocardiography after treadmill testing suggest the occurrence of left ventricular dysfunction persisting after the resolution of chest pain and of the electrocardiographic abnormalities (10). The degree of the wall motion abnormalities seems to be correlated to the intensity and duration of exercise, severity and extension of coronary artery disease and sympathetic stimulation (10). These observations have been extended only to 30 min after exercise. It follows that the abnormalities could also be the consequence of subendocardial ischaemia rather than to a classical stunning and, in any case, seem to be well tolerated.

We examined the occurrence of stunning after 2 h from the exercise test (6) and found that it is a very uncommon phenomenon. When present, however, it has important prognostic implication as a reflection of severe and extensive coronary artery disease.

Acknowledgement The authors thank Miss Roberta Bonetti for the secretarial assistance in preparing the manuscript.

References

1. Braunwald E, Kloner RA (1992) The stunned myocardium: Prolonged, postischemic ventricular dysfunction. Circulation 66: 1146–1149
2. Bolli R (1990) Mechanism of myocardial "stunning". Circulation 82: 723–738
3. Bolli R (1993) Myocardial stunning in man. Circulation 86: 1671–1691
4. Fuster V, Badimon L, Badimon JJ, Chesebro JH (1992) The pathogenesis of coronary artery disease and the acute coronary syndromes. N Engl J Med 326: 242–250, 310–318
5. Gottlieb SO, Weisfeldt ML, Ouyang P, Mellits ED, Gerstenblith G (1986) Silent ischemia as a marker for early unfavorable outcomes in patients with unstable angina. N Engl J Med 314: 1214–1219
6. Ferrari R, La Canna G, Giubbini R, Milan E, Ceconi C, de Giuli F, Berra P, Alfieri O, Visioli O (1994) Left ventricular dysfunction due to stunning and hibernation in patients. Cardiovasc Drugs Ther 8: 371–380
7. Patel B, Kloner RA, Przyklenk K, Braunwald E (1988) Postischemic myocardial "stunning": a clinically relevant phenomenon. Ann Intern Med 108: 626–628
8. Braunwald E (1989) Unstable angina: a classification. Circulation 80: 410–414
9. Ferrari R, Alfieri O, Curello S, Ceconi C, Cargnoni A, Marzollo P, Pardini A, Caradonna E, Visioli O (1990) Occurrence of oxidative stress during reperfusion of the human heart. Circulation 81: 201–211
10. Homans DC, Laxson DD, Sublett E, Pavek T, Crampton M (1991) Effect of exercise intensity and duration on regional function during and after exercise-induced ischemia. Circulation 83: 2029–2037

115–116
© Steinkopff Verlag 1996

L. H. Opie

Chronic stunning: The new switch in thought

Key words Stunning – ischemia – hibernation – calcium

One picture may be worth a thousand words, as they say, but I was asked to write the thousand words and not to provide the picture. My major point can in fact be made in even fewer words. Despite the unanimous acceptance of the standard definition of stunning (1), it appears that this includes vastly different experimental and clinical conditions. Regarding the definition – according to Bolli (1), it is a state in which myocardial blood flow is fully restored following prior ischemia and during which time myocardial mechanical function is depressed. A further feature is that there is no evidence of myocardial necrosis.

The range of experimental conditions covered by this definition is demonstrated by Lavellee et al. (7) who showed progressive recovery following 1 h of coronary artery occlusion in a dog, and a state of stunning lasting at least 2 weeks. As expected with such prolonged periods of ischemia, where there must be some necrosis, mechanical recovery was incomplete. Presumably, however, there was no necrosis in the segments that did recover. In contrast, Du Toit and Opie (4) used an isolated rat heart model with 20 min of global ischemia in which stunning lasted for only about 1 h. Other workers using dog models (11) have described intermediate durations of stunning of some hours, even following a short period of coronary occlusion such as 15 min.

Prof. L. H. Opie (✉)
Heart Research Unit
University of Cape Town
Medical School
Observatory
7925 Cape Town, South Africa

Likewise, clinical stunning may last for only short periods, such as following the severe ischemia caused by balloon inflation during angioplasty which causes transient diastolic dysfunction (8). It is likely that the transient dysfunction observed after an attack of angina pectoris also falls into the short-term category of stunning. At the other extreme is prolonged ischemia over hours, days and possibly weeks following thrombolytic therapy or cardioplegic bypass (3, 8).

In principle it seems unlikely that the same processes would be at work in a short-term, self-correcting phenomenon as in a more complex, long-term, and only partially self-remedying phenomenon. It therefore seems appropriate to distinguish between acute short-term and chronic long-term stunning.

Acute short-term stunning

Short-term ischemia, such as that of 15 – 20 min, is followed by acute short-term stunning in a variety of animal models. There is no question that recovery is quick and can be hastened by a variety of interventions, including the use of calcium antagonists (4), a sodium/proton inhibitor (5), and a host of free radical scavengers (2, 6). The relative merits of the "calcium hypothesis" and the "free radical hypothesis" were intensely debated earlier until it was realized that these are not mutually exclusive. For example, calcium overload can cause mitochondrial damage which in turn promotes the formation of free radicals. Conversely, excess free radicals can interact with the calcium release channel of the sarcoplasmic reticulum, again causing excess release of calcium. In the end, it is clear that abnormalities of calcium ion control must be the ultimate signal responsible for certain aspects of reperfusion injury, such as reperfusion arrhythmias, but this does not necessarily rule out a role for free radicals in the genesis of the cytosolic calcium overload.

Despite a vast amount of experimental work there is as yet no compound that can be given to patients with the specific therapeutic aim of lessening acute stunning.

Because stunning is so extremely varied in its form of clinical expression (2), it is perhaps unrealistic even to think of trials with stunning as an end-point in patients. The one exception is post-cardioplegic stunning, a definite and clearcut entity that needs much more active investigation. It is probably in this type of short-term stunning that the first agents to be approved for human use will appear.

Chronic long-term stunning

In chronic long-term stunning, substantial left ventricular remodeling occurs over a period of days or weeks, with altered protein synthesis likely to play a role. Here the concept of Schaper (9) is attractive. He proposed that acute ischemia can induce altered gene expression by a variety of processes. The postulated initiating factors are release of catecholamines and/or nonspecific damage to the sarcolemma and sarcoplasmic reticulum. The role of long-term protective substances has been taken further by the work of Yellon's group in relation to heat shock proteins. The concept of these workers is that similar metabolic changes can provoke a "second window of opportunity" occurring about 1 day after a brief period of preconditioning ischemia (1).

It is this prolonged recovery from ischemia, probably involving protein metabolism and protective proteins, that appears to explain the delayed recovery of left ventricular function following thrombolysis.

Chronic stunning may explain hibernation

Even more surprising is the role of repetitive short term ischemia in causing chronic stunning, and preliminary evidence suggests that the latter may explain at least some aspects of hibernation. Experimentally, Shen and Vatner (10) used chronic coronary stenosis in conscious pigs, in which episodes of excitement precipitated ischemia followed by prolonged periods of ventricular mechanical dysfunction, although the resting coronary flow was normal. Some observers feel that this finding rules out true hibernation, which in their view is characterized by a chronic although mild reduction in coronary blood flow. Nevertheless, also in man hibernation may be accompanied by virtually normal coronary blood flow and largely unchanged glucose metabolism (12): "Despite nearly normal resting flow and oxygen consumption, these collateral-dependent segments exhibit chronically depressed wall motion and demonstrate marked ultrastructural alterations on morphological analysis." The concept of repetitive ischemia causing prolonged stunning and masquerading as hibernation therefore becomes attractive. The clue to the altered way of thinking is the new possibility that stunning may be chronic.

References

1. Baxter GF, Marber MS, Patel VC, Yellon DM (1994) Adenosine receptor involvement in a delayed phase of myocardial protection 24 hours after ischemic preconditioning. Circulation 90: 2993–3000
2. Bolli R (1990) Mechanism of myocardial "stunning". Circulation 82: 723–738
3. Braunwald E (1990) The stunned myocardium: newer insights into mechanisms and clinical applications. J Thorac Cardiovasc Surg 100: 310–311
4. Du Toit EF, Opie LH (1992) Modulation of severity of reperfusion stunning in the isolated rat heart by agents altering calcium flux at onset of reperfusion. Circ Res 70: 960–967
5. Du Toit EF, Opie LH (1994) Inhibitors of Ca^{2+}-ATPase pump of sarcoplasmic reticulum attenuate reperfusion stunning in isolated rat heart. J Cardiovasc Pharmacol 24: 678–684
6. Hearse DJ (1991) Stunning: a radical review. Cardiovasc Drugs Ther 5: 853–876
7. Lavallee M, Cox D, Patrick TA, Vatner SF (1983) Salvage of myocardial function by coronary artery reperfusion 1, 2 and 3 hours after occlusion in conscious dogs. Circ Res 53: 235–247
8. Patel B, Kloner RA, Przyklenk K, Braunwald E (1988) Postischemic myocardial "stunning": a clinically relevant phenomenon. Ann Intern Med 108: 626–628
9. Schaper W (1991) Molecular mechanisms in "stunned" myocardium. Cardiovasc Drugs Ther 5: 925–932
10. Shen Y-T, Vatner SF (1995) Mechanism of impaired myocardial function during progressive coronary stenosis in conscious pigs. Hibernation versus stunning? Circ Res 76: 479–488
11. Triana JF, Li XY, Jamaluddin U, Thornby JI, Bolli R (1991) Postischemic myocardial "stunning". Identification of major differences between the open-chest and the conscious dog and evaluation of the oxygen radical hypothesis in the conscious dog. Circ Res 69: 731–747
12. Vanoverschelde J-L, Wijns W, Depre C, Essamri B, Heyndrickx GR, Borgers M, Bol A, Melin JA (1993) Mechanisms of chronic regional post-ischemic dysfunction in humans. New insights from the study of noninfarcted collateral-dependent myocardium. Circulation 87: 1513–1523

Ischemic Preconditioning

119 – 122

K. A. Reimer
R. B. Jennings

Ischemic preconditioning: a brief review

Key words Myocardial ischemia – reperfusion – infarct size – ischemic energy metabolism – protein kinase C – K^{+}_{ATP}-channels

Background and definition(s)

Myocardium which has been subjected to one or several brief period(s) of ischemia, of insufficient duration to cause myocyte necrosis, rapidly (within minutes) develops markedly increased resistance to myocyte injury when subjected to a subsequent episode of ischemia. This rapid adaptation to ischemic stress was first described and termed "ischemic preconditioning" (10) based on studies in which a 40-min test episode of ischemia in dogs was preceded by four 5-min episodes of ischemia, each separated by 5 min of reperfusion. Infarct size in the preconditioned dogs was only 25 % of the size expected from a simple 40-min test episode of ischemia followed by reperfusion. We subsequently observed a similar marked limitation of infarct size using a single 15-min episode of ischemia prior to a 40-min test episode. Similar cardioprotection can be observed using a 60-min test episode. Ischemic preconditioning has been observed in several species in addition to dogs, including rats, rabbits, and pigs. Clinical studies suggest that it most likely occurs in patients with ischemic heart disease (23).

It should be noted that subsequent reports have extended the use of the term "ischemic preconditioning" to include several endpoints in addition to the originally described phenomenon of infarct limitation in intact animals. Thus, it has been reported that preconditioning protects against dysrhythmias, post-ischemic contractile dysfunction in isolated, perfused rat or rabbit hearts, autonomic nerve dysfunction, and microvascular dysfunction. However, our discussion of ischemic preconditioning will emphasize results relating to its infarct-limiting facet. However, it should be noted that until the mechanism(s) underlying all facets of ischemic preconditioning is known, it cannot be assumed that the mechanism of each facet is the same.

The adaptive response to preconditioning occurs quickly (within minutes as demonstrated in the aforementioned protocols) but is relatively short lived. If the duration of reperfusion between preconditioning and the sustained 40- or 60-min test period of ischemia is increased to 2 h, the protective effect is largely lost (12). Recent evidence suggests that there may be a slower adaptive response which also is initiated by preconditioning ischemia which results in a second window of protection ("SWOP") detectable in some experimental models at 24 h (7). The cardioprotection seen in the SWOP phenomenon is not as great and probably is explained by a molecular mechanism which is different from that of the early, classic preconditioning response.

Substantial progress has been made toward elucidation of the mechanism of the early preconditioning response by work in a large number of laboratories. These studies have focused on 1) the possible signaling pathway(s) through which rapid adaptation to ischemic stress occurs,

Dr. K. A. Reimer (✉) · R. B. Jennings
Department of Pathology
Box 3712
Duke University Medical Center
Durham, NC 27710, USA

and 2) identification of the resultant intracellular changes which make myocytes more resistant to ischemic injury.

Reduced energy demand

In regard to the second aspect, our studies have shown that the protective effect in dogs is associated with a marked slowing of the rate of energy metabolism (11). We observed that dogs with repeated 10-min episodes of ischemia had a much slower rate of decline of ATP and a much slower production of purine nucleosides and bases during later ischemic episodes vs. the first episode (15). Moreover, we observed that both the rate of ATP depletion and the rate of accumulation of purine nucleosides and bases and catabolites of anaerobic glycolysis during a sustained 40-min period of ischemia occurred much more slowly during ischemia following ischemic preconditioning (11). These metabolic changes were not explained by an increase in collateral blood flow. That ATP depletion occurs more slowly, despite the fact that high energy phosphate (HEP) production via anaerobic glycolysis must also be slowed, indicates a marked reduction in high energy phosphate utilization during ischemia following ischemic preconditioning.

The metabolic slowing that we have observed in dogs also has been observed by others in a variety of animal species. In pigs, preconditioning slows both the rate of ATP utilization and the rate of development of intra- and extracellular acidosis (3, 5). In rat hearts studied either in vivo or in vitro, preconditioning has been reported by several groups to result in a reduction of tissue acidosis and in glycogen utilization during the prolonged ischemic test period (1, 22). Thus, preservation of ATP despite depressed glycogen utilization is a common feature of the preconditioned state whether studied in hearts of large or small animal species, and whether studied during regional ischemia, in vivo, or total ischemia, in vitro in canine myocardium. Recently, it was reported that preconditioning attenuated the rate of ATP loss during ischemia of human myocardium, based on sequential biopsies obtained following repeated brief episodes of global ischemia (preceding coronary bypass surgery) (23).

The cause of the reduced rate of HEP utilization is uncertain but current information can be summarized as follows:

First, we have observed that, although preconditioned myocardium is concurrently "stunned", the energy sparing effect of preconditioning is not related to the reduction in contractile force at the onset of the test episode of ischemia (12). Secondly, although the mitochondrial ATPase is a major cause of ATP depletion during ischemia, and would be even more important in large mammalian species such as dogs and humans if not for the presence of an endogenous inhibitor, the energy sparing effect of preconditioning is not due to earlier inhibition of this reaction (20). Thirdly, since adrenergic stimulation of myocardium increases myocardial metabolism, ischemic preconditioning could occur through an anti-adrenergic mechanism (21). One hypothetical scenario involves the release of adenosine from ischemic myocytes during the preconditioning episode of ischemia. Adenosine, through activation of an inhibitory G protein (G_i), both inhibits exocytotic release of norepinephrine from cardiac nerve endings and counteracts, in cardiac myocytes, the stimulatory effect of β-adrenergic receptor stimulation on adenylate cyclase and hence on protein kinase A-dependent reactions. There is evidence both for and against this scenario (21). Yet another hypothesis to explain both the cardioprotective and metabolic effects of ischemic preconditioning involves ATP-dependent K^+ (K^+_{ATP}) channels (4). It has been proposed that preconditioning may accelerate or enhance the opening of these channels. Activation of K^+_{ATP} channels does occur during ischemia. The decrease in ATP opens the channel and results in an efflux of potassium which decreases the duration of the plateau phase of the cardiac action potential. Thus, the time during which inward flux of Ca^{++} occurs is shortened. This decreases contractile effort, and at the subcellular level reduces the amount of high energy phosphate required to support cellular Ca^{++} cycling. The K^+_{ATP} channel is the second most abundant channel present in the sarcolemma and there is substantial evidence from several laboratories supporting the hypothesis that the mechanism of preconditioning involves either opening of more channels or sustained opening of these channels.

Possible signaling mechanisms

Possible signaling mechanisms through which ischemic preconditioning could be coupled to its metabolic and infarct-limiting effects have been extensively investigated in rodents. The preponderance of recent evidence suggests that the mechanism of preconditioning may involve activation of the protein kinase C (PKC) regulatory pathway (2). Activation of phospholipase C or phospholipase D in the cell membrane leads to the formation of the second messenger, diacylglycerol (DAG). DAG activates protein kinase C (PKC) which phosphorylates a variety of other cellular proteins, with diverse functions (13). A growing number of isoforms of PKC have been identified. At least four different isoforms are present in cardiac muscle, including α, δ, ε and zeta. The activation of PKC occurs through the translocation of the enzyme from the cytosol to the cell membrane via microtubules (17). Several surface receptors are known to induce activation of cardiac PKC, including α_1-adrenergic, muscarinic, endothelin, angiotensin II, and adenosine A_1 receptors (17). Many proteins are phosphorylated by PKC and such phosphorylation modulates the activities of several enzyme systems including adenylate cyclase, L-type calcium channels, the Na^+/Ca^{++} exchanger, AMP deaminase and at least one K^+ channel. Whether and how PKC also modulates the activity of the K^+_{ATP} channel is less clear. It is known that these channels are coupled via a G_1 protein to the adenosine A_1 receptor and to myocardial muscarinic receptors.

Several pathways modulated by the PLC-PKC system, such as sensitization of adenylate cyclase (18), would likely increase, rather than decrease energy utilization. In addition, phospholipase C produces not only diacyl glycerol (DAG), but another second messenger, inositol triphosphate (IP3), which is known to enhance calcium mobilization. Thus, it is not known if or how the consequences of activating the PLC-PKC pathway might result in reduced ischemic metabolism and consequent cardioprotection.

Nevertheless, it has been reported that preconditioning episodes of ischemia are sufficient to induce the translocation and activation of PKC in rat or rabbit hearts (9, 24). Ischemic preconditioning and direct activators of PKC both limit myocardial infarct size, and the infarct-limiting effects of both preconditioning and direct PKC activators could be blocked by inhibitors of PKC (6, 16, 19, 24). In contrast, some studies of the possible role of PKC activation in the mechanism of ischemic preconditioning in large animal models have had negative results (14).

Clinical implications

The results of many clinical studies support the now generally accepted view that morbidity and mortality from myocardial infarction are related directly to the size of a myocardial infarct. Thus, elucidation of mechanisms of ischemic injury has important clinical ramifications in that such knowledge should permit the development of methods to delay the onset of irreversibility that could be applied as adjunctive therapy pending reperfusion. That ischemic preconditioning does result in slower injury during a subsequent period of ischemia is proof that the process of ischemic injury can be delayed.

The phenomenon of preconditioning may have clinical implications in the following respects: First, it is possible that patients who suffer a sustained coronary occlusion after one or more brief episodes of ischemia (e.g. as might occur in unstable, preinfarction angina), may undergo infarction in a setting of spontaneous preconditioning. In such patients, infarction should develop more slowly than occurs following an abrupt occlusion. Second, if the mechanism of preconditioning can be elucidated, it might prove possible to exploit this knowledge to develop pharmacologic agents which mimic the preconditioning response. Such therapy could be used to enhance cardioplegia for myocardial protection during surgery, or to delay myocardial injury in patients with acute myocardial infarction, pending reperfusion. Although these clinical possibilities remain speculative, it must be emphasized that in experimental models, ischemic preconditioning has been consistently reproducible and that this endogenous cardioprotective mechanism has more potent infarct-limiting efficacy than any of a myriad of pharmacologic interventions tested to date as possible adjuncts to early reperfusion (8).

References

1. Asimakis GK, Inners-McBride K, Medellin G, Conti VR (1992) Ischemic preconditioning attenuates acidosis and postischemic dysfunction in isolated rat heart. Am J Physiol 263: H887–H894
2. Bogoyevitch MA, Parker PJ, Sugden PH (1993) Characterization of protein kinase C isotype expression in adult rat heart. Protein kinase C-epsilon is a major isotype present, and it is activated by phorbol esters, epinephrine and endothelin. Circ Res 72: 757–767
3. Fleet WF, Johnson TA, Graebner CA, Gettes LS (1985) Effect of serial brief ischemic episodes on extracellular K^+, pH, and activation in the pig. Circulation 72: 922–932
4. Hearse DJ (1995) Activation of ATP-sensitive potassium channels: A novel pharmacological approach to myocardial protection? (Review). Cardiovasc Res 30: 1–17
5. Kida M, Fujiwara H, Ishida M, Kawai C, Ohura M, Miura I, Yabuuchi Y (1991) Ischemic preconditioning preserves creatine phosphate and intracellular pH. Circulation 84: 2495–2503
6. Liu Y, Ytrehus K, Downey JM (1994) Evidence that translocation of protein kinase C is a key event during ischemic preconditioning of rabbit myocardium. J Mol Cell Cardiol 26: 661–668
7. Marber MS, Latchman DS, Walker JM, Yellon DM (1994) Cardiac stress protein elevation 24 hours after brief ischemia or heat stress is associated with resistance to myocardial infarction. Circulation 1264: 1272

8. Marber M, Walker D, Yellon D (1994) Editorial. Ischaemic preconditioning. Br Med J 308: 1–2
9. Mitchell MB, Meng X, Ao L, Brown JM, Harken AH, Banerjee A (1995) Preconditioning of isolated rat heart is mediated by protein kinase C. Circ Res 76: 73–81
10. Murry CE, Jennings RB, Reimer KA (1986) Preconditioning with ischemia: A delay of lethal cell injury in ischemic myocardium. Circulation 74: 1124–1136
11. Murry CE, Richard VJ, Reimer KA, Jennings RB (1990) Ischemic preconditioning slows energy metabolism and delays ultrastructural damage during a sustained ischemic episode. Circ Res 66: 913–931
12. Murry CE, Richard VJ, Jennings RB, Reimer KA (1991) Myocardial protection is lost before contractile function recovers from ischemic preconditioning. Am J Physiol (Heart Circ Physiol) 260: H796–H804
13. Nishizuka Y (1992) Intracellular signaling by hydrolysis of phospholipids and activation of protein kinase C. Science 258: 607–614
14. Przyklenk K, Sussman MA, Simkhovich BZ, Kloner RA (1995) Does ischemic preconditioning trigger translocation of protein kinase C in the canine model? Circulation 92: 1546–1557
15. Reimer KA, Murry CE, Yamasawa I, Hill ML, Jennings RB (1986) Four brief periods of myocardial ischemia cause no cumulative ATP loss or necrosis. Am J Physiol 251: H1306–H1315
16. Speechly-Dick ME, Mocanu MM, Yellon DM (1994) Protein Kinase C: Its role in ischemic preconditioning in the rat. Circ Res 75: 586–590
17. Stable S, Parker PJ (1991) Protein kinase C. Pharmacol Ther 51: 71–95
18. Strasser RH, Braun-Dullaeus R, Walendzik H, Marquetant R (1992) α_1-Receptor-independent activation of protein kinase C in acute myocardial ischemia: Mechanisms for sensitization of the adenylyl cyclase system. Circ Res 70: 1304–1312
19. Tsuchida A, Liu Y, Liu GS, Cohen MV, Downey JM (1994) α_1-adrenergic agonists precondition rabbit ischemic myocardium independent of adenosine by direct activation of protein kinase C. Circ Res 75: 576–585
20. Vander Heide RS, Hill ML, Reimer KA, Jennings RB (1996) Effect of reversible ischemia on the activity of the mitochondrial ATPase: Relationship to ischemic preconditioning. J Mol Cell Cardiol (in press)
21. Vander Heide RS, Schwartz LM, Jennings RB, Reimer KA (1995) Effect of catecholamine depletion on infarct size in dogs. Role of catecholamines in ischemic preconditioning. Cardiovasc Res 30: 656–667
22. Wolfe CL, Sievers RE, Visseren FL, Donnelly TJ (1993) Loss of myocardial protection after preconditioning correlates with the time course of glycogen recovery within the preconditioned segment. Circulation 87: 881–892
23. Yellon DM, Alkhulaifi AM, Pugsley WB (1993) Preconditioning the human myocardium. Lancet 342: 276–277
24. Ytrehus K, Liu Y, Downey JM (1994) Preconditioning protects ischemic rabbit heart by protein kinase C activation. Am J Physiol 266: H1145–H1152

123–125

L. M. King
L. H. Opie

Preconditioning – a reappraisal of protection

Key words Preconditioning – ischemia – reperfusion – necrosis

Preconditioning – not always beneficial?

Preconditioning has been described as the most potent form of protection against myocardial necrosis yet described (5). The protection conferred by preconditioning has been found against most of the deleterious effects induced by ischaemia and reperfusion, and in most animal models as well as in humans. While preconditioning undoubtedly delays infarct development, and offers intriguing mechanisms of endogenous protection, a word of caution is required before assuming that preconditioning could be the basis of a new-found therapy for patients. We attempt to take a critical look at the literature and to emphasise that the reduction of infarct size, often praised as an important consequence of preconditioning, has two important limitations. First, it is a delay in the development of necrosis that is achieved; thus preconditioning buys time but does not cheat death. Secondly, almost all the models used in the studies of infarct size reduction use regional ischaemia followed by reperfusion, so that the benefits of preconditioning could have occurred in either the ischaemic or in the reperfusion period, which is an important distinction. We will emphasise that preconditioning can have different end-points, and that not all of its effects are favourable. Specifically, there may be adverse effects during the ischaemic period, which differ from those on reperfusion.

Dr. L. King (✉) · Dr. L. Opie
Medical Research Council
University of Cape Town
Ischaemic Heart Disease Research Unit
Observatory
7925 Cape Town, South Africa

The mechanism of preconditioning – no consensus after 10 years of research

Many proposals as to the mechanism of preconditioning have been made, without consensus being reached. Many diverse routes to preconditioning have been proposed, including limitation of glycolysis, maintenance of high-energy phosphate compounds, enhanced activity of ATP-sensitive potassium channels, and increased activity of the inhibitory G protein (5), besides an extensive literature implicating adenosine and protein kinase C activity. Although the role of adenosine has been well studied, and it was one of the first major hypotheses for preconditioning, it can be eliminated as the mechanism in the rat (2), and it therefore cannot be the universal mediator. Another tenable hypothesis involves protein kinase C translocation. However, the particular isoenzyme involved has not been identified; each may have very different actions and different responses to preconditioning ischaemia. Thus in the absence of any agreed single mechanism it becomes important to examine carefully the experimental conditions chosen for the various studies and to understand their limitations.

Variability of protection

A major problem with attaining a consensus on preconditioning is reproducibility. Some authors claim that preconditioning is highly reproducible and very protective; others find the results so variable and that to obtain a consistent model, a number of different protocols must be tested. Such an attempt has been described by Weselcouch et al. (12) who reported that four episodes of preconditioning each of 5 min ischaemia followed by 5 min reperfusion were required, before any noticeable protection could be achieved. This is in contrast to previous reports using rat hearts, which suggested that one episode of ischaemia was as efficacious as two episodes (1).

Indices of protection – infarct size vs stunning and functional recovery

A major point of difficulty lies in the choice of end points. Preconditioning was originally shown to reduce infarct size by 75 % compared to control hearts (6). This observation has been confirmed in many subsequent studies and is indeed the most consistent, and most potent effect of preconditioning. While a reduction in infarct size is very important, in the context of the shorter laboratory experiment, recovery of function has generally been used. Preconditioning can be said to delay the time to onset of necrosis such that at any given time during the sustained ischaemic period (between onset of injury and final development of total necrosis) if the heart is reperfused, recovery of function would be expected to be greater because of a smaller infarct (see Fig. 1). The results, however, have been very contradictory.

Preconditioning does not protect against stunning, the reversible component of injury, but rather delays the development of necrosis (4). A possible point of confusion lies in the definition of functional recovery. Stunning is defined as a transient postischaemic condition in which the cells have full viability, but are poorly functioning. This is usually associated with reperfusion after short term ischaemia. Once there is a component of irreversible injury, as after long-term ischaemia, then preconditioning may be more protective.

However, in larger animals (pigs and dogs), no improvement in recovery of function with preconditioning has been reported to our knowledge, despite a significant reduction in infarct size. Preconditioning prior to short periods of ischaemia (15 min coronary occlusion) showed no benefit on functional recovery (7). Shizukuda et al. used a 60-min period of coronary occlusion, and showed that segment shortening during reperfusion was not improved by ischaemic preconditioning, despite a reduced ultimate infarct size (10). Some studies in rabbits found no improvement in functional recovery (11) despite reduced infarct size after 30 min ischaemia (a time which would be expected to induce at least some necrosis). Other studies have recorded improved function in rabbits (3), but after 5 to 20 min sustained coronary occlusion, which would be expected to produce more stunning and less necrosis. We

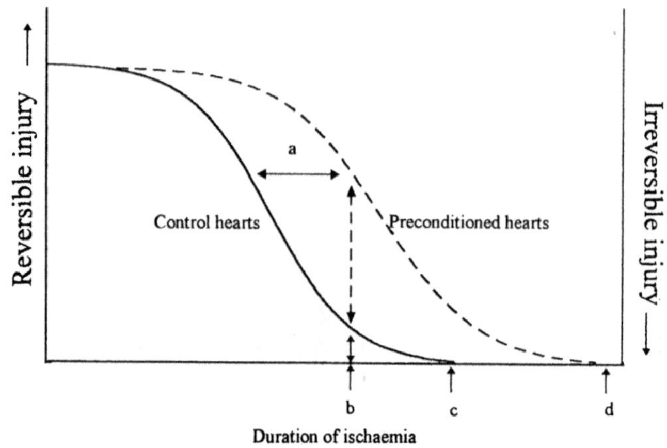

Fig. 1A Effect of preconditioning on degree of residual function in the tissue with duration of ischaemia, as a ratio of reversible to irreversible injury
a – rightward shift in preconditioned hearts of protection against irreversible injury
b – at point b residual function is much greater in preconditioned hearts
c – at point c control hearts have no residual function, with total infarction
d – at point d the duration of tolerated ischaemia has increased but preconditioned hearts end up with the same degree of infarction as control hearts.

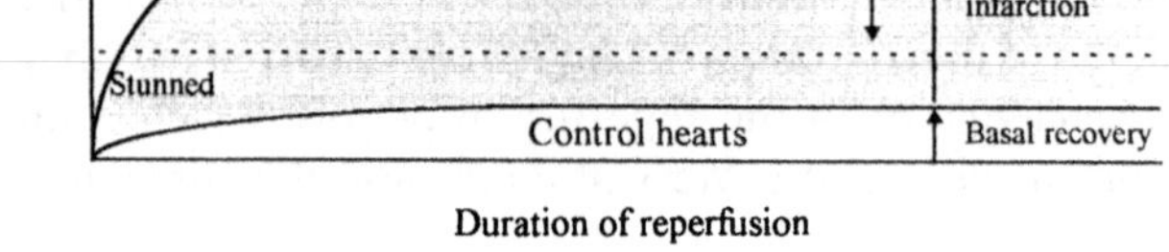

Fig. 1B Persumed recovery of function if control or preconditioned hearts are reperfused at point b. There would still be a component of stunned myocardium, which may not be affected by preconditioning. If overall functional recovery is improved, this may be attributed to reduced infarction; alternatively, if infarct size is reduced, there should be better recovery of function. However, this does not always hold true, and raises concerns as to the validity of preconditioning as a therapy.

have found that preconditioning is not always protective against reperfusion mechanical dysfunction in a rat heart model. Thus, unlike the effects on infarct size, preconditioning does not consistently induce benefits on postischaemic mechanical function.

Ischaemic contracture

The importance of the end-point selected for preconditioning is emphasised by the finding that preconditioning exacerbates ischaemic contracture (1) even when functional recovery is improved. Infarct size is generally measured after a period of reperfusion, which implies that both the components of ischaemia and reperfusion injury are present. Preconditioning may actually exacerbate ischaemic injury by increased contracture, but be beneficial in reperfusion by stimulation of the Na/H exchanger (8). The mechanism for this difference may lie in the following speculative sequences:

1) the preconditioning ischaemic period depletes the heart of glycogen
2) ischaemic contracture is therefore more likely to occur
3) the mechanism may involve inhibition of the sodium pump, which would explain the increased cell sodium values found by Ramasamy et al. (8)
4) in the reperfusion period sodium and proton exchange is enhanced, so that calcium-mediated necrosis would be diminished and the ultimate infarct size after reperfusion would be less.

Effects in absence of full reperfusion

Reduction in infarct size can be found even in the apparent absence of reperfusion, when there is an initial period of total ischaemia followed by low flow ischaemia (9). Two comments are appropriate: firstly, the low flow ischaemia does represent reperfusion when compared with no flow; secondly, during the subsequent low flow ischaemia there was a substantially reduced work index which could have contributed to infarct size reduction.

Concluding comments

While the undoubted benefits of preconditioning on reduction of infarct size after reperfusion are important, it would be prudent to maintain a degree of circumspection because of the variability of the protocol and the differing results according to the end-points chosen. Preconditioning is not always beneficial, and may have some detrimental effects especially in the ischaemic as opposed to the reperfusion period. Thus there should be due care in extrapolating from experiments to any possible clinical application.

References

1. Asimakis GK, Inners-McBride K, Medellin G, Conti VR (1992) Ischemic preconditioning attenuates acidosis and postischemic dysfunction in isolated rat heart. Am J Physiol 263: H887–H894
2. Cave AC, Collis CS, Downey JM, Hearse DJ (1993) Improved functional recovery by ischaemic preconditioning is not mediated by adenosine in the globally ischaemic isolated rat heart. Cardiovasc Res 27: 663–668
3. Cohen MV, Liu GS, Downey J (1991) Preconditioning causes improved wall motion as well as smaller infarcts after transient coronary occlusion in rabbits. Circulation 84: 341–349
4. Jenkins DP, Pugsley WB, Yellon DM (1995) Ischaemic preconditioning in a model of global ischaemia: infarct size limitation, but no reduction in stunning. J Moll Cell Cardiol 27: 1623–1632
5. Lawson CS, Downey JM (1993) Preconditioning: state of the art myocardial protection. Cardiovasc Res 27: 542–550
6. Murry CE, Jennings RB, Reimer KA (1986) Preconditioning with ischaemia: a delay of lethal cell injury in ischaemic myocardium. Circulation 74: 1124–1136
7. Ovize M, Pryzklenk K, Hale SL, Kloner R (1992) Preconditioning does not attenuate myocardial stunning. Circulation 85: 2247–2254
8. Ramasamy R, Liu H, Anderson S, Lundmark J, Schaefer S (1995) Ischemic preconditioning stimulates sodium and proton transport in isolated rat hearts. J Clin Invest 96: 1464–1472
9. Schulz R, Post H, Sakka S, Wallbridge DR, Heusch G (1995) Intraischemic preconditioning. Increased tolerance to sustained low-flow ischaemia by a brief episode of no-flow ischaemia without intermittent reperfusion. Circ Res 76: 942–950
10. Shizukuda Y, Mallet RT, Lee SC, Downey HF (1992) Hypoxic preconditioning of ischaemic canine myocardium. Cardiovasc Res 26: 534–542
11. Thornton J, Striplin S, Liu GS, Swafford A, Stanley AWH, Van Winkle DM, Downey JM (1990) Inhibition of protein synthesis does not block myocardial protection afforded by preconditioning. Am J Physiol 259: H1822–H1825
12. Weselcouch EO, Baird AJ, Sleph PG, Dzwonczyk S, Murray HN, Grover GJ (1995) Endogenous catecholamines are not necessary for ischaemic preconditioning in the isolated perfused rat heart. Cardiovasc Res 29: 126–132

126 – 129

W. Schaper

Ischemic preconditioning, remembrances of things past and future

Key words Adenosine – Insulin-like growth factor – heatshock proteins – K^+-Channel

North Carolina was the birthplace of ischemic preconditioning: in the early 1980s most of the players of today had stayed in or passed through the departments of Pathology, Cardiology and Cardiac Surgery of Duke University or had given seminars at Borroughs-Wellcome Research laboratories, that fountain of knowlegde in nucleotide chemistry that was honored a few years later when the Noble Prize was awarded to Gertrud ("Trudy") Elion, at that time Research Director emeritus of BW.

I remember a seminar at BW that Jim Downey presented; Trudy was present and we discussed, among many other topics, the merits of adding adenosine to the cardioplegic solution. She was adamently against it, because half a gram of adenosine (and that much was felt necessary), if it would be released into the systemic circulation, would represent a significant and damaging urate load for the kidney.

We all were inspired at that time by the finding of Zimmer's (23) and of Reimer's group (12) that *de novo* synthesis of ATP following partial depletion by ischemia takes such a long time. The Holmes-Swain group and we in Bad Nauheim were frantically competing in finding ways to stimulate salvage synthesis of ATP but neither group made a breakthrough (10).

Prof. Dr. W. Schaper (✉)
Max-Planck-Institut for Physiological and Clinical Research
W. G. Kerckhoff-Institute
Department of Experimental Cardiology
Benekestraße 2
61231 Bad Nauheim, FRG

Multiple occlusions protect the ATP-pool

It was at that seminar at BW-laboratories in the winter of 1982/83 that I had the idea that if ATP-depletion is nearly irreversible because of slow resynthesis, repeated occlusions should have a cumulative effect and that it should be possible to create complete depletion (and hence cell death) without a permanent coronary occlusion. Almost immediately, I started the experiments with my collaborators Mauser and Hoffmeister, but much to our consternation, we had to accept that the concept was wrong: brief occlusions, even if repeated 40 times, had no cumulative effect on ATP depletion, caused no cell death and produced measurable amounts of adenosine only during the first two occlusions (5). We concluded that multiple occlusions had a protective effect on the ATP-pool but we somehow missed performing the right experiment, i.e., to test if protection of the ATP-pool is also preventing cell death. That experiment was cleverly designed and carried out by Murry and Reimer (11), and they deserve every ounce of credit they receive.

Adenosine, the magic bullet?

It was quite obvious even at that time that nucleosides may play a significant part in the molecular mechanisms of myocardial protection and a hypothesis that we all agree upon now is that adenosine plays an important but not entirely well understood role. Adenosine is an enigmatic compound that has fascinated scientists since 1928, when it was discovered by Albert Szent-György. It played a prominent role in the early 1960s when it was believed that it is the regulator of coronary blood flow and drugs were designed that potentiated and prolonged its action. Neither the drugs nor the hypotheses were entirely convincing. Now adenosine is the presumed protector of ischemic myoardium.

Most convincing within the context of ischemic preconditioning are the studies that were carried out with adenosine-A_1-agonists and antagonists, and that is understandable because adenosine itself is so rapidly metabolized and hence difficult to work with. It is indeed an enigma how such a shortlived intermediate can exert such profound and relatively long-lasting effects.

A true paradox is the correlation between the amount of tissue damage and the amount of adenosine released: a significant amount of adenosine is only produced during the first occlusion (in the pig and dog), but very little is produced in the following long ischemia. However, without preconditioning, adenosine production during the long occlusion is high. A "naïve" mind cannot escape the conclusion that adenosine is bad for the heart, because if its tissue concentration is high, infarcts are large and vice versa. Although this is probably untenable, however we look at it, it poses a true dilemma. On the other hand, Schulz et al.(16) observed a rise in adenosine tissue concentration with the long occlusion following preconditioning in canine hearts.

The following observation is also disturbing: four 5 min occlusions are necessary in our pig model for protection (and not two) but only the first two produce adenosine. May be adenosine is only the co-variant of the unknown attractor?

The dilemma becomes even more acute when we realize that certain mammals like the guinea pig do not produce significant amounts of adenosine in hypoxia and ischemia because the metabolic pathway favors inosine production via IMP and even nucleoside transport inhibitors do not change the inosine-adenosine ratio (18). It would be interesting to know whether the guinea pig heart can be preconditioned. If yes, that could be the kiss of death for the adenosine hypothesis.

Refractoriness to good and bad

An interesting characteristic of IP is the fact that the heart becomes two times refractory: at first it becomes refractory toward ischemia, secondly it becomes refractory against renewal of the preconditioning stimulus. Whenever in classical receptor pharmacology repeated stimuli produce decremental effects, we know that the receptor is either downregulated or the receptor-ligand complex is internalized or the receptor-effector signaling is uncoupled or "desensitized". It should be interesting to analyze the A_1-receptor for that.

We have chosen a different hypothesis, namely that the amount of ligand is exhausted. As stated above, the production of adenosine greatly declines after the first short occlusion and additional short occlusions, when the myocardium had become refractory, will also not produce meaningful amounts of adenosine. The local infusion of an A_1-agonist, however, restores responsiveness (22). Although this finding restored our faith in the role of adenosine, one must bear in mind that A_1-agonists always seem to protect under all conditions and that this may not be specific for the refractory phase. The refractoriness can also be overcome by K_{ATP}-channel openers and that may or may not have something to do with adenosine.

A "unifying" theory causes dissent

Jim Downey must be lauded for his courage to formulate the unifying field theory of ischemic preconditioning because it provided a model that is testable (4). According to his theory, PKC becomes activated and translocated to the cell membrane where it phosphorylates an unknown effector. Our own studies showed that PKC activity in the myocardium is low in comparison to brain, from which we conclude that PKC may be more important in the brain (3). The prevailing isoforms in the pig heart are PKC α, δ and ε, and there is indeed translocation of activity to the membrane fraction following short ischemia (+30 %). However, inhibition of PKC activity with specific drugs (bisindolyl maleimide, staurosporin) does not prevent preconditioning; on the contrary, these inhibitors reduce infarct size by themselves, whereas stimulators of PKC (phorbolesters) do not protect (19). Furthermore, A_1-agonists in protecting concentrations do not lead to PKC translocation or activation.

Apart from our findings a few arguments exist that make it rather unlikely that the protection is mediated via PKC, i.e., 1) an accepted pathway from inhibitory G-proteins to PKC-translocation and -activation had not been described so far, and 2) the Na^+/H^+ exchanger is activated by PKC which increases the damage rather than protecting.

The "heart's own insulin" mimicks preconditioning

Cardiac myocytes are, like neurons, terminally differentiated cells, and they may need (like neurons) trophic factors for survival since they are unable to renew by cell division. In our screening program for trophic factors, we found IGF-2 mRNA overexpressed in situations of reversible ischemia and surgical trauma (7). The intramuscular infusion of the IGF-2 peptide directly into the myocardium protects against a 60-min coronary occlusion just like ischemic precondititoning, and this effect could be abolished by the simultaneous infusion of the IGF binding protein IGFBP-5 (20).

The molecular mechanism of the growth factor is its insulin-like action on glucose uptake and insulin itself has a similar action, and lavendustin, a tyrosinkinase inhibitor, inhibits the protection by both hormones. The protective role of increased glucose uptake is not new, but it is often overlooked that glucose uptake (but not its supply) is the limiting factor. Trials with increased glucose supply are hampered by the fact that infusion of glucose increases viscosity to such a degree that flow, and hence supply, are reduced. Increased glucose uptake is also partially or wholly responsible for the protective action of adenosine (8).

A new unifying theory?

Downey's concept of translocation of an enzyme as the basis for memory is very useful even if PKC may be the wrong candidate and, to cite Judah Folkman, "it often matters less that a hypothesis is right or wrong than it is fruitful!". There are more enzymes than PKC that are translocated and the situation prevailing during the first hour of reperfusion can perhaps be called "reprograming of the myocyte cell membrane". The following changes manifest themselves during early reperfusion at the sarcolemma:

- translocation of PKC (present but not useful)
- translocation of the glucose transporter (in response to IGF-2 and adenosine)
- translocation NO-synthetase (in myocytes and endothelium (2))
- translocation of 5′-nucleotidase (in response to ischemia (6))
- opening of K^+-channels (in response to adenosine and G_i)
- closure of Na^+-channels (pharmacologic evidence)
- closure of the Na^+/H^+ exchanger (pharmacologic evidence (14))
- closure of the Na^+/Ca^{++} exchanger (pharmacologic evidence).

It is probably not realistic to assume that ischemic preconditioning is caused by a single factor, especially not in view of the fact that ischemia is such a nonspecific stimulus. It is therefore not astonishing that other naturally occurring compounds are being tested. Our own preliminary results with the local infusion of endothelin (binds to a Gi-coupled receptor) were not encouraging, our results with bradykinin were disappointing (no protection even at concentrations that produced spillover), and they were disastrous with noradrenaline (speeded up cell death). Pharmacologic compounds that inhibit neutral peptidases (phosphoamidon) and that are supposed to prolong the actions of peptides with a trophic function showed no protection in our hands (Iltun, unpublished).

The most probable molecular mechanism of protection is the activation of an inhibitory G-protein with a potassium channel opening action, not a farfetched idea since G-proteins exhibit structural homology with ion channels. Protection could be abolished by local infusion of pertussis toxin (21).

Second windows and new molecules

Yellons group described that short occlusions, in addition to their acute protective effect, also exhibit effects about 24 h later (the "second window of protection") (9). The mechanism of protection is believed to reside in heat-shock proteins that are synthesized in response to ischemia. We were among the first to show that hsps gene expression is increased by short occlusions and that the increase in the tissue mRNA concentration is a complicated mix of transcriptional and posttranscriptional activity (1). We found however that by the time of hsp protein synthesis the acute protection was already over. When at 24 h the hsp protein expression was presumed maximal, no second window of protection was found (13). It was furthermore shown that induction of hsps by heat did not lead to cross-protection against ischemia (15). The second window may primarily depend on the species studied because it was clearly shown to be present in the mouse, rabbit and rat but not in the pig and dog.

A report by the Downey group (17) had shown that IP is not dependent on protein synthesis because treatment of rabbits with cycloheximide had no influence on acute protection. Although at first sight a convincing experiment, no evidence was provided of complete inhibition of protein synthesis and of superinduction of immediate early genes, a typical sign of translational inhibition.

Conclusion

Myocardial protection by ischemic preconditioning is probably caused by more than one mechanism, one of which involves most certainly an inhibitory G-protein and opening of a K^+-channel. Additionally, a wide-ranging reprograming of the cellmembrane involving ion-channels, receptors, ligands and the translocation of cytosolic enzyme systems is probably necessary to achieve myocardial protection.

References

1. Andres J, Sharma HS, Knöll R, Stahl J, Sassen LMA, Verdouw PD, Schaper W (1993) Expression of heat shock proteins in the normal and stunned porcine myocardium. Cardiovasc Res 27: 1421–1429
2. Balligand JL, Ungureanu-Longrois D, Simmons WW, Pimental D, Malinski TA, Kapturczak M, Taha Z, Lowenstein CJ, Davidoff AJ, Kelly RA, Smith T, Michel T (1994) Cytokine-inducible Nitric Oxide Synthase (iNOS) Expression in Cardiac Myocytes. J Biol Chem 269: 27580–27588
3. Barancik M, Vogt AM (1995) Differential activation of the mitogen activated protein kinase cascade with prolonged ischemia. Circulation (in press)
4. Cohen MV, Downey JM (1993) Ischemic preconditioning: can the protection be bottled? The Lancet 342: 6
5. Hoffmeister HM, Mauser M, Schaper W (1986) Repeated short periods of regional myocardial ischemia: effect on local function and high energy phosphate levels. Basic Res Cardiol 81: 361–372
6. Kitakaze M, Hori M, Takashima S, Sato H, Inoue M, Kamada T (1993) Ischemic preconditioning increases adenosine release and 5′-nucleotidase activity during moycardial ischemia and reperfusion in dogs. Circulation 87: 208–215
7. Kluge A, Zimmermann R, Münkel B, Verdouw P, Schaper J, Schaper W (1995) Insulin-like growth factor II is an experimental stress inducible gene in a porcine model of brief coronary occlusions. Cardiovasc Res 29: 708–716
8. Law WR, McLane MP (1991) Adenosine enhances myocardial glucose uptake only in the presence of insulin. Metabolism 40: 947–952
9. Marber MS, Latchman DS, Walker JM, Yellon DM (1993) Cardiac stress protein elevation 24 hours after brief ischemia or heat stress is associated with resistance to myocardial infarction. Circulation 88: 1264–1272
10. Mauser M, Hoffmeister HM, Nienaber C, Schaper W (1985) Influence of ribose, adenosine, and "AICAR" on the rate of myocardial adenosine triphosphate synthesis during reperfusion after coronary artery occlusion in the dog. Circ Res 56: 220–230
11. Murry CE, Jennings RB, Reimer KA (1986) Preconditioning with ischemia: a delay of lethal cell injury in ischemic myocardium. Circulation 74: 1124–1136
12. Reimer KA, Hill ML, Jennings RB (1981) Prolonged depletion of ATP and of the adenine nucleotide pool due to delayed resynthesis of adenine nucleotides following reversible myocardial ischemic injury in dogs. J Mol Cell Cardiol 13: 229–239
13. Sack S, Mohri M, Arras M, Schwarz ER, Schaper W (1993) Ischaemic preconditioning – time course of renewal in the pig. Cardiovasc Res 27: 551–555
14. Sack S, Mohri M, Schwarz ER, Arras M, Schaper J, Ballagi-Pordány G, Scholz W, Lang HJ, Schölkens BA, Schaper W (1994) Effects of a new NA^+/H^+ antiporter inhibitor on postischemic reperfusion in pig heart. J Cardiovas Pharmacol 23: 72–78
15. Schott RJ, Nao B, Strieter R, Groh M, Kunkel S, McClanahan T, Schaper W (1990) Heat shock does not "precondition" canine myocardium. Circulation 82 (Suppl III): 1840 (abstr)
16. Schulz R, Rose J, Post H, Heusch G (1995) Involvement of endogenous adenosine in ischaemic preconditioning in swine. Pflügers Arch 430: 273–282
17. Thornton J, Striplin S, Liu GS, Swafford A, Stanley AW, Van-Winkle DM, Downey JM (1990) Inhibition of protein synthesis does not block myocardial protection afforded by preconditioning. Am J Physiol 259: H 1822–1825
18. Van Belle H, Wynants J, Goossens F (1985) Formation and release of nucleosides in the ischemic myocardium. Is the guinea pig the exception? Basic Res Cardiol 80: 653–660
19. Vogt A, Barancik M, Weihrauch D, Arras M, Podzuweit T, Schaper W (1994) Protection of ischemic porcine myocardium from infarction by an A_1-receptor agonist is not mediated by protein kinase C. Circulation 90 (Part 2): 1991 (abstr)
20. Vogt AM, Ando H, Arras M, Kluge A, Zimmermann R, Schaper W (1995) Insulin-like growth factor-II, the heart's own insulin, protects ischemic myocardium. J Mol Cell Cardiol, in press
21. Vogt AM, Böhm M, Ando H, Erdmann E, Schaper W (1995) Pertussis toxin prevents ischemic preconditioning in pig hearts in vivo. J Am Coll Cardiol, submitted (abstr.)
22. Vogt AM, Podzuweit T, Ando H, Elsässer A, Thomas S, Müller A, Htun P, Arras M, Schaper W (1995) Lack om myocardial adenosine production causes refractoriness after ischemic preconditioning's protection has waned. Cardiovasc Res (submitted)
23. Zimmer HG, Gerlach E (1978) Stimulation of myocardial adenine nucleotide biosynthesis by pentose and pentitols. Pflügers Arch 376: 223–227

130–133

M. Connaughton
D. J. Hearse

Three questions about preconditioning

Key words Preconditioning – ischemia – infarct size – adenosine – angioplasty

The recent explosive growth in preconditioning has led to some rather extravagant claims and some equally optimistic projections as to its eventual impact on the management of cardiovascular disease. This short article seeks to place this enthusiasm into a broader cardiovascular perspective.

Preconditioning joins an exclusive coterie of cardiovascular phenomena that although long recognised were largely ignored until they were given a 'catchy' name. Rahimtoola (15) often cites his failure to attract research funding for 'abnormal LV function at rest due to chronic painless, resting, persistent severe myocardial ischemia and which was reversible' until it was renamed 'hibernation'. Likewise the work of Heyndrickx (4) on 'prolonged impairment of regional myocardial function' was little recognised until it was dubbed 'stunning' by Braunwald and Kloner in 1982 (1). In a similar vein, Parratt has claimed (13) that he and others had been working on the phenomenon of 'preconditioning' long before it was 'discovered' by Murry and colleagues (12). It is amazing how a change to a simple and attractive name can result in a surge of research interest[1].

1 Although the 'discovery' of preconditioning is often attributed to Murry and colleagues (12) these authors have never made such a claim.

Dr. M. Connaughton MRCP (✉) · D. J. Hearse
Cardiovascular Research
The Rayne Institute
St. Thomas' Hospital
London SE1 7EH, United Kingdom

Excitement about preconditioning and its potential clinical relevance has resulted in some remarkable claims including: 'the most powerful form of protection known to date' and 'once its mechanism is known it might be bottled and provide a unique approach to the management of ischaemic heart disease'. Are these claims justified?

Is preconditioning the most powerful protection known to date?

Even the greatest proponent of preconditioning would accept that reperfusion is the only means by which ischaemic tissue can be salvaged. Indeed, in fairness to those investigators who are active in the field, the fact that preconditioning only delays cell death was recognised at a very early stage. Acceptance of this crucial limitation is of considerable importance since it has avoided a repeat of the conceptual mistakes of the 1970s where dozens of pharmaceutical agents were proposed as being capable of preventing cell death and limiting infarct size even in the absence of reperfusion.

In seeking to assess the true power of preconditioning to slow ischaemic injury, a critical comparison should be made with the large number of pharmacological interventions which are also able to delay the onset of irreversible injury and thus limit the extent of necrosis occurring during an ischaemic period of fixed duration. Certainly, if the duration of ischaemia is judiciously selected (say 60 to 90 min of regional ischaemia in a dog heart, or 15 to 45 min in a rabbit heart) preconditioning is able to afford a striking protective effect in relation to the size of an infarct measured at the end of reperfusion. Figure 1A shows examples that are typical of many studies in the literature where infarct size expressed as a percentage of the area at risk can be reduced from its control value of 30 ± 4 % to 4 ±

1 % in the dog (9) and from 29 ± 7 % to 3.0 ± 1 % in the rabbit (2).

Of course, if longer periods of ischaemia had been selected, the ability of preconditioning to limit infarct size would have rapidly declined. Although data derived with single ischaemic durations are available from many studies, no-one has carefully characterised the relationship between infarct size and ischaemic duration in the presence and absence of preconditioning. The only really meaningful index of protective efficacy would be the extent to which preconditioning (or any other intervention) can shift this relationship to the right. In the absence of such characterisation, the protective power of preconditioning relative to 'conventional pharmacology' can only be assessed by comparing studies carried out under similar conditions. Figure 1B shows such an example (11) where preconditioning in dogs with 60 min of regional ischaemia reduces infarct size from 29 ± 5 % to 10 ± 3 % of the area at risk.

However, in the same study the ATP-sensitive potassium channel opener bimakalim, given before and during ischaemia, reduced infarct size from the same control level by some 50 % to 14 ± 3 % of the area at risk. This similarity of protection hardly supports the claim that preconditioning has a uniquely powerful ability to limit infarct size.

Protagonists of preconditioning may shout 'foul' at the selection of the above example, arguing that preconditioning may act, in part at least, through the ATP-sensitive potassium channel. However, the literature reveals a rich diversity of agents with apparently comparable protective properties for which no such claims have been made. For instance, Jolly and colleagues have shown that superoxide dismutase (5) can reduce infarct size by over 50 % in dogs following 90 min of regional ischaemia. Significant protection has likewise been reported with agents such as verapamil (16) and acadesine (6). Thus, while it is true that preconditioning is a very powerful means of myocardial protection, current evidence hardly justifies presenting it as greatly superior to the protection afforded by 'conventional pharmacology'.

What is the difference between 'pretreatment' and 'preconditioning': Is it just a question of semantics?

A characteristic feature of preconditioning, whether it be achieved by ischaemia or by pharmacological mimetics such as adenosine, is that there is an intervening period of a few minutes between the preconditioning stimulus and the period of ischaemia under study. This may take the form of a 5 min period of reperfusion or a similar period during which the administered drug is given the opportunity to be washed out of the heart. Although it has recently been shown that reperfusion is not essential before preconditioning against low-flow ischaemia (17), it does appear mandatory to have at least 30 – 60 s of reperfusion when preconditioning against zero-flow ischaemia. In contrast, it has not been shown that drug washout is an

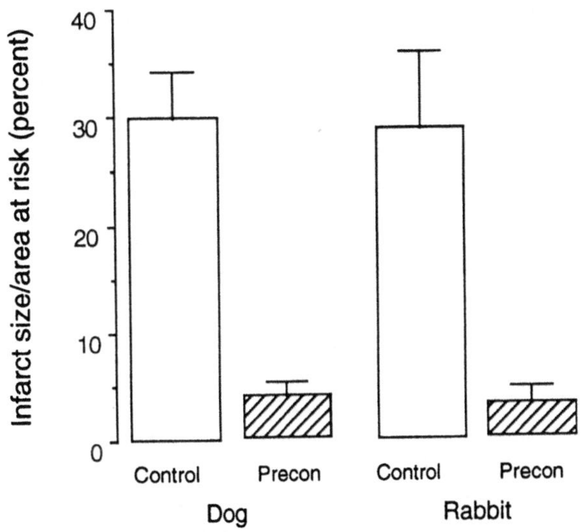

Fig. 1A The ability of preconditioning to reduce infarct size in the dog (60 min regional ischaemia) (9) and the rabbit (20 min regional ischaemia) (2)

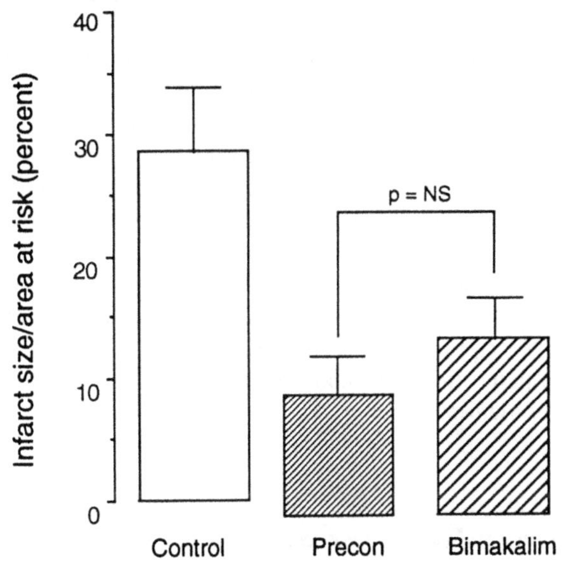

Fig. 1B Dog heart study (11) showing that both preconditioning and bimakalim reduce infarct size by a similar amount (p = NS between preconditioning and bimakalim groups)

essential component for effective pharmacological preconditioning. Indeed it has not even been shown that the washout period incorporated into pharmacological preconditioning is always sufficient to clear a drug from the tissue or its receptors. In the light of this, the devil's advocate might be tempted to question the real difference between pharmacological *preconditioning* and pharmacological *pretreatment*. The literature abounds with studies where drugs such as acadesine (6), verapamil (16) or superoxide dismutase (5) are administered 5 or 10 min before ischaemia and a reduction of infarct size or an enhancement of post-ischaemic function is observed. If the extent of, or need for, drug washout has not been characterised, it becomes difficult to claim that the pretreatment is distinct to pharmacological preconditioning. Indeed, one might even argue to the converse that, in some instances at least, 'old fashioned' pretreatment studies might in fact be working by some preconditioning-mediated mechanism. Intriguing possibilities might include the studies of Lasley and colleagues (7, 8) where adenosine was administered to isolated rat hearts prior to global ischaemia and functional recovery was improved – the manuscript made no mention of 'preconditioning'.

To some extent, the solution to this conundrum will rely on whether we choose to define preconditioning as an observed phenomenon (such as reduction of infarct size) or as a series of biochemical signals (however incompletely known at present), which adapt the cell to withstand a subsequent insult more effectively. If we accept the former, then any intervention must be regarded as truly preconditioning if the same end-point is achieved. The latter definition may allow distinction of mechanism, and thus of nomenclature, even if the same end-point is reached.

In summary, as studies of preconditioning move away from ischaemia as the triggering event into the search for pharmacological mimetics, the distinction between preconditioning and pretreatment may blur. Although not cited by those working with α-receptors and preconditioning, repeated doses of catecholamines were shown over a quarter of a century ago to increase the resistance of isolated cardiac muscle to anoxia (14). This, and many other studies, form a rich literature which significantly predates the descriptions of preconditioning and may well help shed light on the mechanisms underlying this fascinating phenomenon.

Will preconditioning ever make a clinical impact?

At first sight, the profound effect of preconditioning on a number of end-points with considerable clinical relevance makes it potentially a very attractive therapeutic tool. However, translating theoretical promise into clinical reality makes several demands of preconditioning. First, human myocardium must be shown to be capable of being preconditioned in a clinically acceptable and ethical manner. Furthermore, the temporal envelope of the protection must be clinically relevant and the degree of protection therapeutically worthwhile. Lastly, it should be demonstrable that patients proposed for such treatment are not already preconditioned. It is surprisingly difficult to comply rigorously with these demands. Although the evidence from contexts as diverse as cardiac surgery, coronary angioplasty, *in vitro* studies on human tissue and observational studies all suggest that human myocardium is most likely to be amenable to preconditioning, no conclusive evidence yet exists that unequivocal preconditioning occurs in a relevant setting.

Whether the extent and the type of protection afforded are worthwhile remains a moot question. Early or 'classic' protection probably lasts at best no more than 90 min. Except in situations where the timing of both preconditioning stimuli and the subsequent ischaemia is controllable, it is not easy to see how this early envelope of protection may be used to clinical advantage. The so-called 'second window of protection' is much less well characterised (10), but current evidence suggests it may last as long as 24 – 72 h following the initial stimulus and this has much more clinical appeal.

Clinically acceptable methods of inducing preconditioning are unlikely to pose a problem. True ischaemia can readily be induced during cardiac surgery or coronary angioplasty, and many of the agents used experimentally to mimic preconditioning are already established in the pharmacopoeia. However, fundamental problems remain in viewing preconditioning as a practical anti-ischaemic intervention. *Preconditioning of itself does nothing to promote reperfusion of ischaemic tissue,* and ischaemic myocardium must eventually be reperfused or die. Moreover, by the time a patient has given notice of their acute ischaemia it will, of necessity, be too late to precondition and early reperfusion assumes the highest priority. Even if advance warning of acute ischaemia were possible, it would almost always be preferable to reperfuse rather than to precondition.

A further property of preconditioning which is likely to be problematical involves the induction of tolerance. It has been demonstrated in rabbits that repetitive preconditioning over a 48 h period is no longer capable of inducing protection (3). Patients with chronic stable angina may find themselves in an analogous situation, and be unable to benefit from exogenous preconditioning stimuli even if their ischaemia became acute.

These intrinsic limitations with the induction, protection and duration of the protection afforded by preconditioning may significantly limit its clinical potential. Its best chance of establishing itself as a therapeutic tool may lie in settings such as cardiac surgery or high-risk coronary angioplasty in which the induction and termination of the ischaemic challenge is in the hands of the clinician, rather than dependent on pre-existing pathology.

Concluding comments

It is not the intention of this article to denigrate in any way the current high level of interest or activity in the field of preconditioning. Indeed, both authors have published research in the area and continue to do so. It is, however, a plea for a more reasoned evaluation of the phenomenon – our hope being that the current euphoria for the wonders of preconditioning should not lead to a loss of credibility in a field that promises to teach us much about the mechanisms underlying ischaemic injury.

References

1. Braunwald E, Kloner RA (1982) The stunned myocardium: Prolonged, post-ischemic ventricular dysfunction. Circulation 66: 1146–1149
2. Cohen MV, Liu GS, Downey JM (1992) Preconditioning causes improved wall motion as well as smaller infarcts after transient coronary occlusion in rabbits. Circulation 84: 341–349
3. Cohen MV, Yang XM, Downey JM (1994) Conscious rabbits become tolerant to multiple episodes of ischemic preconditioning. Circ Res 74: 998–1004
4. Heyndrickx GR, Millard RW, McRitchie RJ, Maroko PR, Vatner SF (1975) Regional myocardial functional and electrophysiological alterations after brief coronary artery occlusions in conscious dogs. J Clin Invest 56: 978–985
5. Jolly SR, Kane WJ, Bailie MB, Abrams GD, Lucchesi BR (1984) Canine myocardial reperfusion injury. Its reduction by the combined administration of superoxide dismutase and catalase. Circ Res 54: 277
6. Kingma Jr JG, Simard D, Rouleau JR (1994) Timely administration of AICA riboside reduces reperfusion injury in rabbits. Cardiovasc Res 28: 1003–1007
7. Lasley RD, Mentzer RM (1992) Adenosine improves recovery of post-ischemic myocardial function via an adenosine A1 receptor mechanism. Am J Physiol 263: H1460–H1465
8. Lasley RD, Rhee JW, Van Wylen DG, Mentzer RM (1990) Adenosine A1 receptor mediated protection of the globally ischemic isolated rat heart. J Mol Cell Cardiol 22: 39–47
9. Li GC, Vasquez BS, Gallagher KP, Lucchesi BR (1990) Myocardial protection with preconditioning. Circulation 82: 609–619
10. Marber MS, Latchman D, Walker J, Yellon DM (1993) Cardiac stress protein elevation 24 hours after brief ischemia or heat stress is associated with resistance to myocardial infarction. Circulation 88: 1264–1272
11. Mizumura T, Nithipatikon K, Gross GJ (1995) Bimakalim, an ATP-sensitive potassium channel opener, mimics the effects of ischemic preconditioning to reduce infarct size, adenosine release and neutrophil function in dogs. Circulation 92: 1236–1245
12. Murry CE, Jennings RB, Reimer KA (1986) Preconditioning with ischemia: a delay of lethal cell injury in ischemic myocardium. Circulation 74: 1124–1136
13. Parratt JR (1993) Letter to the Editor. Cardiovasc Res 27: 688
14. Poupa O (1969) New pharmacological property of isoproterenol: Increased resistance of isolated cardiac muscle to acute anoxia in IPRO-treated animals. Symposium International; Nancy 499–506
15. Rahimtoola SH (1989) The hibernating myocardium. Am Heart J 117: 211–221
16. Reimer KA, Jennings RB (1985) Effects of calcium-channel blockers on myocardial preservation during experimental acute myocardial infarction. Am J Cardiol 55: 107B–115B
17. Schulz R, Post H, Sakka S, Wallbridge DR, Heusch G (1995) Intraischaemic preconditioning: increased tolerance to sustained low-flow ischemia by a brief episode of no-flow ischemia without intermittent reperfusion. Circ Res 76: 942–950

134–137

A. C. Cave
C. S. Apstein

Preconditioning-induced protection against post-ischemic contractile dysfunction: Inhibitory effect of tissue washout

Key words Preconditioning – ischemia – hypoxia – contractile function

Background

Ischemic preconditioning provides powerful anti-ischemic protection. Murry et al. (10), first reported that preconditioning with 4 cycles of 5 min of ischaemia and reperfusion significantly reduced infarct size in dogs. Subsequent studies have shown similar protection against ischaemia- and reperfusion-induced arrhythmias (7) and contractile dysfunction (1). Furthermore, recent studies have demonstrated that preconditioning-induced protection can be activated by preconditioning stresses other than ischemia. For example, preconditioning with low-flow ischaemia and hypoxia (14), by stimulation of adenosine (A_1), adrenergic (α_1) and muscarinic receptors (9), or by opening of ATP-dependent potassium channels (5, 6) have all been demonstrated to induce protection against a subsequent period of zero flow ischaemia in different models and species.

Dr. A. C. Cave (✉)
Department of Radiological Sciences
18th Floor of the Guy's Tower
Guy's Hospital
London SE1 9RT, United Kingdom

C. S. Apstein
Cardiac Muscle Research Laboratory
Whitaker Cardiovascular Institute
Boston University School of Medicine
80 East Concord Street
Boston, Massachusetts 02118, USA

Can preconditioning provide protection in the presence of residual coronary flow?

Most studies of preconditioning have demonstrated protection against severe or zero flow ischemia. Severe ischemia can cause tissue injury because of tissue hypoxia (i.e., a decrease in the provision of oxygen) as well as by the absence or marked reduction of tissue perfusion which normally provides substrate delivery and metabolite washout. For example, an ischemic decrease in the washout of CO_2 and protons results in tissue acidosis which can be injurious independently of oxygen deprivation.

To determine which component of ischemic injury (oxygen deprivation or reduced tissue perfusion per se) was mitigated by ischemic preconditioning, we recently compared the protective effects of ischemic preconditioning against a subsequent period of zero-flow ischemia with its protective efficacy against an equivalent period of hypoxia (i.e., continued perfusion with "near-anoxic" buffer). Our results suggest that ischemic preconditioning protects against the loss of tissue perfusion per se, rather than against a period of oxygen deprivation (3).

The results of these studies are summarized in Fig. 1. In these experiments isolated buffer-perfused isovolumic (balloon-in-LV) rat hearts were perfused by the Langendorff technique. All preconditioned hearts had an ischemic preconditioning protocol consisting of 5 min of zero-flow ischemia and 5 min of reperfusion. Such preconditioned hearts were compared to non-preconditioned hearts in terms of their recovery from sustained periods of either zero-flow ischemia, substrate-free hypoxia or hypoxia with provision of substrate (5.5 mM glucose + 1.0 mM lactate).

Panel A of Fig. 1 demonstrates the ability of preconditioning to protect against the loss of contractile function caused by 25 min. of zero-flow ischemia. At the end of the 30 min. reperfusion period the preconditioned hearts had

Fig. 1 Preconditioning-induced protection against loss of contractile function: ischemic vs. hypoxic injury. Groups of isolated buffer-perfused isovolumic rat hearts (n = 6/group) underwent either 25 min of ischemia (Panel A), 25 min of substrate-free hypoxia (Panel B), 60 min of hypoxia with substrate provided (Panel C) or 90 min of hypoxia with substrate provided (Panel D). Preconditioned hearts underwent one 5 min cycle of ischemia (I)-reperfusion (R) prior to the sustained ischemic or hypoxic period and are reported as open symbols (□, △, ○). Non-preconditioned hearts are reported as filled symbols (■, ▲, ●). Preconditioning protected against loss of contractile function only for ischemic injury (Panel A) and not for hypoxic injury (Panels B, C, D). Data are presented as means ± SEM $^*p < 0.05$. (adapted from Cave et al., 1994.)

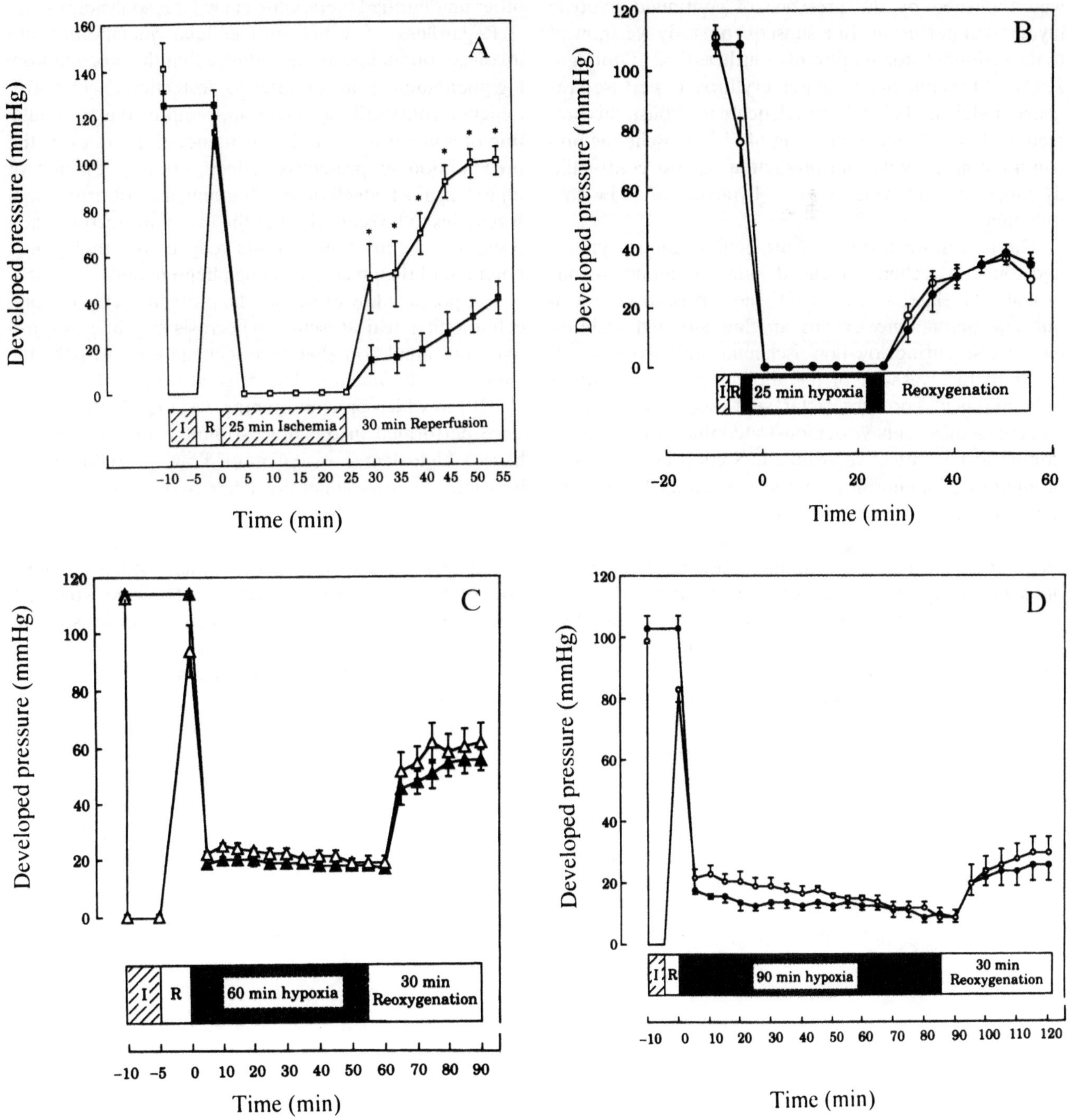

recovered twice the contractile function of the non-preconditioned group (66 ± 6 vs 31 ± 4 %, $p < 0.05$). By contrast, Panels B, C, and D show the lack of preconditioning protection against post-hypoxic contractile dysfunction either after 25 min of substrate-free hypoxia (Panel B), 60 min of hypoxia with substrate provided (Panel C), or 90 min of hypoxia with substrate provided (Panel D). These results show that the anti-ischemic protective effect of preconditioning against post-ischemic contractile dysfunction was abolished by the presence of continued hypoxic myocardial perfusion. In a subsequent study we showed that a residual coronary flow of as little as 0.32 ml/min/gm (10 % of baseline in an isolated erythrocyte perfused rat heart model, see below), was adequate to abolish this protective effect of preconditioning (4). Thus, ischemic preconditioning provided no protection against contractile dysfunction following either hypoxia or low-flow ischemia.

The reason for this loss of protection against hypoxic and low-flow ischemic induced injury is unknown, but probably is related to effects of tissue perfusion and washout. The maintenance of coronary flow, although at different levels, during low-flow ischemia and hypoxia will result in the washout of metabolites produced during ischemia such as protons, lactate and adenosine. Downey and colleagues (8) have demonstrated that, for preconditioning to be protective against infarction in the rabbit, occupation of adenosine receptors is essential during both the preconditioning ischemia and the prolonged ischemic insult. A similar prerequisite has not yet been demonstrated in other species or against other parameters of injury, but such a mechanism is consistent with our results.

A small amount of tissue washout, which did not effectively ameliorate ischemic intracellular acidosis, nonetheless abolished the protective effect of preconditioning in our model. Our studies of low-flow ischemia (4), employed the erythrocyte-perfused isolated rat heart as a model. As a result, coronary flow at baseline was at a physiological level of approximately 2–3 ml/min/gm. Consequently, the average flow during the ischemic period was 0.32 ± 0.01 ml/min/gm. At this level of flow, washout of protons (and probably of other metabolites, such as adenosine), was incomplete: intracellular pH decreased to similar levels as with zero flow ischemia, i.e., after 30 min of this degree of low-flow ischemia, intracellular pH was 6.1 (2), indicating that washout of protons was minimal. Partial lactate washout occurred during this degree of low-flow ischemia, but upon reperfusion, a large lactate peak was seen, indicating that a considerable amount of lactate remained in the tissue during the low-flow ischemic period and was washed out only at reperfusion. Thus it is possible that differences in the degree of tissue lactate accumulation may influence the efficacy of preconditioning, as has been suggested by Murry et al. (11), or other unidentified metabolites may be responsible.

Regardless of which intracellular metabolites are involved, our observations indicate that the preconditioning phenomenon, as it relates to protection against post-ischemic contractile dysfunction, requires the accumulation of a factor in the ischemic tissue, either to exert the preconditioning protective effect, or as a "factor of injury" against which preconditioning affords protection. It remains to be seen whether the loss of protection when residual ischemic flow persists reduces the therapeutic potential of the preconditioning phenomenon.

It is possible however, that the protective effect of preconditioning against ischemic necrosis may be less sensitive to residual flow than its effect against post-ischemic contractile dysfunction. The original studies of Murry et al. (10) in which preconditioning was first demonstrated were performed in the dog. Although this species can have a high degree of collateral flow the reduction of ischemic necrosis generally decreased in regions with mean transmural collateral flow of less than 0.3 ml/min/gm. In a subsequent study in which preconditioning protected against ischemic necrosis animals with a collateral flow of greater than 0.15 ml/min/g (11) were excluded. Similarly, the reduction of infarct size in swine by ischemic preconditioning occurred in risk regions with ischemic perfusion levels of 0.12 – 0.16 ml/min/gm or less, representing ≤ 20 – 25 % of baseline (12, 13). Thus the observed reduction of ischemic necrosis by preconditioning in these studies occurred in the context of relatively severe ischemia, as defined by the absolute perfusion level, although the percent reduction from baseline could be considered as "moderate ischemia". Thus, the influence of residual flow on preconditioning-induced protection against ischemic necrosis still needs to be further assessed.

References

1. Cave AC, Hearse DJ (1992) Ischemic preconditioning and contractile function: Studies with normothermic and hypothermic global ischemia. J Mol Cell Cardiol 24: 1113–1123
2. Cave AC, Eberli FR, Ngoy S (1993) Increased glycolytic substrate protects against ischemic diastolic dysfunction: ^{31}P-NMR studies in the isolated blood perfused rat heart. Circulation 88: I-43 (Abstract)
3. Cave AC, Horowitz GL, Apstein CS (1994) Can ischemic preconditioning protect against hypoxia-induced damage: Studies on contractile function in isolated perfused rat hearts. J Mol Cell Cardiol 26: 1471–1486
4. Cave AC, Silverman AS, Apstein CS (1995) Preconditioning against contractile dysfunction is abolished in the presence of residual flow in the isolated blood perfused rat heart. J Mol Cell Cardiol 27: A145 (Abstract)
5. Cave AC (1995) Preconditioning induced protection against post-ischemic contractile dysfunction: Characteristics and mechanisms. J Mol Cell Cardiol 27: 969–979
6. Gross GJ, Auchampach JA (1992) Blockade of ATP-sensitive potassium channels prevents myocardial preconditioning in dogs. Circ Res 70: 223–233
7. Lawson CS, Coltart DJ, Hearse DJ (1993) "Dose"dependency and temporal characteristics of protection by ischemic preconditioning against ischemia-induced arrhythmias in rat hearts. J Mol Cell Cardiol 25: 1391–1402
8. Liu GS, Thornton J, Van Winkle DM, Stanley AWH, Olsson RA, Downey JM (1991) Protection against infarction afforded by preconditioning is mediated by A_1 receptors in rabbit heart. Circulation 84: 350–356
9. Liu G, Downey JM (1992) Acetylcholine preconditions rabbit heart; further evidence for G_1 protein coupling in preconditioning. Circulation 86 (SI): I-174 (Abstract)
10. Murry CE, Jennings RB, Reimer KA (1986) Preconditioning with ischemia: a delay of lethal cell injury in ischemic myocardium. Circulation 74: 1124–1136
11. Murry CE, Richard VJ, Reimer KA, Jennings RB (1990) Ischemic preconditioning slows energy metabolism and delays ultrastructural damage during a sustained ischemic episode. Circ Res 66: 913–931
12. Schulz R, Rose J, Heusch G (1994) Involvement of activation of ATP-dependent potassium channels in ischemic preconditioning in swine. Am J Physiol 267 (Heart Circ. Physiol 36): H1341–H1352
13. Schulz R, Rose J, Post H, Heusch, G (1995) Involvement of endogenous adenosine in ischaemic preconditioning in swine. Pflugers Arch-Eur J Physiol 430: 273–282
14. Zhai X, Lawson CS, Cave AC, Hearse DJ (1993) Preconditioning and postischemic contractile dysfunction: The role of impaired oxygen delivery versus extracellular metabolite accumulation. J Mol Cell Cardiol 25: 847–857

138–140

T. Miura

Adenosine and bradykinin: Are they independent triggers of preconditioning?

Key words Preconditioning – adenosine – bradykinin – microdialysis

Almost a decade has passed since Murry et al. (8) first reported that myocardial tolerance against ischemic necrosis is markedly enhanced by a brief exposure to ischemia in the dog. This phenomenon has been shown to occur in many animal species, and cardioprotection by ischemic preconditioning was found against other types of ischemic myocardial injury, including arrhythmia. Intense investigation into the mechanism of preconditioning has led to a proliferation of theories, and at least four (adenosine, free radicals, bradykinin, opioids) active substances have been proposed to be involved in infarct size limitation by preconditioning. However, the interrelation between these substances in the mechanism of preconditioning remains unclear. The present review discusses the evidence for the roles of adenosine and bradykinin and their possible relationship in preconditioning against infarction.

Adenosine

Adenosine is the most well characterized trigger of preconditioning, and its importance in the mechanism of preconditioning has been supported by experiments on various animal species except for the rat (7). A study using the in vivo microdialysis technique has shown that interstitial adenosine in the heart indeed increases during preconditioning (12), and the results of a number of in vitro and in vivo studies have demonstrated that adenosine (probably A_1 and/or A_3) receptor activation before ischemic insult is necessary for the cardioprotection of preconditioning (1, 7, 10). Furthermore, Thornton et al. (11) found that infarct size limitation by preconditioning with 5 min ischemia was attenuated by approximately 50 % when an adenosine receptor blocker was administered between the preconditioning ischemia and the subsequent sustained ischemia in the rabbit. These data suggest that adenosine receptors must be activated not only during preconditioning but also during the subsequent longer ischemia for the preconditioning effect to be fully expressed.

Bradykinin

Although it has been known for some time that bradykinin is produced in the ischemic myocardium, its significance is not still clear. The contribution of this peptide to preconditioning was first proposed by Wall et al. (13). In their study, infarct size limitation by preconditioning in the rabbit was blocked by Hoe 140, a specific antagonist of bradykinin type 2 receptor (B_2 receptor), and was mimicked by exogenous bradykinin. In support of these findings, we observed that preconditioning was blocked by aprotinin, an inhibitor of kallikrein (T. Miura, unpublished observation). Furthermore, in a preliminary study, we recently found that captopril, a kininase II inhibitor, can lower the threshold of preconditioning without alteration of the arterial bradykinin level (5). This suggests that bradykinin relevant to preconditioning may be locally

Dr. T. Miura (✉)
Second Department of Internal Medicine
Sapporo Medical University School of Medicine
South-1 West-16 Chuo-ku
Sapporo 060, Japan

generated in the heart. However, there are a number of pathways for bradykinin to be generated in the heart from the plasma and tissue kallikrein-kinin systems (2, 9). The precise mechanism of their activation during preconditioning remains unclear.

In contrast to the adenosine receptor, the B_2 receptor does not appear to play a major role during sustained ischemia. In a recent study by Goto et al. (3), Hoe 140 administered between preconditioning and the subsequent ischemic insult failed to block infarct size limitation by preconditioning, although this B_2 receptor antagonist abolished the cardioprotection when given before the preconditioning with a single episode of ischemia. Considering also the results of aprotinin and captopril, the data by Goto et al. (3) suggest that the B_2 receptor is as important as the adenosine receptor for triggering the preconditioning mechanism, but its activation is not necessary during the sustained ischemic insult for the preconditioning to be cardioprotective.

Interrelationship between adenosine and bradykinin?

Are adenosine and bradykinin independent triggers of preconditioning? This question is raised by the findings that preconditioning with a single episode of transient ischemia was abolished by both adenosine receptor blockers (1, 7, 11) and a B_2 receptor blocker, Hoe 140 (3, 13). Accordingly, we hypothesized that B_2 receptor activation may augment adenosine build-up in the cardiac interstitium during preconditioning ischemia, thus lowering the adenosine threshold for triggering the preconditioning mechanism. To test this hypothesis, we examined the effect of Hoe 140 on the interstitial adenosine level during ischemia in the rabbit heart by the in vivo microdialysis technique. Figure 1 shows the time-course of the nucleoside levels before and during 30 min of ischemia. In the control rabbits, the increase of purines in dialysate during ischemia was modest in the present study, as compared with the data obtained in dog hearts by Van Wylen et al. (12). Although we cannot exclude a species difference in the adenosine metabolism, such as ecto-5′-nucleotidase activity, between the rabbit and canine hearts, a more likely explanation for the lower purine level is the lower recovery by the dialysis probe we used (32 % vs. 18 %).

Pretreatment with 2 μg/kg of Hoe 140, which is sufficient for blocking preconditioning with 5 min of ischemia (13, T. Miura, unpublished observation), did not suppress ischemia-induced elevations of adenosine, inosine and hypoxanthine in the microdialysate from the myocardium (Fig. 1). These results do not support our hypothesis, and

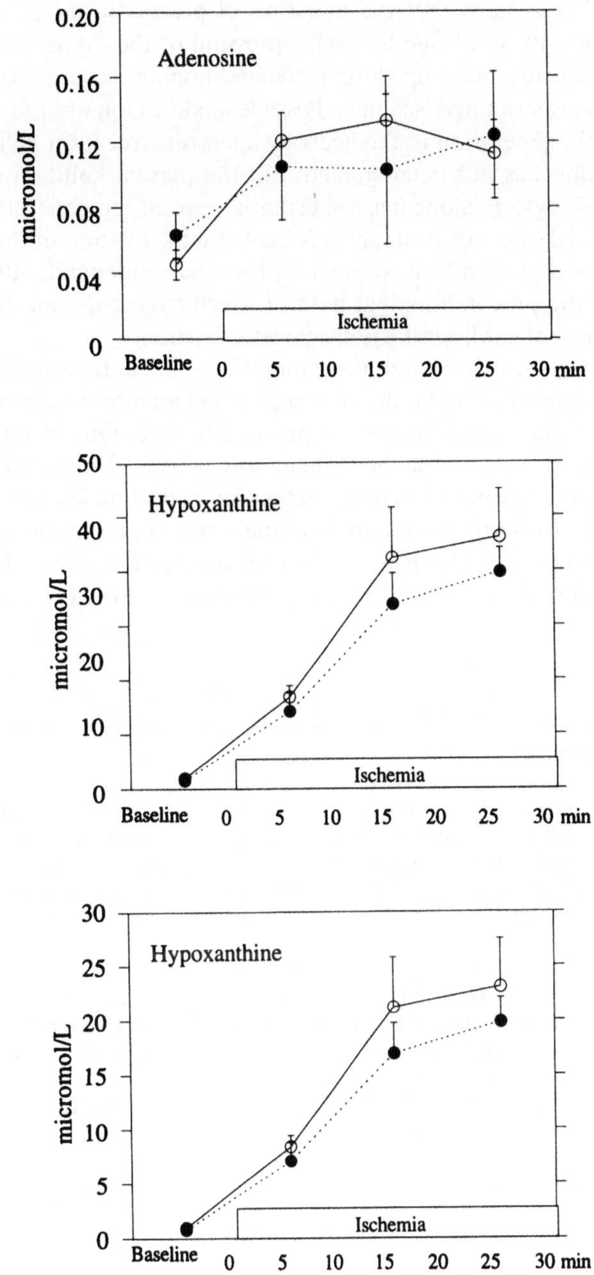

Fig. 1 Profiles of adenosine, inosine, and hypoxanthine in the dialysate before and during 30 min-coronary occlusion. A microdialysis probe (Eicom OP-100-05, Eicom Co., Japan) was inserted into the midmyocardium of the rabbit, and perfused with Ringer solution containing low molecular heparin (10 units/ml) at 2 μl/min. The preparation was stabilized for 2 h before collecting the baseline dialysate samples. Nucleosides in the samples were assayed by reverse phase high performance liquid chromatography. Open circles are data from the controls ($n = 9$) and filled circles are those from the Hoe 140 treated group ($n = 5$). In the Hoe 140 treated group, 2 μg/kg of Hoe 140 was administered intravenously 10 min before ischemia. There was no significant difference in the time-course of the nucleoside levels between the control and Hoe 140 treated groups (p = NS by two-way repeated measures analysis of variance). Bars represent 1 SE.

rather suggest that the abolition of preconditioning by Hoe 140 is not due to the suppression of the interstitial adenosine build-up during preconditioning ischemia or during sustained ischemia. Possible modification of bradykinin generation in the heart by adenosine receptor activation has not been studied, but the plasma kallikrein-kinin system alone has a substantial capacity to generate bradykinin. Accordingly, it is likely that activation of the B_2 receptor and adenosine receptor occurs independently during preconditioning, both of which trigger the mechanism of cardioprotection against infarction.

On the other hand, there might be a link at the subcellular level between the B_2 receptor and adenosine receptor-induced mechanisms of preconditioning. One attractive hypothesis for the cellular mechanism of preconditioning against infarction is activation of protein kinase C (14). Recently, we found that infarct size limitation by A_1 receptor activation is blocked by the protein kinase C inhibitors, staurosporine and polymyxin B (10). A recent study by Goto et al. (3) showed that cardioprotection by exogenous bradykinin was also blocked by the same protein kinase C inhibitors in an isolated rabbit heart preparation. Furthermore, the generation of phosphatidyl inositol triphosphate was demonstrated in cardiac myocytes both after A_1 receptor activation (14) and after B_2 receptor activation (4). Thus, it appears possible that adenosine and bradykinin receptors may share a common pathway, i.e., activation of phospholipase C and subsequent protein kinase C activation, as the subcellular mechanism of their contribution to preconditioning.

In conclusion, both the adenosine receptor and bradykinin (B_2) receptor are important triggers of the mechanism of preconditioning, and their activation is probably independent during preconditioning. The possible interrelationship between the adenosine and B_2 receptor-triggered pathways at subcellular level warrants further investigation.

References

1. Armstrong S, Ganote CE (1994) Adenosine receptor specificity in preconditioning of isolated rabbit cardiomyocytes: evidence of A_3 receptor involvement. Cardiovasc Res 28: 1049–56
2. Carretero OA, Scicli AG (1990) Kinins as regulators of blood flow and blood pressure. In: Laragh JH, and Brenner BM (eds) Hypertension: Pathophysiology. Diagnosis, and Management, Raven Press, New York, pp 805–817
3. Goto M, Liu Y, Yang X-M, Ardell JL, Cohen MV, Downey JM (1995) Role of bradykinin in protection of ischemic preconditioning in rabbit hearts. Circ Res 611–621
4. Kohl C, Linck B, Schmitz W, Scholz H, Scholz J, Toth M (1990) Effects of carbacol and R(-)-N6-phenylisopropyladenosine on myocardial inositol phosphate content and force of contraction. Br J Pharmacol 101: 829–34
5. Miki T, Miura T, Ogawa T, Ura N, Shimamoto K, Iimura O (1995) Captopril, a kininase II, lowers the threshold of preconditioning through B2 receptor mediated mechanism. [Abstract] Circulation 92 (suppl. I): I-455
6. Minshall RD, Nakamura F, Becker RP, Rabito SF (1995) Characterization of bradykinin B2 receptors in adult myocardium and neonatal rat cardiomyoytes. Circ Res 76: 773–780
7. Miura T, Iimura O (1993) Infarct size limitation by preconditioning: its phenomenological features and the key role of adenosine. Cardiovasc Res 27: 36–42
8. Murry CE, Jennings RB, Reimer KA (1986) Preconditioning with ischemia: A delay in lethal injury in ischemic myocardium. Circulation 74: 1124–36
9. Nolly H, Carbini LA, Scicli G, Carretero OA, Scicli AG (1994) A local kallikrein-kinin system is present in rat hearts. Hypertension 23: 919–923
10. Sakamoto J, Miura T, Goto M, Iimura O (1995) Limitation of myocardial infarct size by adenosine A_1-receptor activation is abolished by protein kinase C inhibitors in the rabbit. Cardiovasc Res 29: 682–688
11. Thornton JD, Thornton CS, Downey JM (1993) Effect of adenosine receptor blockade: preventing protective preconditioning depends on time of initiation. Am J Physiol 265: H504–H508
12. Van Wylen DGL (1994) Effect of ischemic preconditioning on interstitial purine metabolite and lactate accumulation during myocardial ischemia. Circulation 89: 2283–2289
13. Wall TM, Sheehy R, Hartman JC (1994) Role of bradykinin in myocardial preconditioning. J Pharmacol Exp Ther 270: 681–689
14. Ytrehus K, Liu Y, Downey JM (1994) Preconditioning protects ischaemic rabbit heart by protein kinase C activation. Am J Physiol 266: H1145–52

141–144
© Steinkopff Verlag 1996

M. Kitakaze
T. Minamino
K. Node
K. Komamura
M. Hori

Activation of Ecto-5′-nucleotidase and cardioprotection by ischemic preconditioning

Key words Adenosine – protein kinase C – myocardial infarction – α_1-adrenoceptor – ischemia

Introduction

Since Jennings and his colleagues found that preceding brief periods of myocardial ischemia limit infarct size following sustained ischemia and reperfusion (11), termed as "ischemic preconditioning", many basic and clinical researchers have focused on the cellular mechanisms of this potent cardioprotection. Downey and his colleagues (10) observed that 8-sulfophenyltheophylline blunts the infarct size-limiting effect of ischemic preconditioning in the rabbit heart. This evidence may point to two hypotheses: 1) adenosine makes the myocardium resistant against the lethal ischemic injury (adenosine as a trigger substance); and 2) ischemic preconditioning makes adenosine act more effectively during the lethal ischemic insult (adenosine as a mediator substance). Since adenosine is known to have many different beneficial cardiovascular effects against ischemia and reperfusion injury (1, 3), we hypothesized the latter mechanism as a candidate of the cellular mechanism of ischemic preconditioning.

Dr. M. Kitakaze (✉) · T. Minamino · K. Node
K. Komamura · M. Hori
The First Department of Medicine
Osaka University School of Medicine
2-2 Yamadaoka, Suita 565, Japan

Enhanced release of adenosine: Role of activation of ecto-5 -nucleotidase

To test our hypothesis, we measured adenosine release during reperfusion following 40 min of ischemia with and without ischemic preconditioning (four times 5 min of coronary occlusion with a 5-min interval) (4). We observed that the coronary venous adenosine concentration during early reperfusion with ischemic preconditioning increases 2–3 times higher compared with the group without ischemic preconditioning (4). To seek the mechanisms for this enhanced release of adenosine, we mueasured 5′-nucleotidase activity, the enzyme responsible for adenosine production, with and without ischemic preconditioning. We found that ecto-5′-nucleotidase activity is markedly increased in the group of ischemic preconditioning (4, 5). To elucidate the cause-effect relationship between activation of ecto-5′-nucleotidase and the infarct size-limiting effect, we blocked the activity of ecto-5′-nucleotidase using, α, β-methylenedenosine 5′-diphosphate (AOPCP), and measured adenosine release during reperfusion and infarct size 6 h following reperfusion. First, in the in vitro experiments, 50 μM AOPCP, which corresponds to the dose of 80 μg/kg/min (ic) AOPCP, almost completely blocked ecto-5′-nucleotidase without changing cytosolic 5′-nucleotidase activity. We also revealed that this dose of AOPCP blunts the infarct size-limiting effect of ischemic preconditioning as well as the enhanced release of adenosine. These results support the hypothesis that the cardioprotection of ischemic preconditioning is mediated by enhanced release of adenosine during lethal ischemic and reperfusion injury through activation of ecto-5′-nucleotidase.

However, we should carefully consider the data showing the decreases in myocardial interstitial adenosine levels during ischemia and reperfusion in the group of ischemic preconditioning, which may contradict our hypothesis. To interpret this discrepancy, we simultaneously measured adenosine concentrations in the coronary venous blood and myocardial interstitial fluid during coronary hypoperfusion (3 % of the control flow) with and without ischemic preconditioning. When we measured adenosine levels in the interstitial fluid and coronary venous blood during 90 min of myocardial ischemia, we also observed the marked increases in adenosine release in coronary venous blood and slight decreases in interstitial adenosine levels sampled by the microdialysis method during ischemia and reperfusion in the group of ischemic preconditioning compared with the control group. One possibility to understand this difference is that ecto-5′-nucleotidase in the endothelial cells is mainly activated by ischemic preconditioning, which may reflect high adenosine levels in the coronary venous blood. However, we also observed that ecto-5′-nucleotidase in the rat cardiomyocytes is activated due to hypoxic stress, suggesting that ischemic stress due to ischemic preconditioning may activate ecto-5′-nucleotidase of canine cardiomyocytes as well. Another possibility is that the scavenging system of adenosine in the interstitial space of the myocardium, i.e., activity of adenosine kinase and deaminase, and AMP deaminase, and transporter of adenosine, may be also increased, which may attenuate the enhanced production of adenosine due to activated ecto-5′-nucleotidase. Even if this were the case, since both ecto-5′-nucleotidase and adenosine receptors are located at the same cellular surface membrane, produced adenosine can easily stimulate adenosine receptors in the microenvironmental condition before being scavenged. In any case, we believe that the signal transduction due to the stimulation of adenosine receptors during myocardial ischemia and reperfusion mediates cardioprotection of ischemic preconditioning.

How is ecto-5′-nucleotidase activated by ischemic preconditioning?

We have previously observed that prazosin, an α_1-adrenoceptor antagonist, attenuates the release of adenosine from canine ischemic myocardium (2), which has been confirmed by several investigators. We also observed using rat cardiomyocytes that activation of protein kinase C due to α_1-adrenoceptor stimulation increases adenosine production in hypoxic conditions via activation of ecto-5′-nucleotidase (7); both methoxamine and 12,13-phorbol myristate ester (PMA) activated ecto-5′-nucleotidase, and enhanced production of adenosine due to methoxamine, and PMA was blunted by AOPCP in the hypoxic condition. Therefore, we tested the role of activation of α_1-adrenoceptor stimulation and protein kinase C on activation of ecto-5′-nucleotidase. In the canine heart, an intracoronary administration of prazosin attenuated the infarct size-limiting effect and activation of ecto-5′-nucleotidase (6). Furthermore, we observed that the activity of protein kinase C in the membrane fraction is increased with slight decreases in the activity of protein kinase C in the cytosol (8). This activation of protein kinase C is Ca^{2+}- and phospholipid-dependent, suggesting that the activation of constitutive protein kinase C is mainly involved in cardioprotection due to ischemic preconditioning (8). Indeed, in the preliminary study, the immunoblotting revealed the translocation of α-protein kinase C to the membrane fraction. We further tested whether an inhibitor of protein kinase C blunts the infarct size-limiting effect as well as the activation of ecto-5′-nucleotidase. GF109203X, a specific inhibitor of protein kinase C, attenuated both the infarct size-limiting effect and the activation of ecto-5′-nucleotidase (8). On the

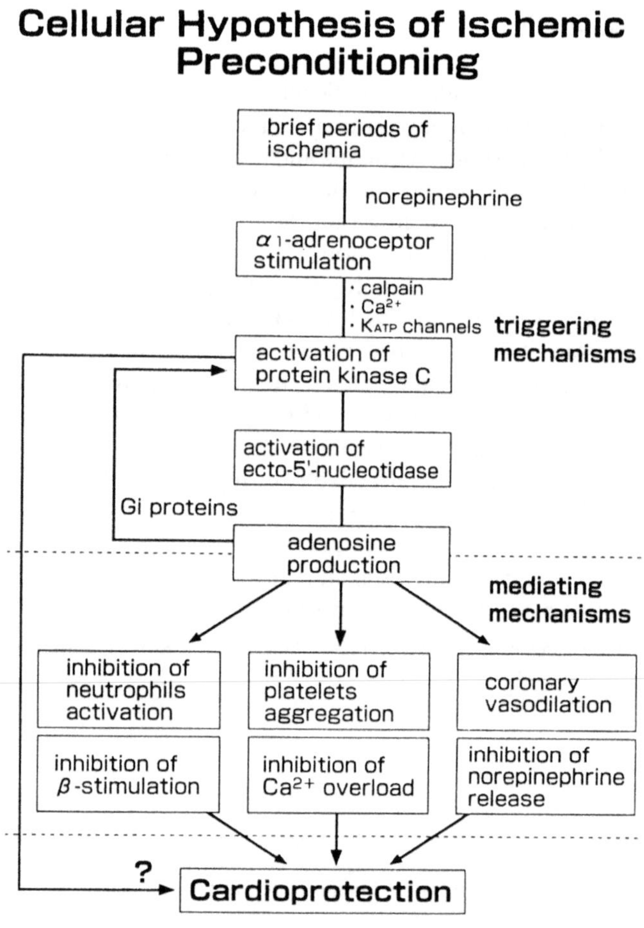

Fig. 1 Our hypothetical scheme of the cellular mechanisms of cardioprotection due to ischemic preconditioning.

other hand, we showed that the intermittent exposures of methoxamine and PMA for four times of 5 min with a 5-min interval, instead of the ischemic preconditioning procedure, activate ecto-5′-nucleotidase and limit infarct size as ischemic preconditioning does (6). Therefore, we strongly suggest that activation of protein kinase C following α_1-adrenoceptor stimulation may be responsible for the infarct size-limiting effect of ischemic preconditioning via activation of ecto-5′-nucleotidase.

Recently, we found that calpain and the opening of ATP-sensitive K^+ channels are involved in the pathway of α_1-adrenoceptor stimulation and protein kinase C activation in ischemic preconditioning. Calpain is a neutral protease, which catalyzes cellular enzymes and proteins, and protein kinase C may be a substrate for calpain. Both calpain inhibitor I, a calpain inhibitor, and glibenclamide, an antagonist of ATP-sensitive K^+ channels, independently inhibited the activation of both protein kinase C and ecto-5′-nucleotidase, and thus, the infarct size-limiting effect in ischemic preconditioning. Figure 1 summarizes our hypothesis of the cellular mechanisms of ischemic preconditioning based on our and others' recent work.

Clinical extensions and application of our hypothesis

Cardioprotection due to preceding anginal attacks has been recently recognized in patients with acute myocardial infarction by several institutes, including ours (9, 12). To obtain cardioprotection without an ischemic attack is ideal for the treatment of coronary artery disease. Since adenosine is a key mediator for cardioprotection, one strategy to obtain cardioprotection is to elevate adenosine levels in the ischemic heart. Adenosine transport inhibitors, such as dilazep and dipyridamole, adenosine-related substances, such as ATP, AP_4A and adenosine itself, and a potentiator of adenosine production, such as acadesine, need to be tested in the acute myocardial infarction. Another possibility is to increase ecto-5′-nucleotidase activity. Cytokines and lipopolysaccharide can increase the transcriptional levels of ecto-5′-nucleotidase, which may be seriously considered for application in the treatment of ischemic heart disease.

As a consequence, we will continue to pursue the clinical applicability of the fruitful results of ischemic preconditioning.

References

1. Hori M, Kitakaze M (1991) Adenosine, the heart and coronary circulation (Brief Review). Hypertension 18: 565–574
2. Kitakaze M, Hori M, Tamai J, Iwakura K, Koretsune Y, Kagiya T, Iwai K, Kitabatake A, Inoue M, Kamada T (1987) α_1-Adrenoceptor activity regulates release of adenosine from the ischemic myocardium in dogs. Circ Res 60: 631–639
3. Kitakaze M, Hori M, Kamada T (1993) The role of adenosine and its interaction with alpha-adrenoceptor activity in myocardial ischemic and repefusion injury (Brief Review). Cardiovasc Res 27: 18–27
4. Kitakaze M, Hori M, Takashima S, Sato H, Inoue M, Kamada T (1993) Ischemic preconditioning increases adenosine release and 5′-nucleotidase activity during myocardial ischemia and reperfusion in dogs: Implication for myocardial salvage. Circulation 87: 208–215
5. Kitakaze M, Hori M, Morioka T, Minamino T, Takashima S, Sato H, Shinozaki Y, Chujo M, Mori H, Inoue M, Kamada T (1994) The infarct size-limiting effect of ischemic preconditioning is blunted by inhibition of 5′-nucleotidase activity and attenuation of adenosine release. Circulation 89: 1237–1246
6. Kitakaze M, Hori M, Morioka T, Minamino T, Takashima S, Sato H, Shinozaki Y, Chujo M, Mori H, Inoue M, Kamada T (1994) Alpha$_1$-adrenoceptor activation mediates the infarct size limiting effect of ischemic preconditioning through augmentation of 5′-nucleotidase activity. J Clin Invest 93: 2197–2207
7. Kitakaze M, Hori M, Morioka T, Minamino T, Takashima S, Okazaki Y, Node K, Komamura K, Iwakura K, Inoue M, Kamada T (1995) Alpha$_1$-adrenoceptor activation increases ecto-solic 5′-nucleotidase activity and adenosine release in rat cardiomyocytes by activing protein kinase C. Circulation 91: 2226–2234
8. Kitakaze M, Node K, Minamino T, Komamura K, Funaya H, Shinozaki Y, Chujo M, Mori H, Inoue M, Hori M, Kamada T. The role of activation of protein kinase C in the infarct size-limiting effect of ischemic preconditioning through activation of ecto-5′-nucleotidase. Circulation (in press)

9. Komamura K, Kitakaze M, Nishida M, Naka K, Tamai J, Uematsu M, Koretsune Y, Nanto S, Hori M, Inoue M, Kamada T, Kodama K (1994) Progressive decreases in coronary vein flow during reperfusion in acute myocardial infarction: A clinical documentation of no-reflow phenomenon following successful thrombolysis. J Am Coll Cardiol 24: 370–377
10. Liu GS, Thornton J, Van Winkle DM, Stanley AHW, Olsson RA, Downey JM (1991) Protection against infarction afforded by preconditioning is mediated by A_1 adenosine receptors in rabbit heart. Circulation 84: 350–356
11. Murry CE, Jennings RB, Reimer KA (1986) Preconditioning with ischemia: A delay of lethal cell injury in ischemic myocardium. Circulation 74: 1124–1136
12. Nakagawa Y, Ito H, Kitakaze M, Kusuoka H, Hori M, Kuzuya T, Higashino Y, Fujii K, Minamino T (1995) Effect of angina pectoris on myocardial protection in patients with reperfused anterior wall myocardial infarction: Retrospective evidence of "preconditioning". J Am Coll Cardiol 25: 1076–1083

145–148
© Steinkopff Verlag 1996

J. R. Parratt
A. Vegh

Endothelial cells, nitric oxide and ischaemic preconditioning

Key words Endothelial cells – nitric oxide – bradykinin – cGMP – ventricular arrhythmias

Introduction

One of the most important, perhaps the most important, consequence of ischaemic preconditioning is the marked suppression of early (phase 1) ventricular arrhythmias that arise from coronary artery occlusion (reviewed in 1). This pronounced protection in species-independent, real (in that arrhythmias are not shifted to a later period during ischaemia; 2) depends on the number and duration of preconditioning occlusions (2), can be demonstrated in blood-free isolated hearts (3) and can be regained and restored after a period of several hours (4). One potential mechanism for this protection, for which there is circumstantial evidence but no direct proof, is that protective substances, derived from endothelial cells, mediate both the early ('classical') and 'delayed' phases of this protection and that this represents an example of 'cross talk' between these vascular cells and cardiac myocytes. The evidence for this hypothesis will now be summarised.

Prof. Dr. J. R. Parratt (✉)
Cardiovascular Research
Department of Physiology and Pharmacology
University of Strathclyde / Royal College
Glasgow GIIXW, United Kingdom

Dr. A. Vegh
Department of Pharmacology
Albert Szent-Györgyi Medical University
Dom ter 12
Szeged, 6701 Hungary

Protective mediators are released, presumably from the endothelium, under conditions of ischaemia

There is good evidence, both experimentally and in patients, for the release of a variety of potentially protective mediators under conditions of ischaemia. These include prostacyclin (5), adenosine, bradykinin and nitric oxide. For example, in patients undergoing coronary angioplasty, sampling from the coronary sinus during the 1-min period of ischaemia results, in some patients, in a 50-fold increase of bradykinin in plasma (Oldroyd, Cobbe, Koide, Zeitlin and Parratt, unpublished). Recent experiments in a canine model of ischaemia have demonstrated that end-products of nitric oxide (nitrite and nitrate) are increased in the coronary vein following graded reductions in coronary flow (6); this release appears to result from α_1-adrenoceptor stimulation. However, we have no evidence that preconditioning modifies the release of these protective mediators. The working hypothesis would suggest i) that these mediators might be released in increased amounts during the period of prolonged ischaemia following 'priming' by short periods of ischaemia and that ii) these mediators are derived from the endothelium and that the release might be impaired under conditions of endothelial dysfunction, for example in patients with atherosclerosis and as a result of vascular damage resulting from balloon angioplasty.

Blockade of the effects of endothelium-derived protective mediators attenuates the antiarrhythmic effect of ischaemic preconditioning

Most of the evidence for a role for nitric oxide, bradykinin and cyclooxygenase products in mediating the antiarrhythmic effects of ischaemic preconditioning comes from studies in the canine in which, either the generation and release of these substances is inhibited, or their effects on relevant receptors prevented. The evidence can be summarised as follows:

Evidence for the involvement of nitric oxide

The antiarrhythmic effect of ischaemic preconditioning in dogs is markedly reduced following inhibition of nitric oxide production by inhibitors of the L-arginine nitric oxide pathway such as N^G-nitro-L-arginine methylester (L-NAME) (7). However, this attenuation of the protective effects of ischaemic preconditioning is incomplete; the effect of ischaemic preconditioning in abolishing ventricular fibrillation (VF) is not modified by this inhibition. In addition, there is no evidence to suggest that infusing L-arginine beneficially modifies ischaemia-induced arrhythmias, or that it reverses the effect of L-NAME.

More persuasive evidence comes from the use of methylene blue, which is both an inhibitor of the L-arginine nitric oxide pathway and or guanylyl cyclase. When infused locally into the coronary circulation it completely reverses the antiarrhythmic effect of ischaemic preconditioning.

Evidence for the involvement of bradykinin

There are two pieces of evidence that bradykinin acts as a mediator of the effects of ischaemic preconditioning in reducing early, phase 1, ventricular arrhythmias. First, the local infusion of bradykinin into the coronary circulation results in a marked suppression of ischaemia-induced arrhythmias and, since this antiarrhythmic effect is prevented by the prior administration of an inhibitor of the L-arginine nitric oxide pathway, this suggests that this effect of bradykinin is mediated through the generation of nitric oxide (discussed in ref (8)). Second, when a drug (icatibant; Hoe 140) that blocks bradykinin B2 receptors is given prior to the preconditioning occlusions the severity of arrhythmias during these occlusions is markedly increased, suggesting that bradykinin is released even during such brief, preconditioning periods of ischaemia. When icatibant is given either before preconditioning, or after preconditioning but prior to the prolonged occlusion, the antiarrhythmic effects of ischaemic preconditioning are markedly attenuated and survival from the combined ischaemia-reperfusion insult is markedly reduced (8). Changes in epicardial ST-segment elevation, and in the degree of inhomogeneity of activation within the ischaemic area, mirror these changes in arrhythmia severity. Such studies suggest that bradykinin acts both as a 'trigger' for preconditioning, and as one of the protective mediator (antiarrhythmic) substances generated by the heart under these conditions.

Recently, there is evidence that bradykinin is involved in the 'delayed' protection afforded by cardiac pacing (9). When dogs are paced for four 5-min periods at a rate of 220 beats min^{-1}, there is protection against coronary artery occlusion-induced arrhythmias both immediately following pacing and also 20 h after termination of the pacing stimulus. The protection disappears between these two times. When icatibant is given prior to the pacing preconditioning stimulus, the number of ventricular premature beats during pacing is increased and the delayed protective effect against arrhythmias 20 h later is markedly attenuated (9). When icatibant is given to paced dogs before coronary artery occlusion 20 h after the preconditioning stimulus, the protective effects are attenuated. This again suggests that early bradykinin release is a trigger not only for the antiarrhythmic effects of 'classical' ischaemic preconditioning, but also for the delayed protective effects of cardiac pacing.

Evidence for the involvement of prostanoids

There is early work (5) suggesting that prostacyclin is released early under conditions of ischaemia and the amount released determines the severity of early phase 1(a) ventricular arrhythmias. This view is supported by the fact that drugs that increase the amount of prostacyclin generated by the ischaemic myocardium (e.g. nafazatrom) are also profoundly antiarrhythmic. The possible role of prostanoids in the antiarrhythmic effects of 'classical' ischaemic preconditioning comes from a study (10) showing that inhibition of the cyclooxygenase pathway with sodium meclofenamate prevents the protective (antiarrhythmic) effect of ischaemic preconditioning in anaesthetised dogs. The difficulty with such studies is that a variety of products arise from activation of the cyclooxygenase pathway, the production of all of which would be inhibited some of these (e.g., thromboxane) are proarrhythmic.

More recent evidence suggests that simultaneously inhibiting both the cyclooxygenase and L-arginine nitric oxide pathways completely abolishes the antiarrhythmic effects of short coronary artery occlusions (11). Indeed, it is extremely difficult to precondition dogs in which both pathways have been blocked.

Evidence for the possible involvement of cGMP in the protective effects of ischaemic preconditioning

This evidence is both direct and indirect. The direct evidence is i) that in rabbits cardiac pacing increases cGMP levels in the myocardium (12); ii) that preconditioning elevates cGMP levels in ischaemic areas of the left ventricle wall compared to those in adjacent, non-ischaemic, regions (13). The indirect evidence comes from studies involving stable analogues of cGMP which can cross cardiac membranes and which are more resistant to breakdown by phosphodiesterase. In some hands, these substances are antiarrhythmic (reviewed in ref. (1)). This is an area for further detailed exploration.

How elevated cGMP levels could modify arrhythmogenesis is illustrated in Fig. 1. The proposal is that there is 'cross talk' between endothelial cells and cardiac myocytes through the liberation of nitric oxide, generated as a result of bradykinin B2 receptor stimulation on the endothelial cell surface. This nitric oxide, which can diffuse rapidly and across quite long distances, stimulates soluble guanylyl cyclase in cardiac myocytes and elevates cGMP. There are three possible effects of cGMP which might then lead to cardiac protection and to suppression of ventricular arrhythmias, remembering that preconditioning leads to less marked ischaemia, as reflected by epicardial ST-segment mapping and by changes in the degree of electrical inhomogeneity within the ischaemic area (2). These possibilities are:

i) Stimulation of a cGMP sensitive phosphodiesterase enzyme which leads to an increased breakdown of cAMP. The suggestion is that it is the balance between cAMP and cGMP which is implicated in early arrhythmogenesis.
ii) Inhibition of calcium entry through L-type calcium channels (reviewed in (1)).
iii) Nitric oxide is known to depress myocardial contractility and is, for example, a major component of myocardial depression in patients with sepsis. This would reduce myocardial oxygen demand, a factor which has been suggested to play an important role in protecting the ischaemic myocardium.

Although such mechanisms might contribute to the protection afforded against ventricular arrhythmias by 'classical' ischaemic preconditioning there is no evidence that they are involved in 'delayed' protection. However, in the canine the protection afforded by pacing is not observed if dexamethasone is administered prior to the pacing preconditioning stimulus (4). This might suggest the induction of nitric oxide synthase (iNOS) within cardiac myocytes or of cyclooxygenase 2. There may be some parallel here with endotoxaemia and sepsis. Under these conditions NOS is induced in cardiac myocytes through cytokine release, an effect which is prevented by dexamethasone. Similarly, endotoxin has protective effects against coronary artery occlusion induced arrhythmias in rats and this protection is also abolished by dexamethasone (14).

We would emphasise that the above is only a working hypothesis. However, as a notable German scientist once stated, "It is more important that a hypothesis is fruitful than that it is true". The endothelial cell, nitric oxide ischaemic preconditioning hypothesis has certainly been fruitful. Whether it is true or not awaits further experimentation.

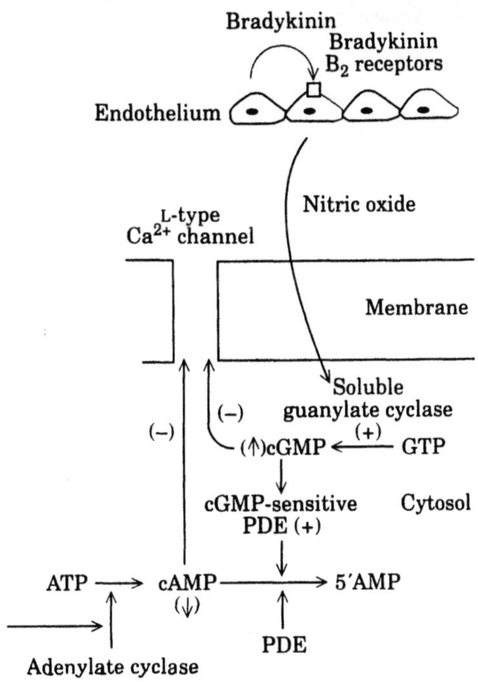

Fig. 1 Role of endothelium derived endogenous protective mediators in ischaemic preconditioning – a hypothesis.
Bradykinin is released, probably from endothelial cells (which have the mechanisms for generating and releasing kinins) which then acts on B2 receptors on the endothelial surface to increase the calcium transient within these cells and to activate the L-arginine nitric oxide pathway. Nitric oxide then 'talks' to the cardiac myocyte, stimulates soluble guanylyl cyclase and elevates cyclic GMP. This stimulates a cGMP sensitive phosphodiesterase (thus reducing cAMP levels), inhibits calcium entry through L-type calcium channels and depresses myocardial contractility. For discussion see text.

Acknowledgements The authors' work in this area was supported by grants from the Royal Society, The Wellcome Trust, the British Council (in collaboration with the Hungarian Committee for Scientific and Technical Development) and by the Hungarian State Government (OTKA). Collaborative research between the two departments in Szeged and Glasgow has also been facilitated by an European Community Network grant, coordinated from Glasgow, on 'Endogenous mechanisms of cardioprotection' (Grant No ERC-CIPA-CT-92-4009).

References

1. Parratt JR, Vegh A (1994) Pronounced antiarrhythmic effects of ischemic preconditioning. Cardioscience 5: 9–18
2. Vegh A, Komori S, Szekeres L, Parratt JR (1992) Antiarrhythmic effect of preconditioning in anaesthetised dogs and rats. Cardiovasc Res 26: 487–495
3. Piacentini L, Wainwright CL, Parratt JR (1993) The antiarrhythmic effect of ischaemic preconditioning in rat isolated hearts involves a pertussis toxin sensitive mechanism. Cardiovasc Res 27: 674–680
4. Vegh A, Papp JGy, Parratt JR (1994) Prevention by dexamethasone of the marked antiarrhythmic effects of preconditioning induced 20 h after rapid cardiac pacing. Br J Pharmacol 113: 1081–1082
5. Coker SJ, Parratt JR, Ledingham IMcL, Zeitlin IJ (1981) Thromboxane and prostacyclin release from ischaemic myocardium in relation to arrhythmias. Nature 291: 323–324
6. Node K, Kitakaze M, Kosaka H, Komamura K, Minamino T, Tada M, Inoue M, Hori M, Kamada T (1995) Plasma nitric oxide end products are increased in the ischemic canine heart. Biochem Biophys Res Commun 211: 370–374
7. Vegh A, Szekeres L, Parratt JR (1992) Preconditioning of the ischaemic myocardium; involvement of the L-arginine nitric oxide pathway. Br J Pharmacol 107: 648–652
8. Vegh A, Papp JGy, Parratt JR (1994) Attenuation of the antiarrhythmic effects of ischaemic preconditioning by blockade of bradykinin B2 receptors. Br J Pharmacol 113: 1167–1172
9. Vegh A, Kaszala K, Papp JGy, Parratt JR (1995) Delayed myocardial protection by pacing-induced preconditioning; a possible role for bradykinin. Br J Pharmacol (in press)
10. Vegh A, Szekeres L, Parratt JR (1990) Protective effects of preconditioning on the ischaemic myocardium involves cyclo-oxygenase products. Cardiovasc Res 24: 1020–1022
11. Kis A, Vegh A, Papp JGy, Parratt JR (1995) Dual blockade of the cyclo-oxygenase and L-arginine-nitric oxide pathways prevents the antiarrhythmic effects of preconditioning. J Molec Cell Cardiol 27: A159
12. Szilvassy Z, Jakab I, Lonovics J, Papp JGy (1992) Is rapid pacing-induced preconditioning related to changes of myocardial cyclic nucleotide content? J Mol Cell Cardiol 24 (Supp V): S99
13. Parratt JR (1995) Possibilities for the pharmacological exploitation of ischaemic preconditioning. J Mol Cell Cardiol 27: 991–1000
14. Wu Song, Furman BL, Parratt JR (1994) Endotoxin protection against ischaemia-induced ventricular arrhythmias is attenuated by dexamethasone. Br J Pharmac 113: 1083–1084

149 – 152

G. J. Gross
D. A. Mei
J. J. Schultz
T. Mizumura

Criteria for a mediator or effector of myocardial preconditioning: Do K_{ATP} channels meet the requirements?

Key words Preconditioning criteria – threshold – memory – K_{ATP} channels – species dependency

Introduction

Although a number of mediators (7) have been shown to mimic the protective effect of ischemia to precondition the heart, i.e., adenosine, acetylcholine, bradykinin, phorbol esters, and several end effectors or targets (7) of these substances have been identified, i.e., specific receptors, (A_1, adenosine; M_2 muscarinic; B_2, bradykinin) ATP-sensitive potassium channels (K_{ATP}), protein kinase C (PKC), no strict criteria have been developed which are necessary to confirm that a substance or effector is an important component of the preconditioning response. This review is an attempt to develop such criteria and to summarize data which suggest that the K_{ATP} channel fits most of these criteria and meets the requirements necessary for it to qualify as a common pathway in the cardioprotective effect produced by a variety of stimuli in different species or models. Infarct size reduction will be the end point used to define preconditioning since this parameter is the one which was used to originally demonstrate this fascinating phenomenon in canine hearts by Murry et al. (6).

Dr. G. J. Gross (✉) · D. A. Mei · J. J. Schultz · T. Mizumura
Department of Pharmacology & Toxicology
Medical College of Wisconsin
8701 Watertown Plank Road
Milwaukee, Wisconsin 53226, USA

Criteria for mediator or effector of preconditioning (see Table 1)

The criteria which have been proposed to be important for determining if a mediator or effector is an important component of the cardioprotective response of ischemic preconditioning (PC) are the following: 1) Ischemic PC should be blocked by specific pharmacological antagonists of the proposed mediator or end effector; 2) Pharmacological agonists in the same class as the mediator or which stimulate the end effector should mimic the effect of ischemic PC to reduce infarct size; 3) Other stimuli which produce a PC-like effect should be blocked by specific antagonists of the end effector or final common pathway; 4) The time-course of the ischemic PC response ("memory") should be mimicked or blocked by agonists

Table 1 Criteria for a mediator or effector of ischemic preconditioning (PC)

- Ischemic PC should be blocked by specific pharmacological antagonists of the proposed mediator or end effector
- Pharmacological agonists in the same class as the mediator or which stimulate the end effector should mimic the effect of ischemic PC to reduce infarct size
- Other stimuli which produce a PK-like effect should be blocked by specific antagonists of the end effector or final common pathway
- The time-course of the ischemic PC response ("memory") should be mimicked or blocked by agonists or antagonists of the end effector
- Pharmacological agonists of receptors or the end effector should decrease the threshold of time necessary to precondition the heart by ischemia
- The mediator or effector of PC should be common to all species including man

or antagonists of the end effector; 5) Pharmacological agonists of receptors or the end effector should decrease the threshold of time necessary to precondition the heart by ischemia; 6) The mediator or effector of PC should be common to all species including man. Because of space limitations, the following discussion will be limited to the evidence supporting a role for the K_{ATP} channel as a final common pathway in the PC response primarily using studies performed in dogs in our laboratory for illustrative purposes.

Ischemic PC – Pharmacological antagonists

The strongest evidence for a role of K_{ATP} channels in ischemic PC is based on studies using pharmacological antagonists, particularly glibenclamide. Our original work in dogs (2) showed that administration of glibenclamide before or immediately after the ischemic PC stimulus totally blocked its protective effect which suggested that the K_{ATP} channel may be involved in both triggering and sustaining the beneficial effect of PC in dogs. Subsequently, we also showed that sodium 5-hydroxydecanoic acid (5-HD), a K_{ATP} antagonist structurally unrelated to glibenclamide and possessing ischemia selectivity also abolished ischemic PC in dogs (1). Glibenclamide and 5-HD have also been shown to block ischemic PC in a number of related studies performed in pigs, rabbits and rats although there is some controversy in the latter two species.

Pharmacological agonists mimic ischemic PC

Several studies in dogs have shown that K_{ATP} channel openers mimic the effect of ischemic PC to reduce infarct size (4, 5). Most recently, Mizumura et al. (5) compared the effects of bimakalim, a K_{ATP} opener, and 5 min of ischemic PC to reduce infarct size, affect adenosine release from the ischemic area and affect neutrophil infiltration into the ischemic-reperfused area. Interestingly, bimakalim and ischemic PC, reduced infarct size, adenosine release and neutrophil infiltration to a nearly equal extent which suggests, but does not unequivocally prove, that these two stimuli may be acting via a common mechanism to reduce ischemic injury in the canine heart. Similar comparative studies have not been performed in other species and are necessary to strengthen the idea that K_{ATP} activation and ischemic PC share similar mechanisms of cardioprotection in all species.

PC mimetics blocked by specific antagonists of the end effector

Recent work by Yao and Gross (10) and Mei and Gross (3) has shown that other mediators or stimuli can produce a PC-like effect to reduce infarct size in dogs via activation of the K_{ATP} channel. Intracoronary administration of adenosine or acetylcholine have been shown to reduce infarct size in canine hearts similar to that produced by ischemic PC, and these protective effects were blocked by glibenclamide or 5-HD (10). Similarly, Mei and Gross (3) recently showed that 5 min of hypoxia was as effective as 5 min of ischemia to precondition the canine heart, and this effect of hypoxia was also abolished by pretreatment with glibenclamide. Hartman and colleagues at Upjohn have also shown that glibenclamide blocks bradykinin-induced PC in rabbits (personal communication). Therefore, it appears that the K_{ATP} channel may serve as a common effector in dogs and rabbits to various pharmacological or pathophysiological stimuli which induce a PC-like effect on infarct size.

Time-course or memory of ischemic PC – Mimicked or blocked by agonists or antagonists of the end effector

One of the most interesting aspects of ischemic PC is the observation that there is a limited time following the PC stimulus during which the heart remembers that it is preconditioned. This phenomenon has been termed acute memory and has been shown to last for approximately 2 h in dogs (6).

In this regard, recent evidence from our laboratory indirectly supports a role for the K_{ATP} channel as a necessary component of the acute memory phase of ischemic PC (12). We observed that glibenclamide, administered 50 min after the ischemic PC stimulus totally abolished the protective effect of ischemic PC which was still present 1 h following preconditioning. We also found that a 10-min intracoronary infusion of both adenosine and bimakalim together produced a cardioprotective effect similar to that of 10 min of ischemic PC to reduce infarct size 60 min after the PC stimulus, whereas, either adenosine or bimakalim administered alone had no sustained cardioprotective effect in this canine model (12). Taken together, these results suggest that myocardial K_{ATP} channels may be an essential component of the acute memory phase of PC. Recent evidence from our laboratory (unpublished results) also suggests that monophosphoryl lipid A (MLA), an endotoxin analogue, can produce a delayed (24 h later) cardioprotective response to reduce infarct size in dogs and rabbits similar to that of acute ischemic

PC and that this delayed protective effect is mediated via the K_{ATP} channel. Further work is necessary to determine if other stimuli known to produce a delayed cardioprotective response, i.e., ischemia, hypoxia, heat shock, adenosine, also act via the K_{ATP} channel.

Pharmacological agonists of receptors or end effectors lower the threshold for ischemic PC

In addition to ischemic PC having the property of memory, there is also a finite period of time or "threshold" required for ischemic PC to produce its cardioprotective effect. Generally, 2 – 3 min of ischemia are necessary for the cardioprotective effect of PC to be manifest in various species including the dog. In this regard, recent results from our laboratory have shown that 3 min of ischemia is not sufficient to precondition the canine heart (11), however, when 0.3 μg/min of the K_{ATP} opener bimakalim was infused simultaneously during the 3-min occlusion period, infarct size was reduced to an extent similar to that of 5 or 10 min of ischemic PC. These results further support the hypothesis that the K_{ATP} channel is an essential component in triggering as well as maintaining the PC response.

Mediators or effectors of PC common to all species including man

There is evidence to support the idea that the K_{ATP} channel is involved in ischemic PC in all species tested although most studies with glibenclamide performed in rats have been negative. Perhaps more importantly, although infarct size was not the end point, a recent study of Tomai et al. (9) showed that glibenclamide blocked a PC-like effect produced by consecutive periods of angioplasty in man. Furthermore, results of Speechly-Dick et al. (8) in human atrial trabeculae preconditioned by hypoxia also suggest a key role for the K_{ATP} channel in mediating PC in man.

Conclusions

A set of criteria have been presented which we feel need to be met before one can assign an important role for a particular endogenous mediator, ion channel or enzyme as an important component of ischemic PC and evidence has been presented to suggest that the K_{ATP} channel meets most of the criteria listed. Obviously, this list is not all conclusive and other important factors will evolve as we increase our understanding of this fascinating phenomenon of ischemic PC.

Acknowledgements The authors wish to thank Ms. Carol Knapp for the excellent assistance in typing this manuscript. The work described was supported by NIH Grant HL 08311.

References

1. Auchampach JA, Grover GJ, Gross GJ (1992) Blockade of ischemic preconditioning in dogs by the novel ATP-dependent potassium channel antagonist sodium 5-hydroxydecanoate. Cardiovasc Res 26: 1054–1062
2. Gross GJ, Auchampach JA (1992) Blockade of ATP-sensitive potassium channels prevents myocardial preconditioning in dogs. Circ Res 70: 223–233
3. Mei DA, Gross GJ (1995) Evidence for the involvement of the ATP-sensitive potassium channel in a novel model of hypoxic preconditioning in dogs. Cardiovasc Res 30: 222–230
4. Mizumura T, Nithipatikom K, Gross GJ (1995) Effects of nicorandil and glyceryl trinitrate on infarct size, adenosine release and neutrophil infiltration in the dog. Cardiovasc Res 29: 482–489
5. Mizumura T, Nithipatikom K, Gross GJ (1995) Bimakalim, an ATP-sensitive potassium channel opener, mimics the effects of ischemic preconditioning to reduce infarct size, adenosine release and neutrophil function in dogs. Circulation 92: 1236–1245
6. Murry CE, Jennings RB, Reimer KA (1986) Preconditioning with ischemia: a delay of lethal cell injury in ischemic myocardium. Circulation 74: 1124–1136
7. Parratt JR (1995) Possibilities for the pharmacological exploitation of ischemic preconditioning. J Mol Cell Cardiol 27: 991–1000
8. Speechly-Dick ME, Grover GJ, Yellon DM (1995) Does ischemic preconditioning in the human atrium involve protein kinase C and the ATP-dependent K channel? Studies of contractile function in an in vitro model. Circ Res 77: 1030–1035

9. Tomai F, Crea F, Gaspardone A, Versaci F, DePaulis R, Penta de Peppo A, Chiariello L, Gioffre PA (1994) Ischemic preconditioning during coronary angioplasty is prevented by glibenclamide, a selective ATP-sensitive K^+ channel blocker. Circulation 90: 700–705
10. Yao Z, Gross GJ (1993) Acetylcholine mimics ischemic preconditioning in dogs: role of nitric oxide, muscarinic receptors and the K_{ATP} channel. Circ Res 73: 1193–1201
11. Yao Z, Gross GJ (1994) Activation of ATP-senstive potassium channels lowers threshold for ischemic preconditioning in dogs. Am J Physiol 267: H1888–H1894
12. Yao Z, Mizumura T, Mei DA, Gross GJ (1996) Myocardial K_{ATP} channels may play a role in the memory of ischemic preconditioning in anesthetized dogs: Evidence for a synergistic effect between adenosine and the K_{ATP} channel. Am J Physiol (in Review)

153–155

J. M. Downey
M. V. Cohen

Preconditioning: Markers vs. epiphenomena

Key words Ischemic preconditioning – adenosine – ST segment – protein kinase C

When the heart is exposed to a brief period of ischemia it becomes protected against infarction during a subsequent period of ischemia. While we now have some insight into the signal transduction system involved in this protective adaptation, the overall mechanism remains enigmatic. If one could merely answer the simple question, "What is different between a preconditioned and a non-preconditioned heart"?, then a key step towards understanding this mechanism will have been taken. The hesitation encountered in answering this question is largely related to the difficulty experienced separating epiphenomena (changes occurring that have no relationship to the protection) from the actual factors that are involved. For example, one sees that glycogen is depleted following a transient period of ischemia. However, most investigators would now agree that glycogen depletion is unrelated to the mechanism of protection. Glycogen is not depleted when the heart is pharmacologically preconditioned with an agent like adenosine and all interventions which deplete glycogen do not precondition. Thus, glycogen depletion appears to be an epiphenomenon.

Dr. J. M. Downey (✉) · M. V. Cohen
Department of Physiology
MSB 3024
University of South Alabama
College of Medicine
Mobile, Alabama 36688, USA

Preconditioning and adenosine release patterns

A similar situation is observed when the amount of adenosine that the heart releases during ischemia is quantitated. While one group has reported that adenosine release is augmented during ischemia in preconditioned dog hearts (6), most observers have actually documented decreased release if the heart has first been preconditioned (13). Most of the adenosine released is thought to derive from ischemically-induced ATP degradation. Could this attenuated relese reflect reduced ATP degradation during ischemia which, in turn, is responsible for the protection? That explanation seems unlikely. Blocking protection of a brief ischemic period with an adenosine receptor antagonist does not prevent the attenuated adenosine release during a second coronary occlusion (4). Additionally, pharmacologic preconditioning of the heart with a brief infusion of adenosine does not lead to attenuation of the amount of adenosine released with a subsequent period of ischemia (4). The heart simply seems to release less adenosine during a second period of ischemia than it does the first time regardless of whether or not it is in a preconditioned state. Therefore, a change in the pattern of adenosine release during preconditioning represents an epiphenomenon.

Preconditioning and ST-segment elevation

Several years ago it was reported that patients undergoing coronary angioplasty showed much less ST-segment elevation on subsequent occlusions of the coronary artery after the first (3). Could this be related to preconditioning's mechanism? Perhaps. The hearts of rabbits and pigs have sparse coronary collaterals, and both show the same pattern of reduced epicardial ST-segment elevation during ischemia if first preconditioned (2, 9). To determine whether this change might also be an epiphenomenon, we again treated rabbits with adenosine antagonists and pharmacologic preconditioning agents to see whether alterations in the magnitude of ST-segment elevation during coronary occlusion tracked with the state of protection of the myocardium. This time rabbits in which protection was blocked by administration of an adenosine receptor antagonist showed equivalent degrees of ST-segment elevation during three successive coronary occlusions (2), that is, blocking protection abolished electrocardiographic evidence of diminished ischemia during later occlusions. Furthermore, pharmacologic preconditioning also abolished the attenuated ST-segment response during the second occlusion because the heart was already protected during the first occlusion and there could be no further reduction in the severity of ischemia as a result of that occlusion (Cohen, M. V., Yang, X.-M., Downey, J. M., unpublished observation). ST-segment elevation is produced where there is a loss of membrane potential in the ischemic region. These data would suggest that the membrane potential is lost more slowly during ischemia if the heart is in a preconditioned state, and that this delay is indeed related to the protective mechanism. Interestingly, preconditioning has been linked to opening of the K_{ATP} channel in the myocytes (5), a major determinant of membrane potential, but it is uncertain how that channel opening could result in preservation of the membrane potential during ischemia.

Adenosine fails to protect the virgin heart

Let us further explore what may be different in naive and preconditioned hearts. From a functional standpoint we would say that in the preconditioned heart a coupling has been established between adenosine receptors and protein kinase C (PKC). Adenosine acting as an agonist of the A_1 receptor was the first autacoid to be proposed as a trigger of the anti-infarct effect of preconditioning (7). Subsequent work by many laboratories has validated that theory. Within a minute or two of the start of a coronary occlusion, adenosine is released in micromolar amounts. This would quickly saturate the A_1 receptors whose K_d is in the nanomolar range. Yet the virgin heart is not protected by all of this adenosine. It has been our experience that adenosine receptor blockers have no effect on infarct size in the non-preconditioned rabbit heart (7). Even when the adenosine concentration has been augmented 100-fold by a deaminase inhibitor, there still was no protection of the non-preconditioned heart (10). On the other hand, if the heart has been preconditioned, then the adenosine that is released becomes very protective. Blocking adenosine receptors after preconditioning but just prior to the long ischemia completely aborts the protection indicating that adenosine receptors must be activated during the long ischemia in order to protect (11).

PKC fails to protect the virgin heart

We now believe that adenosine receptors protect by activating PKC in the myocyte. PKC inhibitors block the protective effect of ischemic preconditioning (14) and agonists of any of the PKC-coupled receptors in the heart (adrenergic α_1, angiotensin II AT_1, endothelin ET_1, bradykinin B_2, muscarinic M_2, and adenosine A_1) can fully mimic preconditioning (1). The timing of PKC activation is also interesting. Blocking PKC in the non-preconditioned rabbit heart has no effect on infarct size (14), just as was seen with adenosine blockers. Protection is also unaffected after exposure of the heart to the PKC blocker staurosporine at the time of the brief preconditioning ischemia (8). But when the long ischemia occurs in the presence of staurosporine, protection is completely blocked (14). The simplest explanation seems to be that in preconditioned myocytes a coupling has been established between the adenosine receptor and PKC which did not previously exist. This newly-established coupling makes the heart's own adenosine become protective.

Phenylephrine can establish the adenosine-PKC coupling

The coupling theory is strongly supported by observations with the α_1-adrenergic agonist phenylephrine. Transient exposure to phenylephrine fully preconditions the heart, but this protection can be aborted if an adenosine blocker is given just prior to the long ischemia (12). On the other hand, blocking adenosine receptors during only the phenylephrine exposure does not block protection (12). Thus, transient activation of α_1 receptors also makes the heart become sensitive to its own adenosine. Coupling to PKC could be illustrated by adding phenylephrine along with the adenosine antagonist during the long ischemia in the above experiment (12). In that case protection returned, presumably because the phenylephrine was able to activate PKC directly despite blockade of the adenosine receptors.

Does the translocation theory explain the data?

The mechanism of the establishment of this coupling between adenosine receptors and PKC is unknown. We have proposed that this coupling may be a result of translocation of a critical PKC isoform into the membranes where it can be quickly activated (1). The attractiveness of the translocation theory is that translocation, the first step in activation, does not involve phosphorylation and can occur in the presence of staurosporine. Experimental evidence for or against this theory is currently sparse, however. We believe that these issues of adenosine-PKC coupling and PKC translocation and activation represent a critical part of the preconditioning puzzle and should receive more attention in future studies.

References

1. Cohen MV, Downey JM (1995) Preconditioning during ischemia: basic mechanisms and potential clinical applications. Cardiol Rev 3: 137–149
2. Cohen MV, Yang X-M, Fletcher JR, Downey JM (1995) Less ST segment elevation during subsequent coronary occlusions indicates preconditioning in rabbit. J Mol Cell Cardiol 27: A144
3. Deutsch E, Berger M, Kussmaul WG, Hirshfeld JW Jr, Herrmann HC, Laskey WK (1990) Adaptation to ischemia during percutaneous transluminal coronary angioplasty: clinical, hemodynamic, and metabolic features. Circulation 82: 2044–2051
4. Goto M, Cohen MV, Van Wylen DGL, Downey JM (1996) Attenuated purine production during subsequent ischemia in preconditioned rabbit myocardium is unrelated to the mechanism of protection. J Mol Cell Cardiol (in press)
5. Gross GJ, Auchampach JA (1992) Blockade of ATP-sensitive potassium channels prevents myocardial preconditioning in dogs. Circ Res 70: 223–233
6. Kitakaze M, Hori M, Takashima S, Sato H, Inoue M, Kamada T (1993) Ischemic preconditioning increases adenosine release and 5′-nucleotidase activity during myocardial ischemia and reperfusion in dogs: implications for myocardial salvage. Circulation 87: 208–215
7. Liu GS, Thornton J, Van Winkle DM, Stanley AWH, Olsson RA, Downey JM (1991) Protection against infarction afforded by preconditioning is mediated by A_1 adenosine receptors in rabbit heart. Circulation 84: 350–356
8. Liu Y, Ytrehus K, Downey JM (1994) Evidence that translocation of protein kinase C is a key event during ischemic preconditioning of rabbit myocardium. J Mol Cell Cardiol 26: 661–668
9. Shattock MJ, Lawson CS, Hearse DJ, Downey JM (1995) Do temporal electrophysiological and collateral flow changes mirror preconditioning-induced infarct size limitation in the pig? J Mol Cell Cardiol 27: A143
10. Silva PH, Dillon D, Van Wylen DGL (1995) Adenosine deaminase inhibition augments interstitial adenosine but does not attenuate myocardial infarction. Cardiovasc Res 29: 616–623
11. Thornton JD, Thornton CS, Downey JM (1993) Effect of adenosine receptor blockade: preventing protective preconditioning depends on time of initiation. Am J Physiol 265: H504–H508
12. Tsuchida A, Liu Y, Liu GS, Cohen MV, Downey JM (1994) α_1-Adrenergic agonists precondition rabbit ischemic myocardium independent of adenosine by direct activation of protein kinase C. Circ Res 75: 576–585
13. Van Wylen DGL (1994) Effect of ischemic preconditioning on interstitial purine metabolite and lactate accumulation during myocardial ischemia. Circulation 89: 2283–2289
14. Ytrehus K, Liu Y, Downey JM (1994) Preconditioning protects ischemic rabbit heart by protein kinase C activation. Am J Physiol 266: H1145–H1152

156–158

D. M. Van Winkle

Limitation of infarct size by myocardial ischemic preconditioning

Key words Ischemia-reperfusion – myocardial infarction – adenosine – ATP-sensitive potassium channels – protein kinase C

Introduction

Myocardial ischemic preconditioning (IP) has caught the attention and imagination of researchers throughout the world (7). And for good reason: the magnitude of protection against ischemic injury conferred by IP is tremendous, far surpassing that offered by past pharmacological therapies. Although the original description of IP focused on limitation of myocardial infarction following acute coronary occlusion and reperfusion, IP may also decrease the incidence of ischemia-induced arrhythmias and improve post-ischemic cardiac function. However, in this article the discussion will be confined to the infarct-limiting effect of IP. Upon suffering a brief episode of ischemia, the myocardium instigates some change in itself which protects it from subsequent ischemic events. On an organ level the visible end-point is a decrease in infarct. This grossly visible change is the result of the cellular transduction of a signal and the institution of an adaptive cellular modification. But what precisely is that cellular process?

Dr. D. M. Van Winkle (✉)
Department of Anesthesiology (UHS-2)
Oregon Health Sciences University
3181 SW Sam Jackson Park Road
Portland, Oregon 97201, USA

How is preconditioning mediated?

Like many processes within the myocardium, IP appears to be mediated by the interaction of endogenous factors with their specific receptors. Typically, receptors elicit a given response by modulating the activity of an effector to which they are coupled; the effector in turn alters the levels of specific second messengers, which then lead to the functional response. Receptor-mediated regulation of effectors (such as phospholipase C [PLC], phospholipase D [PLD], and ion channels) often occurs via G proteins, and second messengers (such as inositol 1,4,5-triphosphate [IP3], phosphatidic acid [PA], and 1,2-diacylglycerol [DAG] often elicit the functional response by activation of protein kinases.

Numerous receptor-mediated agents have been shown to mimic the cardioprotection of IP. These include adenosine and adenosine A_1 receptor (A_1AR) agonists, α-adrenergic agonists, angiotensin II, and bradykinin (2, 5, 6, 13). Although there are species-specific differences in blockade of IP by antagonists of these receptors, this does not necessarily negate the possibility that a given agent is involved in IP. The heart may rely on several stimuli to initiate IP rather than just one, and the initiating events may occur in different proportions in different species. Also, it is possible that the initiating event(s) may be different in different species, but the latter steps in the preconditioning process (effectors, second messengers, phosphorylation targets, etc.) are similar.

Both G protein mediated regulation of effectors, and reliance of second messengers upon protein kinases to elicit the functional response, have been implicated in IP. IP can be abolished by treatment with pertussis toxin, suggesting that it is mediated via a G protein (Gi or Go) (2). Blockade of ATP-sensitive potassium channels (K_{ATP}) eliminates IP and openers of the K_{ATP} channel provide cardioprotection, suggesting that this ion channel may be one of the effectors involved in preconditioning (3). Analogues of DAG induce a cardioprotective state similar to IP; since DAG is formed through the action of PLC or PLD, this suggests that one or both of these effectors are involved in IP. Likewise, since DAG is the endogenous activator of protein kinase C (PKC), this also suggests that PKC may contribute to IP.

Do all the pieces fit together?

One postulated mechanism for the mediation of IP suggests that activation of A_1ARs results in pertussis-toxin sensitive G protein-mediated activation of PLC, resulting in release of DAG, activation of PKC and the subsequent phosphorylation of a target protein (2). Can this be reconciled with other theories, e.g. opening of K_{ATP} channels? Cross-over studies, combining an agonist of one putative mediator of IP with the antagonist of another putative mediator, can help clarify this question. For instance, cardioprotection provided by the A_1 agonist (-)-N^6-2-(phenylisopropyl)-adenosine is abolished by 5-hydroxydecanoate, a blocker of the K_{ATP} channel (11). Since we know that blockade of adenosine receptors blocks IP, we infer that IP may be mediated by adenosine receptor activation followed by opening of the K_{ATP} channel as a subsequent step. Additionally, it has recently been shown that blockade of K_{ATP} channels abolishes the infarct-limiting effect of the DAG-analogue oleyl acetyl glycerol (OAG), furthering the idea that adenosine receptor-G protein-PKC induced cardioprotection (and probably IP as well) occurs via opening of the K_{ATP} channel as a downstream event (12).

For a seamless theory regarding the mechanism of IP, several inconsistencies still need to be clarified:

1) As mentioned above, IP is suggested to occur via A_1AR activation of pertussis toxin sensitive G proteins, leading to activation of PLC. Within the myocardium, the most abundant forms of PLC are PLC-γ and PLC-β, respectively. However, PLC-γ is activated through receptor-associated tyrosine kinases, and PLC-β is activated by pertussis toxin-insensitive Gq proteins. Moreover, although PLC-β has been reported to be linked to α_1-adrenergic, muscarinic, and angiotensin II receptor stimulation, coupling to A_1 receptors has not been described (9).
2) Since many cellular processes occur through protein phosphorylation, the concept that IP occurs via PKC phosphorylation of some target protein is a cogent one. This theory has been supported by studies demonstrating ablation of IP following blockade of PKC with polymyxin B or staurosporine (2, 8). However, these drugs are not selective for PKC and will inhibit other kinases (1) and even the K_{ATP} channel (4). Moreover, use of the PKC-specific inhibitor chelerythrine in rabbits failed to abolish IP, although it did block DAG-analogue induced infarct limitation (12).
3) The occurrence of infarct-limitation with antecedent administration of DAG-analogues or phorbol esters has been used to support the theory that IP is mediated by activation of PKC. Since the conventional (cPKC: α, β, and γ) and novel (nPKC: δ, ε, η, and θ) isoforms of PKC are activated by DAG and phorbol esters but the atypical PKC isoforms (aPKC: ζ, λ, ι, and μ) are not, this suggests that the isoforms relevant for IP are cPKC and nPKC. Immunoreactivity studies suggest that only a few PKC isoforms are present within the adult heart: PKC-δ and PKC-ε in rat hearts, and PKC-ε and PKC-ζ in dog hearts (9). Since PKC-ζ is not activated by DAG/DAG-analogues or phorbol esters, this suggests that the IP-relevant isoform is PKC-ε. However, studies demonstrating increased activity of PKC following brief ischemia have utilized histone as the substrate, which is phosphorylated readily by cPKC but poorly by nPKC isoforms such as PKC-ε (9, 10).

Although much has been learned since the initial description of IP, much is yet to be elucidated. While the concept of receptor-mediated activation of PKC with subsequent phosphorylation of a target protein (e.g., the K_{ATP} channel) is attractive, many details remain to be clarified.

References

1. Casnellie JE (1991) In: August JT, Anders MW, Murad F (eds) Protein kinase inhibitors: probes for the functions of protein phosphorylation. Advances in Pharmacology, Volume 22. Academic Press, Inc., San Diego, pp 167–205
2. Downey JM, Cohen MV, Ytrehus K, Liu Y (1994) Cellular mechanisms in ischemic preconditioning: The role of adenosine and protein kinase C. Ann NY Acad Sci 723: 82–98
3. Gross GJ (1995) ATP-sensitive potassium channels and myocardial preconditioning. Basic Res Cardiol 90: 85–88
4. Harding EA, Jaggar JH, Squires PE, Dunne MJ (1994) Polymyxin B has multiple blocking actions on the ATP-sensitive potassium channel in insulin-secreting cells. Pflügers Arch 426: 31–39
5. Kitakaze M, Hori M, Morioka T, Minamino T, Takashima S, Sato H, Shinozaki Y, Chujo M, Hori H, Inoue M, Kamada T (1994) Alpha$_1$-adrenoceptor activation mediates the infarct size-limiting effect of ischemic preconditioning through augmentation of 5′-nucleotidase activity. J Clin Invest 95: 2197–2205
6. Liu Y, Tsuchida A, Cohen MV, Downey JM (1995) Pretreatment with Angiotensin II activates protein kinase C and limits myocardial infarction in isolated rabbit hearts. J Mol Cell Cardiol 27: 883–892
7. Murry CE, Jennings RB, Reimer KA (1986) Preconditioning with ischemia: a delay of lethal cell injury in ischemic myocardium. Circulation 74: 1124–1136
8. Sakamoto J, Miura T, Goto M, Iimura O (1995) Limitation of myocardial infarct size by adenosine A_1 receptor activation is abolished by protein kinase C inhibitors in the rabbit. Cardiovasc Res 29: 682–688
9. Steinberg SF, Goldberg M, Rybin VO (1995) Protein kinase C isoform diversity in the heart. J Mol Cell Cardiol 27: 141–153
10. Strasser RH, Braun-Dullaeus R, Walendzik H, Marquetant R (1992) α_1-Receptor-independent activation of protein kinase C in acute myocardial ischemia. Mechanisms for sensitization of the adenylyl cyclase system. Circ Res 70: 1304–1312
11. Van Winkle DM, Chien GL, Wolff RA, Soifer BE, Kuzume K, Davis RF (1994) Cardioprotection provided by adenosine receptor activation is abolished by blockade of the ATP-sensitive potassium channel. Am J Physiol 266: H829–H839
12. Van Winkle DM, Kuzume K, Dote K, Wolff RA (1995) Infarct limitation by protein kinase C (PKC) is attenuated by blockade of ATP-sensitive potassium channels. J Mol Cell Cardiol 27: A142 (Abstract)
13. Wall TM, Sheehy R, Hartman JC (1994) Role of bradykinin in myocardial preconditioning. J Pharmacol Exp Ther 270: 681–688

159–161

K. Przyklenk
R. A. Kloner

Role of protein kinase C in ischemic preconditioning: in search of the "pure and simple truth"

Key words Ischemic preconditioning – protein kinase C – translocation – second messengers – signal transduction – myocardial infarction

"The pure and simple truth is rarely pure and never simple"
Oscar Wilde

There is no doubt that brief nonlethal episodes of ischemia protect or "precondition" the heart and render the myocardium resistant to a subsequent more sustained ischemic insult. The vexing question is: what are the cellular mediators and pathways triggered by brief ischemia that initiate this paradoxical yet profound cardioprotection?

One attractive and popular hypothesis, first proposed by Downey and colleagues (4, 11), is that translocation of protein kinase C (PKC) – a family of 11 or more closely related isoenzymes known to participate in the regulation of ionic homeostasis, vascular tone, myocyte contractility, gene expression and hypertrophy via phosphorylation of specific cellular proteins (2) – plays a pivotal role. Specifically: adenosine released during brief ischemia activates adenosine A_1 receptors and, through a pertussis toxin-sensitive G-protein, is proposed to stimulate phospholipase C activity, formation of diacylglycerol, and result in the activation and translocation of PKC from the cytosol to the myocyte membranes. PKC is presumably then strategically positioned to phosphorylate an as yet unidentified membrane-bound effector protein during the early minutes of the subsequent sustained ischemia, and thereby elicit the well-described reduction of infarct size (4, 11).

Does activation and subsequent translocation of PKC represent the "pure and simple truth" behind ischemic preconditioning? Ischemia can indeed trigger the translocation of PKC; for example Strasser et al. (9) have provided compelling biochemical evidence that 10 min of global ischemia in the isolated rat heart results in a modest (approximately 10 %) but significant redistribution of PKC from the cytosol to the particulate cellular components. However, support for the specific concept that translocation of PKC, induced by brief ischemia, mediates infarct size reduction by ischemic preconditioning is largely indirect. For example, in rat and rabbit hearts and isolated rabbit myocytes, treatment with pharmacologic inhibitors of PKC such as staurosporine, polymyxin-B, calphostin C and chelerythrine rendered preconditioning ineffective in limiting myocyte death (1, 3 – 5, 8, 11). The converse was also true: administration of potent PKC activators such as 4β-phorbol 12-myristate 13-acetate (PMA), in lieu of brief ischemia, mimicked the cardioprotection achieved with preconditioning (4, 5, 8, 11). Not all the pharmacologic evidence, however, has been confirmatory: in the dog and pig, PKC inhibitors including polymyxin, H-7, staurosporine, and bisindolylmaleimide – even when given in large intracoronary doses – all failed to attenuate the protective effects of preconditioning (6, 10), and pretreatment with PMA did not protect the porcine heart against infarction (10).

In an effort to resolve these inconsistencies and overcome the inherent limitations of this pharmacologic approach, we expanded our studies and employed biochemical and fluorescence microscopy techniques to

Dr. K. Przyklenk (✉)
Heart Institute/Research
Good Samaritan Hospital
1225 Wilshire Boulevard
Los Angeles, California 90017-2395, USA

directly compare the amount and subcellar distribution of PKC in control versus preconditioned canine myocardium (6). First, we visualized the distribution of *active* PKC by staining subendocardial samples with a novel fluorescent probe – a bisindolylmaleimide PKC inhibitor conjugated to fluorescein – and viewing the tissue sections with a confocal laser scanning microscope. As expected, brief exposure of baseline samples to PMA (the "positive control" for our method) elicited a profound increase in both the overall intensity of fluorescent staining (indicating an increase in PKC activity), and staining specifically associated with membranous structures within the myocytes. In contrast, 4 5-min episodes of coronary occlusion – a regimen known to effectively precondition the canine heart – failed to alter the intensity or distribution of fluorescent staining when compared with baseline (6).

Concern regarding the qualitative nature of the fluorescent staining method prompted us to undertake a second series of experiments in which we biochemically quantified PKC in cytosolic and particulate tissue fractions in dogs subjected to 4 5-min episodes of preconditioning ischemia and time-matched controls. Samples were obtained both after the preconditioning/no intervention period and after a subsequent 10 min of "sustained" coronary artery ligation, while exposure to PMA was once again used as a positive control (6).

PMA produced the anticipated profound translocation of PKC, but, in agreement with our previous qualitative results, we found no quantitative difference in the amount or subcellular distribution of PKC in response to 4 5-min episodes of preconditioning ischemia (6). Interestingly, 10 min of sustained ischemia did trigger a subtle but significant (approximately 10 %) redistribution of PKC to the particulate fraction, reminiscent of the results obtained by Strasser et al. (9) in the isolated rat heart and Vogt et al. (10) in the *in vivo* porcine model. Importantly, however, the same translocation of PKC was observed in both preconditioned dogs and controls that received no intervention prior to the 10 min of sustained occlusion, with no difference in either the amount or subcellular distribution of PKC between the two matched cohorts (6).

How can we reconcile the failure of brief preconditioning ischemia to trigger translocation of PKC with the pharmacologic evidence that PKC angonists and antagonists can, in some models, modulate infarct size? We do not have the answer to this question. Conclusions drawn solely on the basis of the pharmacologic approach are obviously confounded by the known vasoactive consequences of PKC inhibition/activation, deleterious side effects of these agents and their solvents, and the fact that the majority of PKC inhibitors also inhibit other protein kinases in addition to PKC. On the other hand, if only 1 PKC isoenzyme is crucial in ischemic preconditioning, conclusions based exclusively on the biochemical and microscopic assessment of total PKC could arguably be limited by the resolution of these methods. Finally, it is perhaps most tempting to attribute this discrepancy to differences among species: i.e. PKC may play a role in rabbits and rats, but does not mediate preconditioning in dogs or pigs. However, recent quantitative biochemical data from our laboratory indicates that, as in the dog model, brief preconditioning ischemia in the rabbit does not result in the translocation of PKC from the cytosol to the particulate fraction (7). Thus, if activation and translocation of PKC truly plays a role in ischemic preconditioning, its contribution is "rarely pure" and, indeed, "never simple".

References

1. Armstrong S, Downey JM, Ganote CE (1994) Preconditioning of isolated rabbit cardiomyocytes: Induction by metabolic stress and blockade by the adenosine antagonist SPT and calphostin C, a protein kinase C inhibitor. Cardiovasc Res 28: 72–77
2. Johnson JA, Mochly-Rosen D (1995) Inhibition of the spontaneous rate of contraction of neonatal cardiac myocytes by protein kinase C isozymes: A putative role for the ε isozyme. Circ Res 76: 654–663
3. Li Y, Kloner RA (1994) Does protein kinase C play a role in ischemic preconditioning in rat hearts? Am J Physiol 268: H426–H431
4. Liu Y, Ytrehus K, Downey JM (1994) Evidence that translocation of protein kinase C is a key event during ischemic preconditioning of rabbit myocardium. J Mol Cell Cardiol 26: 661–668
5. Mitchell MB, Meng X, Ao L, Brown JM, Harken AH, Banerjee A (1995) Preconditioning of isolated rat heart is mediated by protein kinase C. Circ Res 76: 73–81
6. Przyklenk K, Sussman MA, Simkhovich BZ, Kloner RA (1995) Does ischemic preconditioning trigger translocation of protein kinase C in the canine model? Circulation 92: 1546–1557
7. Simkhovich BZ, Przyklenk K, Hale SL, Kloner RA (1995) Subcellular distribution of protein kinase C is not altered by brief preconditioning ischemia in rabbit myocardium. Circulation 92 (Suppl I): I-137 (abstract)

8. Speechly-Dick ME, Mocanu MM, Yellon DM (1994) Protein kinase C: Its role in ischemic preconditioning in the rat. Circ Res 75: 586–590

9. Strasser RH, Braun-Dullaeus R, Waldendzik H, Marquetant R (1992) α_1-receptor-independent activation of protein kinase C in acute myocardial ischemia: Mechanisms for sensitization of the adenylyl cyclase system. Circ Res 70: 1304–1312

10. Vogt A, Barancik M, Weihrauch D, Arras M, Podzuweit T, Schaper W (1994) Protein kinase C inhibitors reduce infarct size in pig hearts in vivo. Circulation 90 (Suppl I): I-647 (abstract)

11. Ytrehus K, Liu Y, Downey JM (1994) Preconditioning protects ischemic rabbit heart by protein kinase C activation. Am J Physiol 266: H1145–H1152

162 – 164

P. D. Verdouw
B. C. G. Gho
D. J. Duncker

Cardioprotection by organs in stress or distress

Key words Remote protection – partial coronary artery occlusion – ventricular pacing – renal artery occlusion – mesenteric artery occlusion

Introduction

Ischemic preconditioning studies usually employ one or more brief, abrupt, total coronary artery occlusion – reperfusion sequences to protect the myocardium against irreversible damage produced by a subsequent prolonged coronary artery occlusion. Evidence is now accumulating that partial coronary artery occlusions with or without concomitant increments in myocardial oxygen demand can also precondition the myocardium (1). Moreover, in contrast to what was reported earlier (2), partial coronary occlusions appear capable of preconditioning the myocardium without a period of intervening reperfusion (3), provided that the flow reduction is sufficiently severe (4). The severity of the flow reductions during the first stage (preconditioning stimulus) may be more critical for the cardioprotection against the second stage (prolonged occlusion) than the duration of flow reduction. Thus, we have shown that either a 30 min or a 90 min 30 % flow reduction failed to precondition the myocardium, but that both a 30 min and a 90 min 70 % flow reduction limited infarct size produced by a 60 min total coronary occlusion (4). Conversely, Schultz et al. (5) have shown that infarction produced by a prolonged period of low-flow ischemia is reduced when it is immediately preceded by a brief total occlusion without intervening reperfusion. Although these partial occlusion studies (3 – 5) indicate that ischemic preconditioning occurs in situations which mimic the clinical setting more closely than the abrupt occlusion-reperfusion sequences, a new series of observations is now emerging which suggest that myocardial protection can be triggered by (patho)physiological stimuli that do not produce myocardial ischemia.

Myocardial protection by remote ischemic and non-ischemic stress

Przyklenk et al. (6) showed that after a brief coronary artery occlusion in the dog, infarct size was reduced not only in the preconditioned myocardium but also in adjacent "virgin" myocardium ("remote intracardiac preconditioning"). Their study was the first to suggest that myocardium does not require direct exposure to ischemia to become protected against the irreversible damage produced by a prolonged coronary occlusion.

The observations of Przyklenk et al. (6) have generated several studies that investigated whether myocardium can be protected not only by remote *intracardiac* ischemic preconditioning but also by *interorgan* ischemic preconditioning. In a preliminary study in rabbits it was reported that a brief renal artery occlusion limited myocardial infarct size produced by a 45 min coronary artery occlusion (7). We reported similar results in anesthetized rats which under-

Supported by grant 92.144 from the Netherlands Heart Foundation and by grant CIPA-CT-4009 of the European Economic Community. The research of Dr. Dirk J. Duncker has been made possible by a fellowship of the Royal Netherlands Academy of Arts and Sciences.

Dr. P. D. Verdouw (✉) · B. C. G. Gho · D. J. Duncker
Experimental Cardiology, Thoraxcenter
Erasmus University Rotterdam
P.O. Box 1738
3000 DR Rotterdam, The Netherlands

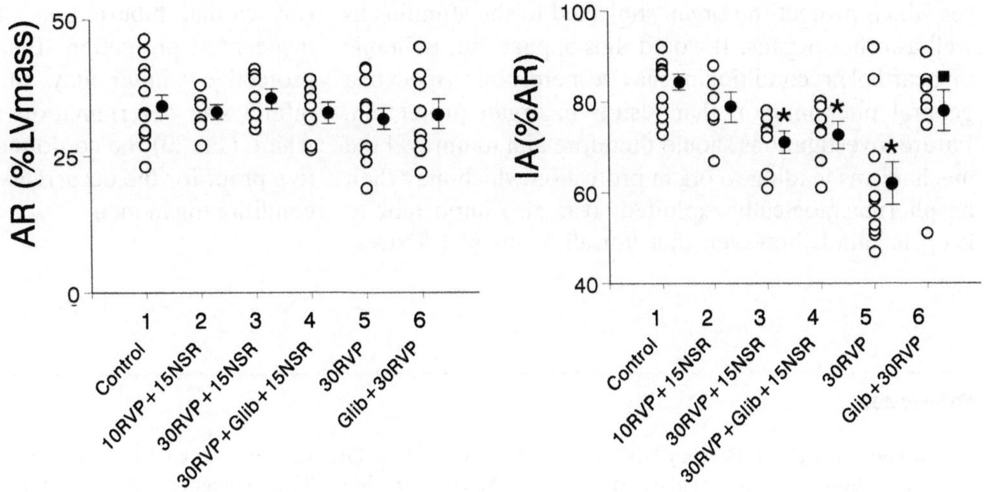

Fig. 1 Area at risk expressed as percentage of the left ventricle (AR) and the infarct area expressed as percentage of the area at risk (IA) are presented for each group. Individual data are indicated by open circles; mean data and SEM of each group are indicated by solid circles and Tbars. ✻ $p < 0.05$ vs control, ■ $p < 0.05$ vs 30 min RVP.

went a 60 min coronary artery occlusion 10 min after release of a 15 min renal artery coronary artery occlusion (8). Shortly thereafter suspicion arose, however, that the results of at least our experiments might have been influenced by the body temperature (9, 10). We therefore repeated our experiments during rigorous temperature control. We now found that a 15 min renal artery occlusion preceding the 60 min coronary artery occlusion reduced infarct size by 30 % during hypothermia (30 – 31 °C), but had no effect on infarct size during normothermia (36 – 37 °C). In contrast, a 15 min mesenteric artery occlusion was as effective as a 15 min coronary artery occlusion in limiting infarct size (by 25 %) during normothermia (unpublished observations from our laboratory).

In several studies it has been shown that various other forms of stress can protect the myocardium against infarction *without* the need for ischemia. Ovize et al. (11) demonstrated that stretch and increased wall stress of the left ventricle produced by acute volume overload decreased infarct size. This observation suggests that stretch of the remote myocardium due to dyskinesis in the ischemic myocardium may have contributed to the occurrence of remote intracardiac preconditioning (6). The mechanisms of interorgan preconditioning, however, remains speculative as myocardial stretch is unlikely to be a contributing factor in interorgan preconditioning.

In support of the observations by Ovize et al. (11) that non-ischemic stimuli can also protect the myocardium, we observed in pigs that 30 min of ventricular pacing at 200 bpm followed by 15 min of normal sinus rhythm reduced infarct size produced by a 60-min coronary occlusion from 84 ± 7 % (mean ± SD) of the area at risk in control animals to 71 ± 6 %. Even smaller infarct sizes (63 ± 13 %) were observed when 30 min of ventricular pacing immediately preceded the 60 min coronary occlusion without an intervening period of normal sinus rhythm (Fig. 1). The protective effect of ventricular pacing was abolished by pretreatment with the K^+_{ATP} channel blocker glibenclamide. K^+_{ATP} channel activation did not appear to be due to myocardial ischemia as indicated by metabolic and contractile functional data such as the absence of post-systolic segment shortening, the normal transmural blood flow distribution and maintenance of myocardial ATP-levels during ventricular pacing and the absence of reactive hyperemia and the immediate recovery of systolic segment shortening after stopping the ventricular pacing (12). Administration of glibenclamide following 30 min of ventricular pacing at the *onset* of 15 min of normal sinus rhythm did not attenuate the protection suggesting that K^+_{ATP} channels did not contribute to the protection that was still present 15 min after cessation of ventricular pacing (Fig. 1). These findings indicate that K^+_{ATP} channel activation was needed to trigger the protection but that, at variance with ischemic preconditioning (13), continued activation was not required once the myocardium was in a protected state.

Conclusion

Several studies now suggest that the myocardium can be protected by forms of stress other than myocardial ischemia. These include stimuli which stress the heart but do not lead to ischemia (stretch, ventricular pacing) and stimuli which cause distress (ischemia) in organs other than the heart. Since ischemia in remote organs such as kidney (14), brains (15), skeletal muscle (16) and liver (17) can also precondition these organs, it is clear that several forms of stress or distress are capable of triggering processes which protect the organ subjected to the stimulus as well as other organs. It would thus appear that ischemic myocardial preconditioning may be merely one aspect of a general phenomenon that results in organ protection. Future investigations should therefore aim to unravel the mechanisms leading to organ protection which may then be pharmacologically exploited. It is also important to keep in mind, however, that not all forms of (di)stress (myocardial hibernation (4), smoking (18)) result in myocardial protection. Finally, these newly recognized protective stimuli may, in addition to problems with infarct size determination in patients as outlined elsewhere (19, 20), be confounding factors in finding definitive proof for the occurrence of ischemic myocardial preconditioning in man.

References

1. Iwamoto T, Bai XJ, Downey HF (1993) Preconditioning with supply-demand imbalance limits infarct size in dog heart. Cardiovasc Res 27: 2071–2076
2. Ovize M, Przyklenk K, Kloner RA (1992) Partial coronary stenosis is sufficient and complete reperfusion is mandatory for preconditioning the canine heart. Circ Res 71: 1165–1173
3. Koning MMG, Simonis LAJ, De Zeeuw S, Nieukoop S, Post S, Verdouw PD (1994) Ischaemic preconditioning by partial occlusion without intermittent reperfusion. Cardiovasc Res 28: 1146–1151
4. Koning MMG, Gho BCG, Van Klaarwater E, Duncker DJ, Verdouw PD (1995) Endocardial and epicardial infarct size after preconditioning by a partial coronary artery occlusion without intermittent reperfusion. Cardiovasc Res (in press)
5. Schulz R, Post H, Sakka S, Wallbridge DR, Heusch G (1995) Intraischemic preconditioning. Increased tolerance to sustained low-flow ischemia by a brief episode of no-flow ischemia without intermittent reperfusion. Circ Res 76: 942–950
6. Przyklenk K, Bauer B, Ovize M, Kloner RA, Whittaker P (1993) Regional ischemic "preconditioning" projects remote virgin myocardium from subsequent sustained coronary occlusion. Circulation 87: 893–899
7. McClanahan TB, Nao BS, Wolke LJ, Martin BJ, Metz TE, Gallagher KP (1993) Brief renal occlusion and reperfusion reduces myocardial size in rabbits. The FASEB Journal 7: A118, 682
8. Gho BCG, Schoemaker RG, Van der Lee C, Sharma HS, Verdouw PD (1994) Cardioprotection by transient renal ischemia, an in vivo study in rats. Circulation 90,4-2: I-476, 2557
9. Chien GL, Wolff RA, Davis RF, Van Winkle DM (1994) "Normothermic range" temperature affects myocardial infarct size. Cardiovasc Res 28: 1014–1017
10. Duncker DJ, Klassen CL, Ishibashi Y, Herrlinger SH, Pavek TJ, Bache RJ (1995) Effect of temperature on myocardial infarction in swine. Am J Physiol (in press)
11. Ovize M, Kloner RA, Przyklenk K (1994) Stretch preconditions canine myocardium. Am J Physiol 266: H137–H146
12. Koning MMG, Gho BCG, Van Klaarwater E, Opstal RLJ, Duncker DJ, Verdouw PD (1995) Rapid ventricular pacing produces myocardial protection by non-ischemic activation of K^{+}_{ATP} channels. Circulation (in press)
13. Gross GJ, Auchampach JA (1992) Blockade of ATP-sensitive potassium channels prevents myocardial preconditioning. Circ Res 70: 223–233
14. Zager RA, Baltes LA, Sharma HM, Jurkowitz MS (1984) Responses of the ischemic acute renal failure kidney to additional ischemic events. Kidney Int 26: 689–700
15. Kitagawa K, Matsumoto M, Tagaya M, Hta R, Ueda H, Niinobe M, Handa N, Fukunaga R, Kimura K, Mikoshiba K, Kamada T (1990) "Ischemic tolerance" phenomenon found in the brain. Brain Res 528: 21–24
16. Mounsey RA, Pang CY, Forrest C (1992) Preconditioning: a new technique for improved muscle flap survival. Otolaryngology-Head and Neck Surg 107: 549–552
17. Lloris-Carsi JM, Cejalvo D, Toledo-Pereyra LH, Calvo MA, Suzuki S (1993) Preconditioning: effect upon lesion modulation in warm liver ischemia. Transplant Proc 25: 3303–3304
18. Zhy BQ, Sun YP, Seevers RE, Glantz SA, Parmley BW, Wolfe CL (1994) Exposure to environmental tobacco smoke increases myocardial infarct size in rats. Circulation 89: 1282–1290
19. Kloner RA, Yellon D (1994) Does ischemic preconditioning occur in patients? J Am Coll Cardiol 24: 1133–1142
20. Verdouw PD, Gho BCG, Duncker DJ (1995) Ischaemic preconditioning: is it clinically relevant? Eur Heart J (in press)

165–167

P. Whittaker

An alternative perspective on ischemic preconditioning derived from mathematical modeling

Key words Gadolinium – ischemia – second messenger systems – signal transduction – stretch receptors

Introduction

The usual roads taken in attempts to determine the mechanism of ischemic preconditioning have employed pharmacologic methods as the primary tool of investigation. Specifically, different agents have been used to either block the protection induced by ischemic preconditioning or agents have been administered prior to ischemia to mimic preconditioning. Although these approaches may yield valuable information, it is important to keep in mind that the actions of the agents employed may not be as discrete as we might think (or hope). For example, cellular second-messenger pathways are complex with multiple entry points and interconnections (5). Therefore a blocker of one receptor or pathway may also block others. Furthermore, many such agents have hemodynamic effects which adds an additional confounding factor when whole animal preparations are used.

Attempts to avoid or minimize such hemodynamic problems may result in completely unforeseen consequences. For example, we tried to examine the cardioprotective ability of adenosine by injecting it directly into cardiac muscle prior to coronary artery occlusion and so avoid the profound hypotension produced by systemic adenosine. This route of administration resulted in a significant reduction in the number of arrhythmias and also in infarct size versus hearts that did not receive injections (8). However, we subsequently found that injection of saline alone was also capable of reducing infarct size. This saline-mediated protection (perhaps due to local cellular stretch) may or may not be related to ischemic preconditioning. Nevertheless, it emphasizes the difficulty of examining any system without inadvertently perturbing it. These problems prompted us to seek an alternative road to examine ischemic preconditioning.

Dr. P. Whittaker (✉)
The Heart Institute
Good Samaritan Hospital
1225 Wilshire Boulevard
Los Angeles, California 90017, USA

Formulating a model

We noticed, in data collected from ischemic preconditioning studies in rat hearts, that infarct size (expressed as a percent of the area at risk) in preconditioned hearts was dependent upon the size of the area at risk; that is, the larger the area at risk, the larger the infarct (7). In contrast, infarct size in control hearts did not increase over the range of risk areas (Fig. 1). In addition, we found that while the lateral distance between the edge of the infarct and the edge of the area at risk was constant in control hearts, in preconditioned hearts this distance decreased as the size of the area at risk increased. We speculated that one possible explanation for these relationships was that the agent(s) responsible for the protection induced by ischemic preconditioning was produced throughout the heart and then transported into the area at risk. In preconditioned hearts with small risk areas, there would be a large area containing the induced protection that would not be subjected to the prolonged period of coronary artery occlusion. This "excess" protection might then be

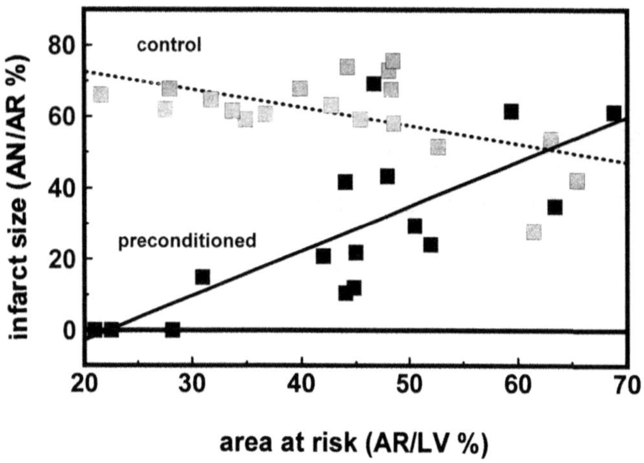

Fig. 1 Infarct size (area of necrosis [AN] expressed as a percent of the area at risk [AR]) plotted as a function of the size of the area at risk (expressed as a percent of the left ventricle [LV]). Data obtained from control hearts (n = 19) subjected to 90 min of coronary artery occlusion are shown in gray, while data from hearts that were preconditioned prior to coronary artery occlusion (n = 16) are shown in black. There was a statistically significant correlaton (solid regression line) between the variables in the preconditioned hearts (r = 0.76, p = 0.0007); infarct size increased as the size of the area at risk increased. In contrast, no such relationship was found in the control hearts. Redrawn from (7).

able to enter most of the risk region where it could protect against the subsequent prolonged period of ischemia. Conversely, in a heart with a large area at risk, the "excess" protection would be less, the distance to the center of the risk region greater and so the infarct would be larger. From these observations, we were able to construct a simple mathematical model which was consistent with our experimental infarct size data in both the preconditioned and control rat hearts (7).

Implications of the model

If this mathematical approach is to be more than a mere intellectual curiosity, then it must provide insight into the problem under consideration, and suggest new experiments to advance understanding. One consequence of our model was that if ischemic preconditioning activated protection throughout the heart, then preconditioning one area should protect a remote region from prolonged ischemia. We tested this hypothesis in dog hearts (6). We used a branch of the circumflex artery for the preconditioning protocol, which consisted of four, 5-min occlusions each followed by 5 min of reperfusion. We then occluded the left anterior descending (LAD) artery for 1 h. Infarct size in the control group, which underwent 1 h of LAD occlusion alone, was significantly greater (16 ± 5 %) than that found in the hearts preconditioned with circumflex occlusions (6 ± 2 %). Thus, preconditioning-mediated protection occurs at sites remote from the initial ischemia, as predicted by the model.

Mechanism of "preconditioning at a distance"?

To explain the hypothesis of global myocardial activation of protection derived from our mathematical model and the observation of preconditioning at a distance, the non-ischemic tissue must be able to "detect" ischemia during the preconditioning regime. Because the left ventricle dilates in response to regional ischemia, we speculated that such detection could be achieved via a stretch-mediated mechanism. This hypothesis was examined in two ways. First, 500 ml of saline was infused into the left ventricle via the left atrium over a 10-min period to stretch the muscle prior to 60 min of LAD occlusion. The infusion resulted in a ventricular dilation of approximately 15 % (versus 19 % after LAD occlusion) and a significant reduction in infarct size versus control hearts (4). Furthermore, the protection induced by saline infusion could be blocked by prior administration of gadolinium chloride, a blocker of stretch-activated ion channels (9). Second, gadolinium chloride was given prior to ischemic preconditioning and found to partially block the reduction in infarct size (4). In fact, gadolinium also blocked the protection induced by intramyocardial saline injection that I mentioned earlier (8).

The precise mechanism of this stretch-activated protection is unknown; however, there are numerous possibilities. For example, cellular stretch can activate several phosphorylation cascades involving protein kinase C, inositol phosphates, and diacyclglycerol to name but three (3). In addition, cellular stretch could affect G proteins (1), which in turn couple adenosine receptors and K_{ATP} channels (2), both implicated as mediators of ischemic preconditioning. Thus cellular stretch has the potential to provide a unified theory capable of linking and reconciling the different pathways that have been suggested to mediate ischemic preconditioning.

Unanswered questions and future directions

Starting from an empiric relationship and a subsequent mathematical model of ischemic preconditioning, we have been able to open up an entirely new line of investigation. However, the mathematical model does not predict the "mediator" of the protection nor how it is transported from the non-ischemic to the ischemic tissue. There are several possible methods of transport including collateral blood flow, lymphatic circulation, and diffusion. In rat hearts, which lack significant collateral flow, our model was consistent with diffusion; however, the distances that must be travelled in a relatively short time appear to rule out passive diffusion by anything other than small molecules or ions. We are currently investigating this aspect of the model in prospective experiments.

Of course, the use of gadolinium chloride to block stretch-activated channels, and possibly also ischemic preconditioning, brings us back to the same main road that we left at the start. Even though our detour along the backroads has returned us to intracellular signalling pathways, we return with a different perspective that may provide us with new ways to advance.

References

1. Hilal-Dandan R, Brunton LL (1995) Transmembrane mechanochemical coupling in cardiac myocytes: novel activation of G_i by hyposmotic swelling. Am J Physiol 269: H798–H804
2. Kirsch GE, Codina J, Birnbaumer L, Brown AM (1990) Coupling of ATP-sensitive K^+ channels to A_1 receptors by G proteins in rat ventricular myocytes. Am J Physiol 259: H820–H826
3. Komuro I, Yazaki Y (1994) Intracellular signalling pathways in cardiac myocytes induced by mechanical stress. Trends Cardiovasc Med 4: 117–121
4. Ovize M, Kloner RA, Przyklenk K (1994) Stretch preconditions canine myocardium. Am J Physiol 266: H137–H146
5. Port JD, Malbon CC (1993) Integration of transmembrane signalling. Cross-talk among G-protein-linked receptors and other signal transduction pathways. Trends Cardiovasc Med 3: 85–92
6. Przyklenk K, Bauer B, Ovize M, Kloner RA, Whittaker P (1993) Regional ischemic "preconditioning" protects remote virgin myocardium from subsequent sustained coronary occlusion. Circulation 87: 893–899
7. Whittaker P, Przyklenk K (1994) Reduction of infarct size in vivo with ischemic preconditioning: mathematical evidence for protection via non-ischemic tissue. Basic Res Cardiol 89: 6–15
8. Whittaker P, Kloner RA, Przyklenk K (1995) Intramyocardial injections and protection against myocardial ischemia: an attempt to examine the cardioprotective actions of adenosine Circulation (in press)
9. Yang XC, Sachs F (1989) Block of stretch-activated ion channels in xenopus oocytes by gadolinium and calcium ions. Science 243: 1068–1071

168 – 170

R. Schulz
G. Heusch

Ischemic preconditioning and myocardial hibernation: Is there a common mechanism?

Key words Myocardial ischemia – reperfusion – myocarial infarction

Myocardial ischemia, even if it persists for a prolonged period of time, does not inevitably induce irreversible damage. Recent studies have identified two phenomena which are characterized by endogenous cardioprotective features, namely ischemic preconditioning (3) and myocardial hibernation (5).

Ischemic preconditioning is characterized by the reduction of infarct size resulting from prolonged and severe myocardial ischemia by one or more preceding short episodes of ischemia and reperfusion. Myocardial ATP and creatine phosphate contents remain somewhat higher and lactate production is attenuated in preconditioned hearts as compared to hearts subjected to prolonged ischemia without ischemic preconditioning (4).

Myocardial hibernation is characterized by ischemic contractile dysfunction of viable myocardium which is fully reversible upon reperfusion (5). Myocardial creatine phosphate content, after an initial reduction, recovers towards control values, myocardial ATP content remains stable at a slightly reduced level, lactate production is attenuated over time, and regional myocardial function can be transiently increased by an inotropic challenge (6, 9). The lower limit of myocardial blood flow which is still compatible with the development of myocardial hibernation amounts to approximately 25 % of baseline in the experimental (9) and clinical setting (2).

Since both, ischemic preconditioning and myocardial hibernation, are characterized by preservation of viability and attenuation of ischemic alterations in metabolism, a common mechanism for both phenomena could be conceived.

In swine, like in most other species, increased levels of endogenous adenosine and activation of ATP-dependent potassium channels are involved in the infarct size-reducing effect of ischemic preconditioning. When the breakdown of endogenous adenosine is increased by intracoronary infusion of adenosine deaminase the infarct size reduction achieved by ischemic preconditioning is attenuated (10). Also blockade of ATP-dependent potassium channels with glibenclamide prevents the infarct size reduction achieved by ischemic preconditioning (Fig. 1) (8).

In contrast, neither increased breakdown of endogenous adenosine nor blockade of ATP-dependent potassium channels prevent the development of myocardial hibernation. Myocardial creatine phosphate content recovers and lactate production is attenuated during ongoing ischemia, regional myocardial function is increased during inotropic stimulation with dobutamine, and myocardial necrosis is absent in placebo swine undergoing 90 min of moderate ischemia as well as in swine undergoing moderate ischemia and receiving adenosine deaminase or glibenclamide (11). Therefore, endogenous adenosine and ATP-dependent potassium channels are involved in the infarct size reducing effect of ischemic preconditioning (8, 10), but do not interfere with the development of myocardial hibernation (11).

Recently, Ferrari and associates demonstrated in isolated buffer-perfused rabbit hearts that an initial stimulus of very severe ischemia is necessary to permit the development of myocardial hibernation during subsequent sus-

R. Schulz · Prof. Dr. G. Heusch (✉)
Abteilung für Pathophysiologie
Zentrum für Innere Medizin
Universitätsklinikum Essen
Hufelandstraße 55
45147 Essen, FRG

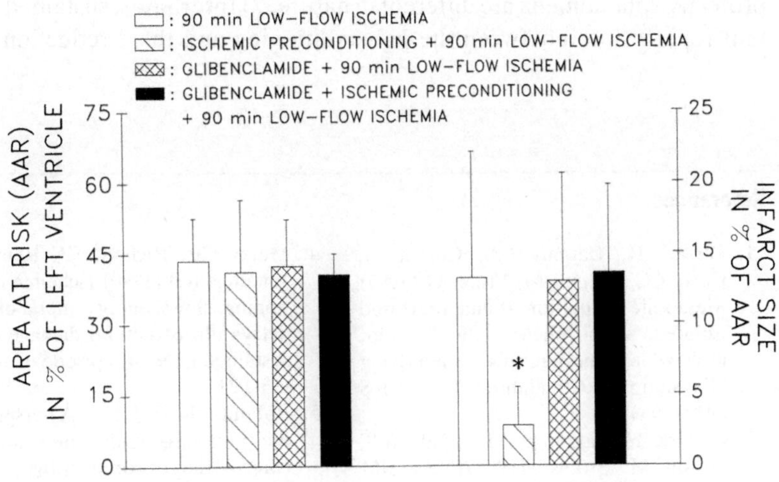

Fig. 1 Effect of blockade of ATP-dependent potassium channels with glibenclamide on infarct size (right panel) in swine undergoing 90 min low-flow ischemia without or with a preceding 10 min preconditioning ischemic period followed by 15 min reperfusion. The area at risk (left panel) was comparable among the groups. In ischemic preconditioned hearts infarct size was reduced. This benefical effect was abolished by glibenclamide. Glibenclamide per se did not increase infarct size. $*p < 0.05$ vs. all other groups. From (8)

tained low-flow ischemia, raising the possibility of a mechanistic link between ischemic preconditioning and myocardial hibernation. In their model, myocardial ATP content was maintained and lactate production was reversed to lactate consumption after sustained low-flow ischemia only when hearts underwent a preceding short episode of no-flow ischemia. Furthermore, in hearts undergoing the initial no-flow ischemic period contractile function rapidly recovered during reperfusion, and only a transient CK release occurred (1).

Also in the anesthetized swine *in situ*, infarct size as a result of a prolonged period of low-flow ischemia is reduced by a preceding short episode of no-flow ischemia, even without intermittent reperfusion. The threshold of subendocardial blood flow for tissue to remain viable is lower in swine with an initial no-flow ischemia than in swine undergoing sustained low-flow ischemia only, indicating an increased ischemic tolerance of the myocardium in swine with the initial no-flow ischemic episode. However, this cardioprotective effect is lost after blockade of ATP-dependent potassium channels with glibenclamide (Fig. 2) (7). Therefore, the underlying mechanism for protection by a brief episode of ischemia without intermittent reperfusion relates to ischemic preconditioning rather than to myocardial hibernation.

In conclusion

1) Despite certain similarities between ischemic preconditioning and myocardial hibernation, these two cardio-

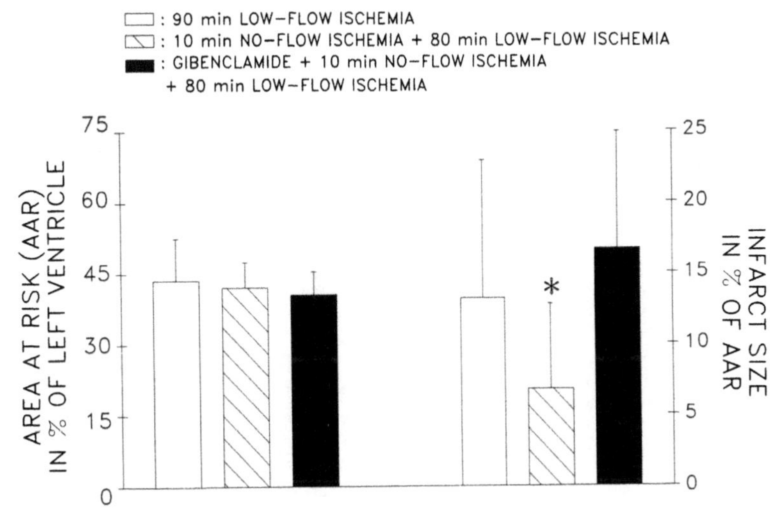

Fig. 2 Effect of blockade of ATP-dependent potassium channels with glibenclamide on infarct size (right panel) in swine undergoing 10 min no-flow ischemia followed by 80 min low-flow ischemia. The area at risk (left panel) was comparable among the groups. In pigs undergoing 10 min of no-flow ischemia followed by 80 min of low-flow ischemia infarct size was reduced compared to pigs undergoing 90 min of low-flow ischemia at comparable subendocardial blood flows. This benefical effect was abolished by glibenclamide. $*p < 0.05$ vs. the two other groups. From (7)

protective phenomena are different in nature. 2) Intermittent reperfusion inbetween the preconditioning and the sustained ischemic period is not necessary for infarct size reduction by ischemic preconditioning.

References

1. Ferrari R, Cargnoni A, Curello S, Ceconi C, Volpini M, Visioli O (1993) Metabolic adaptation of underperfused isolated rabbit heart: insight into molecular mechanisms underlying hibernation. Circulation 88: I-188 (Abstract)
2. Gewirtz H, Fischman AJ, Abraham S, Gilson M, Strauss HW, Alpert NM (1994) Positron emission tomographic measurements of absolute regional myocardial blood flow permits identification of nonviable myocardium in patients with chronic myocardial infarction. J Am Coll Cardiol 23: 851–859
3. Murry CE, Jennings RB, Reimer KA (1986) Preconditioning with ischemia: a delay of lethal cell injury in ischemic myocardium. Circulation 74: 1124–1136
4. Murry CE, Richard VJ, Reimer KA, Jennings RB (1990) Ischemic preconditioning slows energy metabolism and delays ultrastructural damage during a sustained ischemic episode. Circ Res 66: 913–931
5. Rahimtoola SH (1985) A perspective on the three large multicenter randomized clinical trials of coronary bypass surgery for chronic stable angina. Circulation 72 Suppl V: V-123–V-135
6. Schulz R, Guth BD, Pieper K, Martin C, Heusch G (1992) Recruitment of an inotropic reserve in moderately ischemic myocardium at the expense of metabolic recovery: a model of short-term hibernation. Circ Res 70: 1282–1295
7. Schulz R, Post H, Sakka S, Wallbridge DR, Heusch G (1995) Intraischemic preconditioning. Increase tolerance to sustained low-flow ischemia by a brief episode of no-flow ischemia without intermittent reperfusion. Circ Res 76: 942–950
8. Schulz R, Rose J, Heusch G (1994) Involvement of activation of ATP-dependent potassium channels in ischemic preconditioning in swine. Am J Physiol 267: H1341–H1352
9. Schulz R, Rose J, Martin C, Brodde OE, Heusch G (1993) Development of short-term myocardial hibernation: its limitation by the severity of ischemia and inotropic stimulation. Circulation 88: 684–695
10. Schulz R, Rose J, Post H, Heusch G (1995) Involvement of endogenous adenosine in ischemic preconditioning in swine. Pflügers Archiv 430: 273–282
11. Schulz R, Rose J, Post H, Heusch G (1995) Regional short-term hibernation in swine does not involve endogenous adenosine or KATP channels. Am J Physiol 268: H2294–H3201

171 – 174

G. F. Baxter
D. M. Yellon

Delayed myocardial protection following ischaemic preconditioning

Key words Cardioprotection – ischaemia – ischaemic preconditioning – second window of protection

The last two years have brought the realisation that ischaemic preconditioning of myocardium is associated with a biphasic pattern of myocardial protection. In addition to the well-researched early phase of protection ('classic' preconditioning) there is now a considerable body of evidence pointing to a much delayed phase of protection which we have termed the 'second window of protection' (19). That two distinct phase of protection occur in response to transient ischaemic stress suggests that there are at least two different endogenous routes to cytoprotection in myocardium. Both forms of adaptation may be extremely pertinent to our conceptions of the natural history of ischaemic heart disease and both may provide new templates for the development of cardioprotective strategies. Our own feeling is that the second window of protection is an adaptive cytoprotection sharing many of the features of the cellular stress response, widely observed in prokaryotic and eukaryotic cells, and in several mammalian tissues. Here, we outline the evidence for a second window of protection in myocardium, discuss some current concepts concerning underlying mechanisms, and speculate on its pathophysiological relevance.

Dr. G. F. Baxter · Dr. D. M. Yellon (✉)
The Hatter Institute for Cardiovascular Studies
Division of Cardiology
University College London Hospitals
Grafton Way
London WC1E 6DB, United Kingdom

Experimental models of delayed preconditioning and endpoints of injury

Investigation of this aspect of preconditioning protection is still at an early stage. Nevertheless, following the first reports of the delayed anti-infarct effect of preconditioning, several newer aspects of second window tolerance have been described in the last 12 months. As such, a picture is now developing of a form of myocardial adaptation that affords protection against all forms of ischaemia/hypoxia-related injury, including necrosis, ventricular tachyarrhythmias, post-ischaemic contractile dysfunction in the absence of necrosis (stunning), and post-hypoxic creatine kinase release from isolated cardiomyocytes.

Tissue necrosis

The second window of protection was originally described as a period of enhanced tolerance to lethal ischaemia in open-chest rabbit (9) and canine (8) models of coronary artery occlusion 24 h after a preconditioning stimulus of brief repetitive cycles of coronary occlusion. This delayed anti-infarct effect has subsequently been confirmed in two further open-chest rabbit studies (1, 3) and has also been observed 24 h after preconditioning in chronically-instrumented conscious rabbits (18). More recent work from our laboratory suggests that this delayed anti-infarct effect of preconditioning may extend over a period of between 1 and 3 days unlike the early period of protection which is lost within 60 – 90 min (2).

Ventricular arrhythmias

There is evidence also that the delayed protection conferred by preconditioning extends to other indices of ischaemic and post-ischaemic myocardial dysfunction. During an investigation of the second window in a conscious rabbit model we observed abolition of coronary occlusion-induced ventricular fibrillation 24 h after preconditioning (18). Recently Vegh's group reported a delayed anti-arrhythmic effect following preconditioning (15). Four 5-min periods of ventricular rapid pacing in the dog induced a biphasic pattern of protection against coronary occlusion- and reperfusion-induced tachyarrhythmias, with a second window of protection around 20 – 24 h after the pacing stimulus. This group extended the interval between the pacing stimulus and coronary occlusion up to 72 h and found that anti-arrhythmic protection is almost completely lost by 48 h (6), in contrast to the anti-infarct effect in the rabbit which as mentioned above extends to 72 h.

Myocardial stunning

Another endpoint of delayed preconditioning protection has been described by Bolli's group (14). These workers used conscious pigs to investigate post-ischaemic myocardial dysfunction following repeated 2 min coronary artery occlusions: this induced myocardial stunning lasting 3 to 4 h. Repetition of the protocol in the same animals 24 h later revealed that post-ischemic recovery of thickening fraction was significantly accelerated compared with recovery following the initial protocol. It appeared that the initial stunning protocol preconditioned against a subsequent stunning protocol 24 h later. This novel finding is particularly interesting since it describes an index of protection in the second window that is not seen in the early window, there being no conclusive evidence that classic preconditioning confers protection against myocardial stunning in the absence of tissue necrosis.

Hypoxic injury in isolated myocytes

Further evidence for a delayed effect of preconditioning has been obtained in an isolated cardiomyocyte study. Yamashita et al. (17) established that hypoxic preconditioning of rat cardiomyocytes conferred resistance to a subsequent more prolonged hypoxic period 24 h later. This was measured in terms of reduced creatine kinase release after the long hypoxic period.

Mechanisms

The cellular mechanisms through which cardioprotection is manifested in the second window are not clear. One possibility is that preconditioning might open coronary collateral vessels or stimulate angiogenesis, providing collateral support in the ischaemic region. However, whilst collateralisation can undoubtedly provide valuable support to the ischaemic myocardium, this is unlikely to be the primary mechanism of protection. For example, the rabbit is well known to lack preformed collateral coronary vessels and, moreover, this species has a very limited capacity to develop collaterals in response to ischaemia.

Several lines of evidence suggest that the protection is due to direct enhancement of tissue tolerance and could be related to the appearance of new proteins or to alterations in protein activity by post-translational mechanisms. The appearance of a large number of new gene products including proto-oncogenes, intracellular anti-oxidants, heat shock proteins and other regulatory proteins, as well as the post-translational modification of proteins, would be anticipated after sublethal ischaemia as part of the intracellular stress response and as a consequence of the activation of various signalling pathways triggered by the local release of paracrine mediators during preconditioning. The slow onset of appearance and subsequent duration of the second window would be consistent with this proposal. Two early reports raised the possibility that the delayed phase of protection involves a mechanism related to alterations in the activity of superoxide dismutase (SOD) and to myocardial content of the major inducible heat shock protein, HSP70i: both are stress-induced proteins. Hoshida et al. described the temporal dynamics of manganese-SOD activity following preconditioning in canine myocardium and reported a biphasic pattern of enzyme activity over a 24-h period similar to the pattern of ischaemic tolerance (5). Similarly, we found that myocardial content of HSP70i, was elevated 24 h after preconditioning, a time when ischaemic tolerance was observed (9). Relationships between enhanced ischaemic tolerance and stress-inducible cytoprotective protein activity have been pursued most convincingly in gene transfection studies (4, 16), antisense oligonucleotide studies (17) and studies with transgenic mice constitutively over-expressing human HSP70 (10, 13). These studies tend to suggest, but do not confirm, that the appearance of the delayed protection could be related to changes in activities of stress-inducible cytoprotective proteins in the preconditioned myocardium. Furthermore, since the regulation of a large number of proteins is altered by sublethal ischaemia, it is conceivable and indeed, probable, that the second window involves proteins other than these two candidate families (i.e. anti-oxidants and heat shock proteins).

Perhaps a useful key for manipulating this adaptive property of myocardium to therapeutic advantage will come from an understanding of the cell signalling pathways. So far we have ascertained that for the rabbit at least, adenosine receptor activation during preconditioning is an important trigger of delayed protection (3) and that activation of protein kinase C (PKC) is an intermediate step (2). We envisage a critical role for nuclear translocation of PKC, and probably activation of other kinases, in the gene transcription events that are hypothesised to be the basis of this form of adaptation (see ref. (19)). However, since considerable cross-talk exists between PKC and other kinase systems, such as the MAP kinase cascade, a more complex signalling mechanism is likely to underlie this adaptation.

Clinical and pathophysiological considerations

There have been suggestions that preconditioning may be a feature of the natural history of myocardial ischaemic syndromes in man. Although the prognostic significance of angina pectoris before acute myocardial infarction is by no means certain, three recent studies of patients with a history of unstable angina before myocardial infarction suggest a beneficial effect in terms of reduced infarct size (7, 11, 12). In all studies, these beneficial effects appear to be poorly correlated with the extent of coronary collateralisation and previous anti-anginal drug therapies. All three studies suggest that episodes of angina within a critical period before infarction may protect the myocardium in the absence of collateralisation. Notably, the kinetics of this preconditioning effect of angina occur over many hours or days rather than the 1 or 2 h associated with the classic preconditioning phenomenon and would suggest a form of adaptation temporally related to the second window of protection rather than to classic preconditioning. For example in a study by Ottani et al. (12) patients were selected with a 24-h history of angina prior to infarction. The mean time between the last episode of angina and onset of infarction was around 11 h, a time that clearly falls outside the timeframe of experimentally-defined classic preconditioning. In the study by Nakagawa et al. (11) patients in the group that showed benefit had their last episode of angina a mean 25 h before onset of infarction and although greatest benefit was seen in patients who had experienced angina nearer to infarction, none of these patients experienced their last episode of angina within the timeframe of classic preconditioning (60 – 90 min).

It is possible that an understanding of the physiology of delayed preconditioning could shed light on the associations between antecedant angina pectoris and myocardial infarction, and promote the rational development of new therapeutic approaches to cardioprotection in patients with coronary artery disease, especially those about to undergo elective procedures such as coronary angioplasty and cardiac surgery. As we learn more about its characteristics and mechanisms we may find that delayed preconditioning protection has greater potential for therapeutic exploitation than classic preconditioning. Although its investigation may present as many if not more challenges to research than classic preconditioning protection, a fuller appreciation of this innate adaptative capacity of myocardium should contribute to our understanding of myocardial responses to ischaemia and the pathophysiology of ischaemic diseases.

Acknowledgement The authors gratefully acknowledge support for their work in this field by the Wellcome Trust, the British Heart Foundation and the Hatter Foundation.

References

1. Baxter GF, Goma FM, Yellon DM (1995a) Involvement of protein kinase C in the delayed cytoprotection following sublethal ischaemia in rabbit myocardium. Br J Pharmacol 115: 222–224
2. Baxter GF, Goma FM, Yellon DM (1995b) Duration of the 'second window of protection' following ischaemic preconditioning in the rabbit. J Mol Cell Cardiol 27: A162 (abstract)
3. Baxter GF, Marber MS, Patel VC, Yellon DM (1994) Adenosine receptor involvement in a delayed phase of protection 24 hours following ischemic preconditioning. Circulation 90: 2993–3000
4. Heads RJ, Yellon DM, Latchman DS (1995) Differential cytoprotection against heat stress or hypoxia following expression of specific stress protein genes in myogenic cells. J Mol Cell Cardiol 27: 1669–1678
5. Hoshida S, Kuzuya T, Fuji H, Yamashita N, Oe H, Hori M, Suzuki K, Taniguchi N, Tada M (1993) Sublethal ischemia alters myocardial antioxidant activity in canine heart. Am J Physiol 264: H33–H39
6. Kaszala K, Vegh A, Parratt JR, Papp JG (1995) Time course of pacing induced preconditioning in dogs. J Mol Cell Cardiol 27: A145 (abstract)

7. Kloner RA, Shook T, Przyklenk K, Davis VG, Luni L, Matthews RV, Burstein S, Gibson CM, Poole WK, Cannon CP, McCabe CH, Braunwald E (1995) Previous angina alters inhospital outcome in TIMI-4: a clinical correlate to preconditioning? Circulation 91: 37–47
8. Kuzuya T, Hoshida S, Yamashita N, Fuji H, Oe H, Hori M, Kamada T, Tada M (1993) Delayed effects of sublethal ischemia on the acquisition of tolerance to ischemia. Circ Res 72: 1293–1299
9. Marber MS, Latchman DS, Walker JM, Yellon DM (1993) Cardiac stress protein elevation 24 hours after brief ischemia or heat stress is associated with resistance to myocardial infarction. Circulation 88: 1264–1272
10. Marber MS, Mestril R, Chi S-H, Sayen R, Yellon DM, Dillmann WH (1995) Overexpression of the rat inducible 70-kD heat stress protein in a transgenic mouse increases the resistance of the heart to ischemic injury. J Clin Invest 95: 1446–1456
11. Nakagawa Y, Ito H, Kitakaze M, Kusuoka H, Hori M, Kuzuya T, Higashino Y, Fujii K, Minamino T (1995) Effect of angina pectoris on myocardial protection in patients with reperfused anterior wall myocardial infarction: retrospective clinical evidence of "preconditioning". J Am Coll Cardiol 25: 1076–1083
12. Ottani F, Galvani M, Ferrini D, Sorbello F, Limonetti P, Pantoli D, Rusticali F (1995) Prodromal angina limits infarct size: a role for ischemic preconditioning? Circulation 91: 291–297
13. Plumier J-CL, Ross BM, Currie RW, Angelidis CE, Kazlaris H, Kollias G, Pagoulatos GN (1995) Transgenic mice expressing the human heat shock protein 70 have improved postischemic myocardial recovery. J Clin Invest 95: 1854–1860
14. Sun J-Z, Tang X-L, Knowlton AA, Park S-W, Qiu Y, Bolli R (1995) Late preconditioning against myocardial stunning: an endogenous protective mechanism that confers resistance to postischemic dysfunction 24 h after brief ischemia in conscious pigs. J Clin Invest 95: 388–403
15. Vegh A, Papp JG, Parratt JR (1994) Prevention by dexamethasone of the marked antiarrhythmic effects of preconditioning induced 20 h after rapid cardiac pacing. Br J Pharmacol 113: 1081–1082
16. Williams RS, Thomas JA, Fina M et al. (1993) Human heat shock protein 70 (hsp70) protects murine cells from injury during metabolic stress. J Clin Invest 92: 503–508
17. Yamashita N, Nishida M, Hoshida S, Kuzuya T, Hori M, Taniguchi N, Kamada T, Tada M (1994) Induction of manganese superoxide dismutase in rat cardiac myocytes increases tolerance to hypoxia 24 hours after preconditioning. J Clin Invest 94: 2193–2199
18. Yang X-M, Baxter GF, Heads RJ, Yellon DM, Downey JM, Cohen MV (1996) Infarct limitation in the second window of protection in a conscious rabbit model. Cardiovasc Res: in press
19. Yellon DM, Baxter GF (1995) A 'second window of protection' or delayed preconditioning phenomenon: future horizons for myocardial protection? J Mol Cell Cardiol 27: 1023–1034

175 – 181
© Steinkopff Verlag 1996

R. Bolli

The early and late phases of preconditioning against myocardial stunning and the essential role of oxyradicals in the late phase: an overview

Key words Preconditioning – myocardial stunning – oxygen radicals – antioxidants – myocardial ischemia – superoxide dismutase

Although ischemic preconditioning is remarkably powerful in protecting the myocardium against cell death (1), its effects on myocardial stunning are less clear and somewhat controversial. The purpose of this essay is to succinctly review the existing knowledge regarding the influence of preconditioning on myocardial stunning and to reconcile apparently conflicting results into a coherent paradigm. It has recently become apparent that ischemic preconditioning against stunning includes an early phase (which becomes manifest within minutes) and a late phase (which becomes manifest ≤ 12 h after the preconditioning ischemia). Accordingly, the early and the late phases will be discussed separately.

Early phase of preconditioning against stunning

Stunning induced by a single ischemic episode lasting 10 – 15 minutes

All published studies (e.g., 2, 3) have uniformly concluded that preconditioning with brief episodes of ischemia does not attenuate the myocardial stunning induced by a subsequent 15-min coronary occlusion. We performed a systematic investigation of the effects of preconditioning on myocardial stunning in 62 open-chest dogs undergoing either a 15-min or a 10-min coronary occlusion followed by 4 h of reperfusion. Before the 15-min occlusion, dogs received either no intervention (n = 11) or one of the following preconditioning protocols: 5-min occlusion (O)/10-min reperfusion (R) x 1 (n = 8); 2-min O/5-min R x 4 (n = 7); 1-min O/5-min R x 10 (n = 3); or 40-s O/1-min R x 5 (n = 16). Before the 10-min occlusion, dogs received either no intervention (n = 9) or a 5-min O/10-min R cycle (n = 8). We found that none of these preconditioning protocols enhanced the recovery of function after the 15-min or 10-min occlusion. Thus, using a variety of different protocols, we were unable to demonstrate an immediate preconditioning effect of ischemia against the myocardial stunning induced by either a 10-min or a 15-min coronary occlusion in open-chest dogs. Furthermore, pretreatment (intracoronary infusion) with extremely large doses of adenosine (4) or of the adenosine A_1-receptor agonist 2-chloro-N^6-cyclopentyladenosine (CCPA) (5) before ischemia failed to enhance the recovery of function after a subsequent 15-min coronary occlusion, indicating that unlike the protection conferred against cell death (1), adenosine receptor activation does not precondition against postischemic dysfunction. These results emphasize the differences between the pathophysiology of stunning and that of infarction (4, 5).

In summary, brief ischemia does not precondition against the stunning induced by a subsequent 10- or 15-min ischemic episode.

Supported in part by NIH R01 Grants HL-43151 and HL-55757

Dr. R. Bolli (✉)
Division of Cardiology
University of Louisville
Louisville, Kentucky 40292, USA

Stunning induced by a prolonged (≥ 20 min) ischemic episode

All of the published studies (e.g., 6, 7) have demonstrated that preconditioning with brief episodes of ischemia does not attenuate the dysfunction observed in the viable, reperfused myocardium after a prolonged (≥ 20 min) coronary occlusion resulting in subendocardial infarction. In one such study (6), wall motion was improved by preconditioning but this could be explained entirely by the reduction in infarct size.

In summary, brief ischemia does not precondition against the stunning induced by a subsequent ischemic episode lasting > 15 min.

Stunning induced by a sequence of brief (≤ 5 min) ischemic episodes of equal duration

This is an apparently controversial area. Numerous studies have examined the effects of repetitive brief coronary occlusions on myocardial contractile function (e.g., 8, 9; since the number of papers is too large to be quoted here, we refer to ref. 10, in which all of these previous studies are summarized and discussed). Most of these previous studies indicate that repetitive ischemic episodes cause a cumulative decrease in contractility. These same studies, however, have also concluded that the decrement in function resulting from each subsequent ischemic episode becomes smaller with the number of repetitions and that after the first three to five coronary occlusions, subsequent occlusions have little or no effect on postischemic dysfunction (8, 9; reviewed in ref. 10). This has been interpreted as evidence that the initial ischemic episodes precondition against the stunning induced by subsequent ischemic episodes.

We (10) have recently examined this issue in depth in open-chest dogs subjected to a sequence of ten 5-min coronary occlusions interspersed with 10-min reperfusion intervals. In accordance with previous studies (e.g., 8, 9; reviewed in ref. 10), we found that the first occlusion caused the largest decrease in function (Fig. 1), that subsequent occlusions caused only relatively small additional decrements (Fig. 1), and that this pattern could not be explained by the fact that postischemic dysfunction had reached near-maximal levels after the first reperfusion (10). On the basis of these data alone, we would have to conclude, as did the previous studies, that the last nine occlusion-reperfusion cycles did not produce significant additional dysfunction, i.e., that the myocardium was preconditioned up until the 10th occlusion. However, we used a different approach to determine whether there was a preconditioning effect. Instead of measuring the recovery of function a few minutes after reperfusion (as was done in all previous studies), we measured the recovery of function over the entire 4-h reperfusion period after the last occlusion. The results of this analysis differ from those

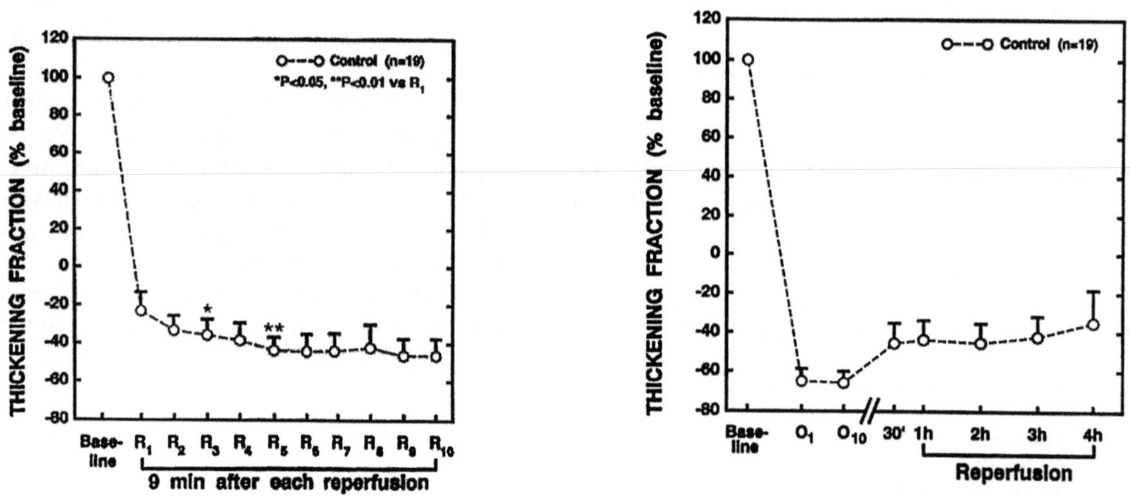

Fig. 1 *Left:* Systolic thickening fraction in the ischemic-reperfused region at baseline and 9 min into each of the ten reperfusion (R) intervals after the 5-min occlusions. Open-chest dogs were subjected to a sequence of ten 5-min coronary occlusion/5-min reperfusion cycles. *Right:* Systolic thickening fraction in the ischemic-reperfused region 4 min into the first LAD occlusion (0_1), 4 min into the tenth LAD occlusion (0_{10}), and at selected times during the final 4-h reperfusion interval. Thickening fraction is expressed as a percentage of baseline values. Data are mean ± SEM. *$p < 0.05$, **$p < 0.01$ vs. R_1. Reproduced from ref. 10.

suggested by Fig. 1 and by the previous studies reviewed in ref. 10. We found that the overall magnitude of postischemic dysfunction (as assessed by the total deficit of systolic wall thickening during the 4-h reperfusion period, which is an integrative measure of the duration and degree of myocardial stunning after reperfusion [10]) was similar after one and three 5-min occlusions (Fig. 2), indicating that the first occlusion did precondition against the next two occlusions. However, the overall magnitude of postischemic dysfunction was approximately 2.5 times greater after ten occlusions than after three (Fig. 2), indicating that the last seven occlusions caused considerable additional injury; that is, the first three ischemic episodes failed to precondition against the next seven episodes. We therefore concluded that in this setting of multiple 5-min coronary occlusions, the protection against stunning afforded by ischemic preconditioning exists but is limited; at some point between the fourth and tenth occlusions, the protection is lost, and recurrent ischemic episodes start to produce a cumulative deterioration of function.

These conclusions are in contrast with those that we would have reached on the basis of the data presented in Fig. 1. *Accordingly, we propose that the magnitude of the injury caused by recurrent ischemic insults cannot be adequately assessed from the magnitude of the dysfunction attained shortly after each insult, and is more accurately reflected in the overall severity of postischemic dysfunction (as measured by the total deficit of wall thickening).*

The loss of protection against stunning after the first three occlusions (Fig. 2) may be due to the fact that the preconditioning effect is limited in its effficacy (i.e., it protects only against a limited ischemic burden, less than that associated with ten 5-min occlusions) or in its duration (i.e., it lasts less than the time [150 min]) necessary to complete the 10-occlusion sequence). In either case, the early phase of preconditioning against stunning resembles the early phase of preconditioning against cell death. The mechanism of the early phase of preconditioning against stunning is not fully understood, but Bunch et al. (11) have provided evidence that it involves stimulation of A_1-

Fig. 2 *Left:* Systolic thickening fraction in the ischemic-reperfused region at baseline, during the first LAD occlusion (0_1), during the tenth LAD occlusion (0_{10}), and at selected times during the final 4-h reperfusion interval in a dog subjected to one 5-min occlusion (top) and in a dog subjected to ten 5-min occlusions (bottom). Thickening fraction is expressed as a percentage of baseline values. In both panels, the dotted area represents the area that is integrated to measure the total deficit of wall thickening after reperfusion. This area is comprised between the thickening versus time line and the baseline (100 % line) over the 4-h period of observation after the last reperfusion. Measurement of this area provides an estimate of the overall magnitude of postischemic dysfunction during the entire reperfusion interval. *Right:* The total deficit of wall thickening after reperfusion after one 5-min LAD occlusion (open bar), three 5-min occlusions (crosshatched bar), and ten 5-min occlusions (hatched bar). The total deficit of wall thickening is expressed in arbitrary units obtained by measuring the area of deficit with a computerized program. Values are mean ± SEM. Reproduced from ref. 10.

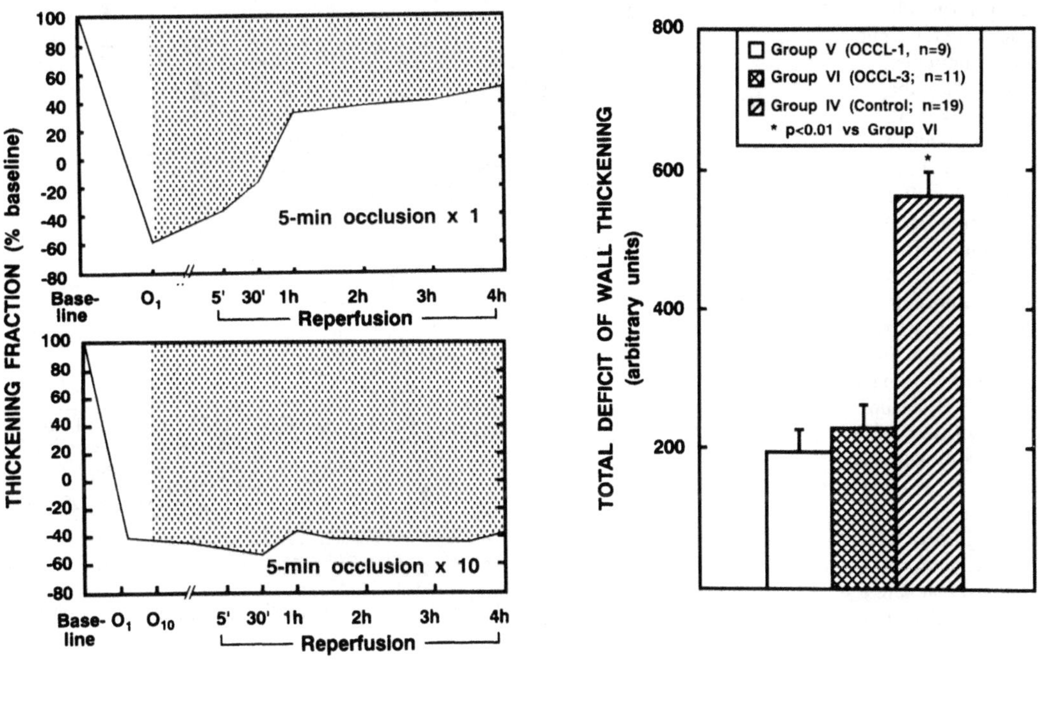

receptors by the adenosine released during the first ischemic episode. We (10) have demonstrated that recurrent brief ischemic episodes result in recurrent bouts of oxygen-derived free radical formation and that the preconditioning effect on function is associated with attenuation of free radical generation after reperfusion.

In summary, when the heart is subjected to a sequence of brief (5 min) ischemic episodes, the first episode preconditions against the stunning induced by the next two episodes, but this protection disappears at some point between the fourth and tenth episode, so that recurrent ischemic episodes start to have a cumulative effect on function.

Late phase of preconditioning against stunning

The phenomenon of late preconditioning against stunning

In all of the studies reviewed above (2–11), the question addressed was whether ischemic preconditioning confers immediate protection against postischemic dysfunction; no information was available regarding the late effects of ischemic preconditioning on myocardial stunning. We hypothesized that the stress of sublethal ischemia may induce cellular adaptations that protect against the development of stunning after subsequent exposure to ischemia, but that these adaptations develop slowly and require several hours to become manifest. We tested this hypothesis in conscious pigs subjected to a sequence of ten 2-min coronary occlusions interspersed with 2-min reperfusion intervals (12). We found that this sequence induced severe myocardial stunning, but when the same sequence was repeated 24 h later, the severity of stunning was markedly reduced (by approximately 50 %) (Figs. 3 and 4). The resistance to stunning was associated with an increase in the myocardial levels of heat stress protein (HSP) 70 (12) – a finding that is compatible with, but does not prove, a role of HSPs in the pathogenesis of the protective effect. The protection dissipated within 10 days after the last ischemic stress, but could be reinduced by another sequence of ten 2-min occlusion/2-min reperfusion cycles (12) (Fig. 4). Unlike early preconditioning against infarction, this form of protection does not appear to be mediated by activation of adenosine receptors, since it is not prevented by 8-p-sulfophenyl theophylline (12) (Fig. 4). We also assessed the time-course of this protective effect (13). We found that preconditioning was not present at 6 h after the last ischemic episode, became manifest at 12 h, lasted for at least 3 days, and disappeared within 6 days from the preconditioning ischemia, a time-course that is consistent with the synthesis and degradation of cardioprotective proteins (13). We (14) have recently

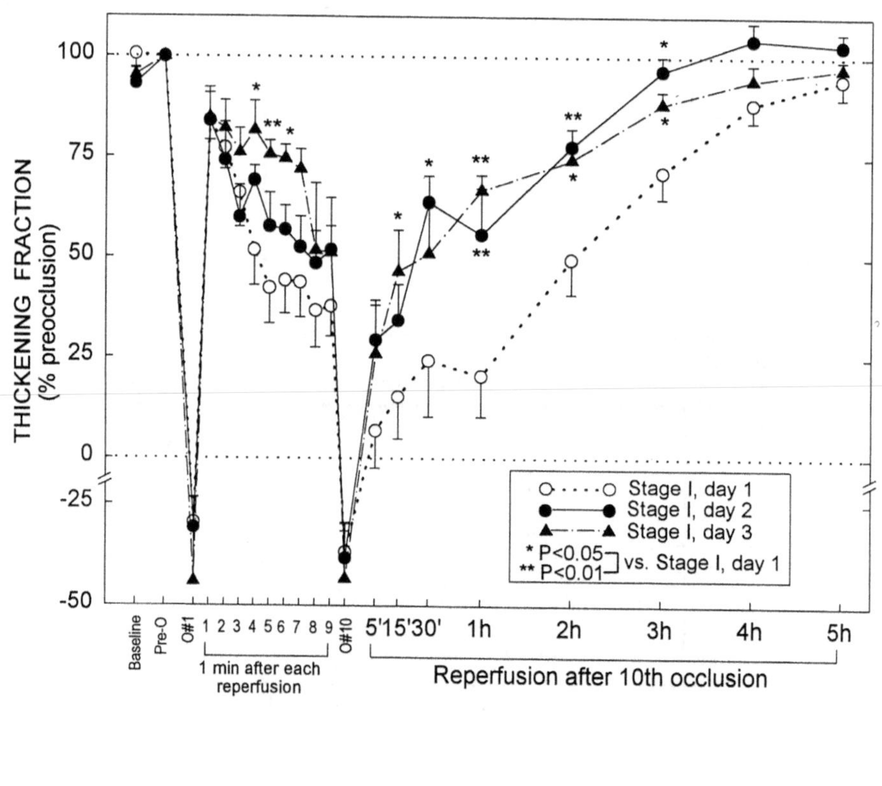

Fig. 3 Systolic thickening fraction in the ischemic-reperfused region of conscious pigs subjected to a sequence of ten 2-min LAD occlusion/2-min reperfusion cycles. Shown are the measurements of thickening fraction obtained at baseline, immediately before the first occlusion (preocclusion, Pre-O), 1 min into the first LAD occlusion (0#1), 1 min into each of the first nine reperfusions, 1 min into the tenth occlusion (0#10), and at selected times during the 5-h reperfusion interval following the tenth coronary occlusion. (- - - o - - -) Measurements taken on day 1 (n = 10); (– ● –) measurements taken on day 2 (n = 9); and (· — · ▲ · — ·) measurements taken on day 3 (n = 8). Thickening fraction is expressed as a percentage of preocclusion values. Data are means ± SEM. Reproduced from ref. 12.

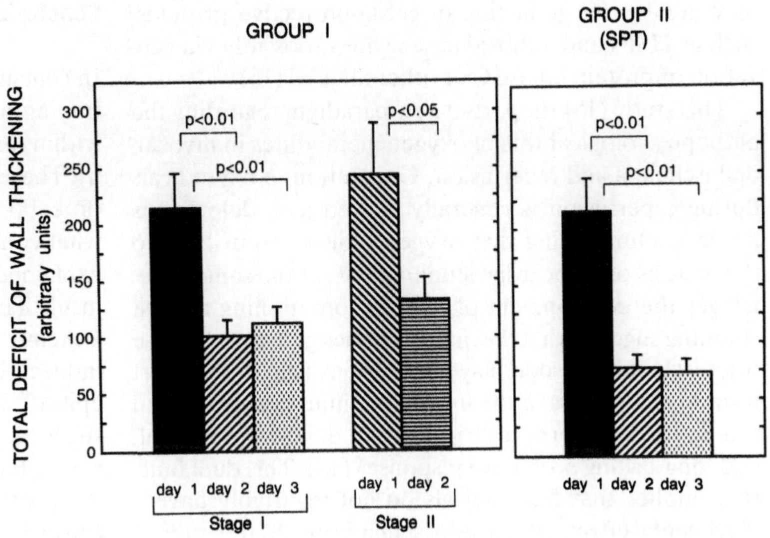

Fig. 4 Total deficit of wall thickening after the tenth reperfusion in conscious pigs in group I, which did not receive SPT, and in group II, which received SPT on day 1. Conscious pigs were subjected to a sequence of ten 2-min LAD occlusion/2-min reperfusion cycles and systolic thickening fraction was measured as in Fig. 3. The total deficit of wall thickening was calculated in a manner similar to that shown in Fig. 2. SPT, 8-*p*-sulfophenyl theophylline. Data are means ± SEM. Reproduced from ref. 12.

observed a similar preconditioning effect (with a similar time-course) in conscious rabbits subjected to a sequence of six 5-min coronary occlusion/5-min reperfusion cycles.

In summary, these studies (12–14) demonstrate, for the first time, that a brief ischemic stress induces a powerful, long-lasting (at least 72 h) adaptive response that renders the myocardium resistant to stunning. This adaptive response disappears within 6 days after the last ischemic stress, but can be reinduced by another ischemic stress. We have termed this response "late preconditioning against stunning" (12).

Essential role of reactive oxygen species (ROS) in late preconditioning against stunning

Recently, we (15) have demonstrated that administration of antioxidant therapy completely prevents the development of late preconditioning against stunning, indicating that the production of ROS is the mechanism whereby ischemia induces this protective response. Using the same model employed previously (12), i.e., conscious pigs subjected to a sequence of ten 2-min occlusion/2-min reperfusion cycles for 3 consecutive days (days 1, 2, and 3), we found that administration of antioxidants (superoxide dismutase plus catalase plus mercaptopropionyl glycine) on day 1 attenuated myocardial stunning on day 1 (indicating that ROS contribute to stunning in the pig), but then resulted in loss of the preconditioning effect on day 2 (i.e., stunning on day 2 was much more severe than on day 1 and similar to that observed on day 1 in control pigs) (Fig. 5). On day 3, antioxidant-treated pigs exhibited a marked attenuation of stunning, indicating that the ischemia produced on day 2 preconditioned the heart against stunning on day 3 (15) (Fig. 5). Taken together, these results (15) indicate that the oxidative stress incurred during brief ischemia and reperfusion triggers a protective response that makes the myocardium resistant to stunning 24 h later. The precise mechanism whereby the exposure to oxygen radicals during the preconditioning ischemia leads to late preconditioning against stunning is unclear, but it

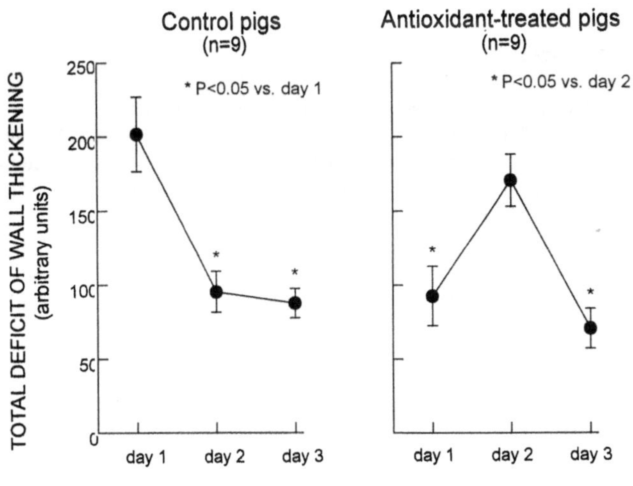

Fig. 5 Total deficit of wall thickening after the tenth reperfusion in conscious pigs on days 1, 2, and 3 in the control group (n = 9) and in the group treated with antioxidants (superoxide dismutase plus catalase plus mercaptopropionyl glycine) (n = 9). The total deficit of wall thickening is an integrated measure of the overall severity of myocardial stunning and is expressed in arbitrary units as described in ref. 12. Note that antioxidant therapy on day 1 prevented preconditioning on day 2 in the treated group. Also note that antioxidant therapy attenuated stunning on day 1 in this group. Data are means ± SEM. Data are from ref. 15.

may involve the induction of cardioprotective proteins, such as HSPs and antioxidant enzymes, possibly via activation of protein kinase C or other kinases (15).

This study (15) supports a new paradigm regarding the pathophysiological role of oxygen metabolites in myocardial ischemia and reperfusion. Generation of oxyradicals during reperfusion is generally viewed as a deleterious process. Our finding that oxygen radicals contribute to the genesis of myocardial stunning but, at the same time, trigger the development of late preconditioning against stunning suggests that the radical species generated after a brief ischemic episode play an injurious role in the short term (as mediators of the immediate injury) and a useful role in the long term (as triggers of a delayed, powerful, and long-lasting protective response) (15). This dual function implies that free radicals do not invariably have a detrimental effect: after a mild ischemic insult, free radical generation could serve as a "warning" signal (primordial in evolutionary terms) that activates a protective response designed to minimize further injury through the upregulation of a family of redox-sensitive genes (antioxidant enzyme genes, HSP genes, and probably other genes). In this manner, the sublethal oxidative stress associated with brief ischemic episodes could act as a transduction pathway signaling an imminent threat and the need to develop cellular defenses against it.

Conclusions

In conclusion, there are two phases of ischemic preconditioning against stunning: an early phase (which begins within minutes) and a late phase (which begins after > 6 h). These two phases have different pathophysiology and probably different mechanisms. The early phase is somewhat controversial, but most of the discrepancies can be explained by differences in the duration of the ischemic insult: That is, the available evidence indicates that a brief ischemic episode preconditions against the stunning induced by a second ischemic episode when the second episode lasts ≤ 5 min but not when it lasts ≥ 10. This suggests that the early preconditioning effect is rather weak. Furthermore, when early preconditioning occurs, the protection is limited to only few ischemic episodes (probably three to five). The duration of the early phase is unknown. In addition to this early phase of protection, brief ischemia induces a late phase of preconditioning against stunning which is long-lasting (at least 72 h), is powerful (approximately 50 % reduction in total dysfunction), and is mediated by the generation of reactive oxygen species during the preconditioning ischemia-reperfusion cycles. Because the late phase offers sustained protection, it is probably more important and more clinically relevant than the early phase.

References

1. Downey JM, Cohen MV, Ytrehus K, Liu Y (1994) Cellular mechanisms in ischemic preconditioning: The role of adenosine and protein kinase C. In: Das DK (ed) Cellular, Biochemical, and Molecular Aspects of Reperfusion Injury. Annals of the Academy of Sciences, New York, NY 723: 82–98
2. Ovize M, Przyklenk K, Hale S, Kloner RA (1992) Preconditioning does not attenuate myocardial stunning. Circulation 85: 2247–2254
3. Miyamae MH, Fujiwara H, Kida M, Yokota R, Tanaka M, Katsuragawa M, Hasegawa K, Ohura M, Koga K, Yabuuchi Y, Sasayama S (1993) Preconditioning improves energy metabolism during reperfusion but does not attenuate myocardial stunning in porcine hearts. Circulation 88: 223–234
4. Sekili S, Jeroudi MO, Tang X-L, Zughaib M, Sun J-Z, Bolli R (1995) Effect of adenosine on myocardial "stunning" in the dog. Circ Res 76: 82–94
5. Jeroudi MO, Tang XL, Abd-Elfattah A, Sun JZ, Bolli R (1994) Effect of adenosine A_1-receptor activation on myocardial stunning in intact dogs. Circulation 90: I-479
6. Cohen MV, Liu GS, Downey JM (1991) Preconditioning causes improved wall motion as well as smaller infarcts after transient coronary occlusion in rabbits. Circulation 84: 341–349
7. Schott RJ, Rohmann S, Braun ER, Schaper W (1990) Ischemic preconditioning reduces infarct size in swine myocardium. Circ Res 66: 1133–1142
8. Nicklas JM, Becker LC, Bulkley BH (1985) Effects of repeated brief coronary occlusion on regional left ventricular function and dimension in dogs. Am J Cardiol 56: 473–478
9. Hoffmeister HM, Mauser M, Schaper W (1986) Repeated episodes of regional myocardial ischemia: effect on local function and high energy phosphate levels. Basic Res Cardiol 81: 361–372
10. Bolli R, Zughaib M, Li X-Y, Tang X-L, Sun J-Z, Triana JF, McCay P (1995) Recurrent ischemia in the canine heart causes recurrent bursts of free radical production that have a cumulative effect on contractile function: A pathophysiological basis for chronic myocardial "stunning". J Clin Invest 96: 1066–1084
11. Bunch FT, Thornton J, Cohen MV, Downey JM (1992) Adenosine is an endogenous protectant against stunning during repetitive ischemic episodes in the heart. Am Heart J 124: 1440–1445

12. Sun JZ, Tang X-L, Knowlton M, Park SW, Qiu Y, Bolli R (1995) Late preconditioning against myocardial stunning: An endogenous protective mechanism that confers resistance to postischemic dysfunction 24 hours after brief ischemia in conscious pigs. J Clin Invest 95: 388–403
13. Tang X-L, Qiu Y, Sun J-Z, Park S-W, Maldonado C, Bolli R (1995) Time-course of late preconditioning against myocardial stunning in conscious pigs. Circulation (Suppl I): I-388
14. Qiu Y, Maldonado C, Tang X-L, Bolli R (1995) Late preconditioning against myocardial stunning in conscious rabbits. Circulation (Suppl I): I-389
15. Sun J-Z, Tang X-L, Park S-W, Qiu Y, Turrens JF, Bolli, R: Evidence for an essential role of reactive oxygen species in the genesis of late preconditioning against myocardial stunning in conscious pigs. J Clin Invest (in press)

GPSR Compliance

The European Union's (EU) General Product Safety Regulation (GPSR) is a set of rules that requires consumer products to be safe and our obligations to ensure this.

If you have any concerns about our products, you can contact us on ProductSafety@springernature.com

In case Publisher is established outside the EU, the EU authorized representative is:

Springer Nature Customer Service Center GmbH
Europaplatz 3
69115 Heidelberg, Germany

Batch number: 10578403

Printed by Printforce, the Netherlands